Calls
for revamp
of RCTs

Case Studies in Innovative Clinical Trials

Drug development is a strictly regulated area. As such, marketing approval of a new drug depends heavily, if not exclusively, on evidence generated from clinical trials. Drug development has seen tremendous innovation in science and technology that has revolutionized the treatment of some diseases. And yet, the statistical design and practical conduct of the clinical trials used to test new therapeutics for safety and efficacy have changed very little over the decades. Our approach to clinical trials is steeped in convention and tradition. The large, fixed, randomized controlled trial methods that have been the gold standard are well understood and expected by many trial stakeholders. However, this approach is not well suited to all aspects of modern drug development and the current competitive landscape. We now see new therapies that target a small fraction of the patient population, rare diseases with high unmet medical needs, and pediatric populations that must wait for years for new drug approvals from the time that therapies are approved in adults. Large randomized clinical trials are at best inefficient and at worst completely infeasible in many modern clinical settings. Advances in technology and data infrastructure call for innovations in clinical trial design.

Despite advances in statistical methods, the availability of information, and computing power, the actual experience with innovative design in clinical trials across industry and academia is limited. This book will be an important showcase of the potential for these innovative designs in modern drug development and will be an important resource to guide those who wish to undertake them for themselves.

This book is ideal for professionals in the pharmaceutical industry and regulatory agencies, but it will also be useful to academic researchers, faculty members, and graduate students in statistics, biostatistics, public health, and epidemiology due to its focus on innovation.

AUDIENCE

Key Features:

- Written by pharmaceutical industry experts, academic researchers, and regulatory reviewers, this is the first book providing a comprehensive set of case studies related to statistical methodology, implementation, regulatory considerations, and communication of complex innovative trial design.
- Has a broad appeal to a multitude of readers across academia, industry, and regulatory agencies.
- Each contribution is a practical case study that can speak to the benefits of an innovative approach but also balance that with the real-life challenges encountered.
- A complete understanding of what is actually being done in modern clinical trials will broaden the reader's capabilities and provide examples to first mimic and then customize and expand upon when exploring these ideas on their own.

Chapman & Hall/CRC Biostatistics Series

Series Editors

Shein-Chung Chow, Duke University School of Medicine, USA
Byron Jones, Novartis Pharma AG, Switzerland
Jen-pei Liu, National Taiwan University, Taiwan
Karl E. Peace, Georgia Southern University, USA
Bruce W. Turnbull, Cornell University, USA

Recently Published Titles

Real World Evidence in a Patient-Centric Digital Era
Edited by Kelly H. Zou, Lobna A. Salem, and Amrit Ray

Data Science, AI, and Machine Learning in Pharma
Harry Yang

Model-Assisted Bayesian Designs for Dose Finding and Optimization
Methods and Applications
Ying Yuan, Ruitao Lin, and J. Jack Lee

Digital Therapeutics: Strategic, Scientific, Developmental, and Regulatory Aspects
Oleksandr Sverdlov and Joris van Dam

Quantitative Methods for Precision Medicine
Pharmacogenomics in Action
Rongling Wu

Drug Development for Rare Diseases
Edited by Bo Yang, Yang Song, and Yijie Zhou

Case Studies in Bayesian Methods for Biopharmaceutical CMC
Paul Faya and Tony Pourmohamad

Statistical Analytics for Health Data Science with SAS and R
Jeffrey Wilson, Ding-Geng Chen, and Karl E. Peace

Design and Analysis of Pragmatic Trials
Song Zhang, Chul Ahn, and Hong Zhu

ROC Analysis for Classification and Prediction in Practice
Christos Nakas, Leonidas Bantis, and Constantine Gatsonis

Controlled Epidemiological Studies
Marie Reilly

Statistical Methods for Health Disparity Research
J. Sunil Rao, Ph.D.

Case Studies in Innovative Clinical Trials
Kristine Broglio and Binbing Yu

For more information about this series, please visit: www.routledge.com/Chapman-Hall-CRC-Biostatistics-Series/book-series/CHBIOSTATIS

Case Studies in Innovative Clinical Trials

Edited by
Kristine Broglio and Binbing Yu

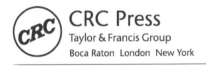

CRC Press
Taylor & Francis Group
Boca Raton London New York

CRC Press is an imprint of the
Taylor & Francis Group, an **informa** business

A CHAPMAN & HALL BOOK

Front cover image: cybermagician/Shutterstock

First edition published 2024
by CRC Press
2385 NW Executive Center Dr, Suite 320, Boca Raton, FL, 33431

and by CRC Press
4 Park Square, Milton Park, Abingdon, Oxon, OX14 4RN

CRC Press is an imprint of Taylor & Francis Group, LLC

ISBN: 978-1-032-26265-9 (hbk)
ISBN: 978-1-032-26518-6 (pbk)
ISBN: 978-1-003-28864-0 (ebk)

DOI: 10.1201/9781003288640

Typeset in Palatino LT Std
by Newgen Publishing UK

Contents

About the Editors

Binbing Yu is a Senior Director in the Oncology Statistical Innovation group at AstraZeneca. He serves as the statistical expert across the whole spectrum of drug R&D, including drug discovery, clinical trials, operation and manufacturing, clinical pharmacology, oncology medical affairs, and postmarketing surveillance. He obtained his PhD in Statistics from the George Washington University. His primary research interests are clinical trial design and analysis, cancer epidemiology, observational studies, PKPD modeling, and Bayesian analysis. He has published three books on immunogenicity, cure modeling, and real-world data/real-world evidence (RWD/RWE).

Kristine Broglio is a Statistical Science Senior Director in the AstraZeneca Oncology Statistical Innovation group with interests in adaptive clinical trials and Bayesian statistics. She earned an MS in Biostatistics from the University of Washington and joined the University of Texas M.D. Anderson Cancer Center, where she specialized in applied statistical analysis relating to the diagnosis, treatment, and long-term outcomes of breast cancer. Later, at Berry Consultants, she led the design, execution, and analysis of well over 100 Bayesian adaptive and complex clinical trials. Ms Broglio is a member of numerous cross-industry working groups through the ASA and DIA and has contributed over 120 papers to the medical and statistical literature.

Contributors

Rochelle Bagatell
Children's Hospital of Philadelphia,
    University of Pennsylvania
Philadelphia, Pennsylvania, USA

Anna Berglind
AstraZeneca
Gothenburg, Sweden

Lydia Ould Brahim
Ingram School of Nursing McGill
    University
Montreal, Quebec, Canada

Joan Buenconsejo
Bristol Myers Squibb
New York, New York, USA

Andy Chi
Takeda Pharmaceuticals
Cambridge, Massachusetts, USA

George Chu
Edwards Lifesciences
Irvine, California, USA

Debarshi Deya
Biogen
Cambridge, Massachusetts, USA

Vladimir Dragalin
Janssen Research & Development
Raritan, New Jersey, USA

Steven G. DuBois
Dana-Farber Cancer Institute
Boston, Massachusetts, USA

Jordan J. Elm
Medical University of South Carolina
Charleston, South Carolina, USA

Samvel B. Gasparyan
AstraZeneca
Gothenburg, Sweden

Emily G. Greengard
University of Minnesota
Minneapolis, Minnesota, USA

Micki Hultquist
AstraZeneca
Gaithersburg, Maryland, USA

Bradley Hupf
Takeda Pharmaceuticals
Cambridge, Massachusetts, USA

Silke Jörgens
Janssen-Cilag
Neuss, Germany

Martin Klein
U.S. Food and Drug Administration
Silver Spring, Maryland, USA

Gary G. Koch
University of North Carolina
Chapel Hill, North Carolina, USA

Elaine K. Kowalewski
University of North Carolina
Chapel Hill, North Carolina, USA

Sylvie D. Lambert
Ingram School of Nursing McGill
    University
St-Mary's Research Centre
Montreal, Quebec, Canada

Qing Li
MorphoSys US Inc
Boston, Massachusetts, USA

Yinpu Li
Florida State University
Tallahassee, Florida, USA

Jianchang Lin
Takeda Pharmaceuticals
Cambridge, Massachusetts, USA

Junjing Lin
Takeda Pharmaceuticals
Cambridge, Massachusetts, USA

Rachael Liu
Takeda Pharmaceuticals
Cambridge, Massachusetts, USA

Yingying Liu
Biogen
Cambridge, Massachusetts, USA

Renee L. Martin
Medical University of South Carolina
Charleston, South Carolina, USA

Erica E.M. Moodie
McGill University
Montreal, Quebec, Canada

Arlene Naranjo
Children's Oncology Group Statistics and
    Data Centre, University of Florida
Gainesville, Florida, USA

Fredrik Öhrn
Quantitative Sciences Consulting (QSC)
Janssen Research & Development,
    Janssen-Cilag
Solna, Sweden
Previously:
AstraZeneca
Gothenburg, Sweden

Doray Sitko
Berry Consultants LLC
Austin, Texas, USA

Hengrui Sun
Food and Drug Administration (FDA)
Silver Spring, Maryland, USA

Jian Wang
AstraZeneca
Gaithersburg, Maryland, USA

Liwen Wu
Takeda Pharmaceuticals
Cambridge, Massachusetts, USA

Tianyu Zhan
AbbVie Inc
Chicago, Illinois, USA

1

Review of Advances in Complex Innovative Trials

Kristine Broglio and Binbing Yu

A whitepaper from the Tufts Center for the Study of Drug Development in 2015 estimated that the time required to develop a new drug for approval in the United States was 10 years (1). Because only 11% of therapies evaluated are ultimately approved for use, the total average cost to bring a new drug to market, inclusive of the cost of the failures, was estimated to be greater than $2.6 billion (1). Trends over time point toward decreasing success rates and increasing duration and costs, which can be attributed in part to drug development moving into increasingly difficult indications (1). One example of this is Alzheimer's disease. The rate of failure in Alzheimer's clinical trials is high and has been attributed to numerous issues such as disease heterogeneity, variability in disease assessments, and the slow progression of the disease making treatment effects difficult to observe (2). Another example is oncology, where advances in our understanding of the biology have driven a surge in therapeutics that target specific processes within tumors and companion diagnostics to match patients to these therapies (3). Oncology is now sliced into small incidence subtypes of cancer and clinical trials must contend with this new paradigm (3).

Clinical trialists have responded to this landscape. Many innovations in clinical trials are focused on making clinical trial designs more efficient and suitable to the more complex clinical questions being asked. This includes innovative trial designs such as Bayesian adaptive designs and master protocol trials. This also includes innovative ways of measuring and analyzing the effects of new treatments, such as the development of novel and surrogate endpoints and more sophisticated statistical modeling of diseases.

The current development landscape has also generated a growing need to leverage real-world data (RWD) and real-world evidence (RWE). RWD/RWE allows us to better target and optimize clinical trial questions as well as augment the evaluation of safety and efficacy beyond what can be learned in a clinical trial setting. There is a corresponding growth in the role of artificial intelligence (AI) and machine learning (ML). These analytical methods are well suited to the large and complex real-world datasets that are now available such as those from electronic health records, medical imaging, genomic data, and continuous monitoring assessments from wearable health sensors (4).

However, innovations have not just been analytical in nature. We also see innovation in the conduct of clinical trials. Many clinical trials were forced to become more decentralized during the COVID-19 pandemic and it is likely that many of these practices will become a more permanent way of conducting trials (5). Decentralization is pragmatic, reduces the burden of clinical trials on clinical trial staff and participants, and can also help to enhance the diversity of the clinical trial population to address important questions about

DOI: 10.1201/9781003288640-1

1

disease and treatment effect heterogeneity (6). This chapter will give a brief overview of each of these key areas of innovation mentioned above and highlights examples of these innovations in practice using examples available from the literature.

1.1 Innovative Trial Designs

1.1.1 Bayesian Adaptive Designs

The gold standard of clinical trials, the randomized controlled double-blinded trial, was born in the 1940s with Bradford Hill's randomized trial evaluating streptomycin in pulmonary tuberculosis (7). By the 1970s, group sequential designs were proposed. This method allowed trials to stop early at an interim analysis for efficacy should the data suggest that the treatment was extremely promising (8). The field of adaptive clinical trials has since grown and by the early 2000s, Bayesian adaptive designs were gaining traction in oncology (9). Today, Bayesian adaptive clinical trials have become increasingly common across multiple different diseases settings (10).

Adaptive designs use interim analyses of the trial's accumulated data and prespecified rules to react to what has been learned within the trial and modify aspects of the trial going forward. Examples of adaptive features include the ability to stop early for success such as in group sequential design, but also include sample size reestimation, dropping poorly performing arms or changing allocation ratios to the trial arms, restricting the inclusion/ exclusion criteria to a subgroup of patients more likely to benefit, or seamlessly shifting from one trial phase to the next. While adaptions are certainly performed under the frequentist statistical paradigm, Bayesian statistics are more often used for more complex adaptive designs. The Bayesian statistical paradigm is natural for adaptive trials because of how it accounts for uncertainty both in the current trial data and the future unobserved data to inform the adaptive decisions. Bayesian statistics also provides intuitive probability statements on the treatment effects and probabilities of trial success that are easily communicated to nonstatisticians. These trials can address more complex clinical trial settings, answer multiple different questions in a single trial, and generate evidence more efficiently (11). There are several case studies comparing the results of a completed clinical trial to the results that could have been produced by a counterfactual Bayesian adaptive trial. Each of these evaluations concluded that the same data, under a Bayesian adaptive design, would have led to the same conclusions but would have done so more quickly or with a smaller sample size (12–14).

The ability to adaptively address multiple different questions makes these innovative trials well suited to the exploratory stages of drug development. Adaptive trials have been used in the confirmatory setting, but more care needs to be exercised due to issues surrounding the characterization of the trial's performance such as the overall Type I error rate and bias in estimation. Additionally, these trials often require extensive computing and simulation to determine the design. Validated commercial software is frequently not available due to the customized nature of many of these trials. The interim analyses in these designs also introduce operational complexity and concerns about operational bias and trial integrity should the interims in some way convey even partial information about the accumulating data so that data confidentiality plans may be necessary.

1.1.2 Bayesian Adaptive Design Case Study

An example of a Bayesian adaptive phase III trial is the DAWN trial (DWI or CTP Assessment with Clinical Mismatch in the Triage of Wake-Up and Late Presenting Strokes Undergoing Neurointervention with Trevo) (15). This was a randomized trial to evaluate endovascular thrombectomy in patients with acute stroke. At the time of trial design, it was unknown whether the benefit of the device would extend to patients with larger infarct sizes on imaging. Therefore, this trial used a Bayesian adaptive design to have the flexibility to modify the infarct size inclusion/exclusion criteria during enrollment. The trial had interim analyses planned to start when 150 subjects were enrolled and after every additional 50 subjects. At each interim analysis, there were prespecified rules to restrict further enrollment in the trial to patients with smaller infarct sizes. Each interim analysis also included the possibility of stopping early for predicted success with the current patients. In this manner, the sample size of the trial was also adaptive. Only the necessary number of patients would be enrolled to show the efficacy of the device based on the effect being observed in the trial. The DAWN trial was ultimately stopped early for efficacy at the interim analysis with 200 patients enrolled. Efficacy was seen across the range of infarct sizes and the adaptive algorithm never restricted the inclusion/exclusion criteria.

1.1.3 Master Protocols

Master protocol trials are an important class of innovative clinical trial designs. Master protocols are clinical trials that are designed to answer multiple questions under a single overarching protocol (16). Consider that within an indication, there may be multiple different drug candidates, or that one drug candidate may be of interest within multiple different indications. Traditionally each of these questions might require its own clinical trial. Looking across the drug development landscape, there are then multiple related trials with redundant elements. A master protocol can be conceived of as collecting these related clinical trials and condensing them into a single clinical trial process, where each independent trial is now considered a substudy under the master protocol, and the redundant elements become a single shared resource across the different substudies.

The literature describes three kinds of master protocol trials, though the nomenclature is not consistent across authors. A basket trial refers to a master protocol trial where one experimental therapy is being administered across multiple different patient populations. A platform trial often refers to a master protocol trial that investigates multiple experimental therapies within a single patient population. An umbrella trial also investigates a single disease but breaks it into important subgroups and investigates therapies within the subgroups. The umbrella trial has some aspects of personalized medicine in that it attempts to match patients to the therapies most likely to benefit them. Master protocols trials may be perpetual in nature, meaning that as substudies complete, new substudies can be added.

Master protocol trials have obvious operational efficiencies in that they consolidate trial infrastructure and processes. They also offer an opportunity for statistical efficiencies. Basket trials can share information across the related patient groups. Such an approach has been shown to improve decision making as compared to evaluating groups independently (17) and can be particularly useful in increasing power in rare disease settings. Platform trials frequently make use of a single common control arm that each experimental arm is compared against. As compared to stand-alone trials, this reduces the total number of patients required, speeds up the time to find an effective therapy, and reduces the total number of patients that must be randomized to control (18). One study estimated that a platform trial approach for a phase II oncology trial would reduce cost by 12–15% and reduce trial duration by 13–18% (19). The impact of the master protocol approach is also seen in the recent recipients of the David Sackett Trial of the Year Award from the Society of Clinical Trials. This award is given to a randomized clinical trial with results published in the previous year that provide the basis for a substantial, beneficial change in healthcare and reflects expertise, methodological excellence, and concern for its participants (20). Recent recipients include the TOGETHER platform trial in 2022, the RECOVERY (Randomized Evaluation of COVID-19 Therapy) platform trial in 2021, and the STAMPEDE (Systemic Therapy in Advancing or Metastatic Prostate Cancer) platform trial in 2017.

Some statistical aspects of master protocols have been controversial (21). For example, in a basket trial that proposes to share information across groups, group-specific control of the Type I error rate will not be possible under all scenarios. Similarly in the platform trial, there is debate about when a multiplicity adjustment for the multiple experimental arms would be necessary. Another debate within master protocols is whether control patients that were not concurrently randomized to an experimental arm can be included in the primary analysis population. Recent FDA guidance related to platform trials in COVID-19 recommends against the use of nonconcurrent controls, but it could be appropriate in other settings where the disease, patient population, and available therapies are more stable over time (22). Other drawbacks of the master protocol approach relate to the increase in operational complexity. While master protocol trials offer a single trial infrastructure for the multiple related substudies, that single infrastructure must be larger and more complex than the traditional trial. Trial processes must be scaled up to be able to handle the multiple different questions and to anticipate and accommodate changes over time. There are also practical issues with a perpetual trial such as how to accommodate changing standard of care over time or how to report one substudy without jeopardizing the integrity of ongoing substudies (21).

1.1.4 Master Protocol Case Studies

The ROAR trial (Rare Oncology Agnostic Research) is an example of a basket trial (23). This is a phase II trial to evaluate dabrafenib plus trametinib in patients across different histologies whose tumors harbored BRAFV600E mutations. This trial planned a maximum of 25 patients in each histology cohort and prespecified an analysis of tumor response rates according to a Bayesian hierarchical model. This analysis approach shares information across the multiple related histology groups and increases study power. Extensive simulations were performed to determine the trial's Type I error and power across different mixtures of the response rates across the histology cohorts. This trial led to the approval of dabrafenib plus trametinib for some of the histologies included in the basket (24).

As mentioned above, the RECOVERY trial is an example of a platform trial (36). RECOVERY was initiated to evaluate therapies for patients hospitalized with suspected or confirmed COVID-19. This platform trial is truly unique in terms of the speed with which it was able to be designed, operationalized, and open for patient accrual. RECOVERY was able to enroll its first patient only 9 days after the first draft of the protocol had been prepared and produced its first conclusion that hydroxychloroquine had no benefit, within approximately 3 months. The RECOVERY trial has since randomized at least 47,000 participants and has evaluated at least 10 therapies and has produced practice-changing results. The most notable of these was the conclusion that dexamethasone could reduce COVID-19 mortality. The RECOVERY trial has been said to stand out in a landscape of smaller underpowered trials in COVID-19 that produced a lot of discrepant and difficult-to-interpret results. The model for the RECOVERY trial was the large, simple cardiology trials of the 1980s (25). This speaks to the idea that platform trials do not have to be overly statistically complex and to the ability to accommodate the additional operational complexities and practical concerns associated with these trials.

1.2 Endpoints and Analysis

Endpoints used for registrational purposes in drug development are those that are clinically meaningful; they measure how a patient feels, functions, or survives. Surrogate endpoints, on the other hand, do not directly measure clinical benefit, but they tend to measure a biomarker of the disease process that is expected to be predictive of clinical outcomes (26). For example, immune response can be used as a surrogate endpoint for the efficacy of a vaccine under the assumption that an appropriate immune response will prevent symptomatic infection. The use of surrogate endpoints is very desirable in drug development because they are usually able to be ascertained sooner during therapy and have less variability than clinical endpoints. A trial tasked with showing an effect on a surrogate will be smaller and faster than a trial tasked with showing an effect on the clinical endpoint. However, it is difficult to establish surrogacy and candidates for surrogacy have a long history of poorly predicting clinical outcomes (27). A large base of evidence is required to show that a benefit on a surrogate endpoint will predict a benefit on the important clinical endpoints (28), and because surrogacy also depends on the treatment being studied, it is rare to have a deep evidence base for a particular class of therapy before drug development has moved into a newer class. However, the FDA has granted accelerated approval based on "reasonably likely" surrogate endpoints with the expectation that additional studies will be conducted to confirm clinical benefit. Due to the benefits in trial efficiency related to surrogates, the development of these endpoints is an active research area. For example, the Healey ALS platform trial features an "endpoint engine," meaning a prospective plan to collect data on candidate surrogate endpoints and clinical endpoints alike in order to be able to perform the analyses required to establish new surrogate endpoints for drug development (29). Wearable technology and the associated digital measurements have also unlocked potential novel endpoints. Wearable technology allows for very frequent and objective measurements to be taken at home in a real-world setting. One example is stride velocity 95th percentile (SV95C). This measures the speed of the fastest strides taken by the device wearer over a recording period of 180 hours and was qualified by the European Medicines Agency (EMA) in 2019 for use as an endpoint in trials for Duchenne's muscular dystrophy (30). The traditional registrational endpoint in this indication is the 6-minute walk test, but this test has numerous known issues including large amounts of variability and changes that depend on factors beyond disease (30). However, SVC95 was shown to correlate with the 6-minute walk test and to have the ability to predict clinical benefit. Trials based on this endpoint can be smaller and shorter than trials based on the 6-minute walk test (30).

Other types of novel endpoints include utility scores and composite endpoints. Utility scores have been proposed to weigh together multiple different endpoints into a single measure. Utility scores incorporate multiple different dimensions of efficacy and safety and represent the tradeoffs between them (31). The DAWN trial described above-used utility scores in place of an ordinal rating scale outcome to reflect that the ordinal categories were not equally spaced in terms of the desirability of the different health states (15). Hierarchical composite endpoints are another way to combine multiple different endpoints into a single measure. An example of the hierarchical composite endpoint is the Alive and Ventilator Free score (AVF) in acute respiratory distress syndrome (ARDS) (32). In this approach each patient is compared with every other patient in the trial and each comparison is categorized as a win, loss, or tie. Comparisons are made according to a prespecified ordering of endpoints from most to least clinically meaningful. For AVF, comparisons are first made on mortality, but if both patients in the comparison are still alive, they are then compared on the number of days they received mechanical ventilation. Based on the number of comparisons won or lost, the patients in the trial can be ranked and these ranks are compared between treatment and control. Approaches such as this are increasingly important in settings where mortality outcomes are improving and other endpoints beyond mortality are important clinically meaningful outcomes themselves.

When novel endpoints are not available, some trials have made use of novel statistical models. The addition of statistical modeling adds efficiency in many settings. For example, dose-response models can increase the power in a phase II dose-finding trial (33), or modeling across patient populations in a basket trial can increase power in small subgroups, as described above. In many progressive diseases, the clinical endpoint is measured at regular intervals longitudinally over the course of treatment and follow-up. The primary analysis may compare groups based on a change from the baseline or a model for repeated measures. However, a class of analysis, the disease progression model, is an alternative analysis method. These models characterize a rate of decline on the clinical endpoint and measure a relative, rather than absolute, improvement (34,35). This analysis method is less problematic in populations where some patients may be at earlier stages of their disease, where absolute changes can be small, and has been shown to have superior power as compared to other standard analysis models (35).

1.2.1 Endpoint and Analysis Case Study

GNE myopathy is a rare disease that causes muscle weakness where different skeletal muscle groups become involved in a particular predictable sequence as the disease progresses. Disease progression is slow, over decades, but results in a significant loss of muscle and causes disability. Quintana et al. used natural history data that included muscle strength measurements collected longitudinally to develop a Bayesian disease progression model that could be used in clinical trials for this indication (36). The model fits the individual patient-level data and estimates disease onset, rate of progression, and the resulting current "disease age" of the individual for each of the six muscle groups. Because a clinical trial population would include patients both early and late in the progression of the disease, and as such progression would be occurring in different muscle groups, the model synthesizes the progression across the six muscle groups to quantify the entire spectrum of the disease. However, muscle strength is considered a surrogate endpoint for the clinical outcome of functioning in daily life. The authors also show that the model-based disease age had a strong correlation with clinical endpoints such as the 6-minute walk test and other functional rating scales. Simulations showed that a clinical trial using the disease progression model for its analysis would require a much smaller sample size than using other endpoints or taking the strategy of limiting the trial population to a more homogenous population. This model and analysis strategy was used in a phase II trial of ManNAc (37). This trial enrolled 12 patients, all treated with ManNAc, and used the disease progression model to compare the treated group to the natural history data. Even with the small sample size, the disease progression model estimated a benefit due to treatment through 18 months. There were some issues noted with the long-term estimation of treatment effect including dropout, noncompliance, and a dysfunction in the device to measure strength for one of the muscle groups.

1.3 Real-World Data/Real-World Evidence

Real-world data (RWD) are data pertaining to a patient's health status and/or the delivery of health care collected from a variety of sources such as electronic health records (EHRs), claims and billing activities, pragmatic clinical trials, product and disease registries, patient-generated data including in home-use settings, and mobile or wearable devices. Real-world evidence (RWE) is the clinical evidence regarding the usage and potential benefits or risks of a medical product derived from the rigorous analysis of RWD with proper analytical methodology (38).

RWD consists of information collected during routine clinical practice, whereas RCTs are conducted in highly selective populations in well-controlled settings. RCTs can provide evidence on the efficacy and safety of a drug or device and have been the gold standard for evidence generation supporting regulatory approval. However, there are several disadvantages of RCTs (39). In addition to the high financial costs and long execution times, RCTs do not account for the broader patient population due to restrictive inclusion and exclusion criteria. Furthermore, RCTs are often of limited study duration and unable to assess long-term safety and effectiveness. Finally, regular follow-up and close monitoring in most clinical trials does not reflect routine clinical practice. It is clear that RWE would complement evidence generated from traditional clinical trials, especially in the assessment of safety and efficacy in real-world settings.

RWD can be used to better target and optimize clinical trial questions by furthering our understanding of the burden and natural history of the disease, identifying prognostic biomarkers and subgroups of patients where there is therapeutic potential, and to assess candidate endpoints (40). Historically, RWD has been used to help determine the treatment effect and sample sizes for powering RCTs. With careful design and patient selection, RWD can be used to emulate the target clinical trials (41). RWD can also be utilized in the planning and execution of clinical trials, including accelerating patient recruitment by applying trial inclusion/exclusion criteria against deidentified patient data from EHR databases to determine eligible patients, using analytics to select fast enrolling sites based on past performance such as the number of protocol violations. Recently, RWD have been used in risk-based monitoring to mitigate data quality issues.

Pragmatic clinical trials (PCTs), conducted in real-world clinical practice settings with typical patients and qualified clinicians, can serve as a bridge between RWE and RCTs (42). In PCTs, investigators often relax inclusion criteria requirements and accept a broader and more representative patient population. However, the patients are still randomized to treatment and control groups. When properly designed and conducted, PCTs can both test the treatment effect and understand the differences in treatment effects in different healthcare settings. They can generate evidence to inform both regulatory and payer decision-making.

RWD can be used to accelerate clinical trials by augmenting or replacing the control arm of a clinical trial, particularly in rare diseases where randomization is considered unethical or not feasible (43). Bayesian dynamic borrowing to form a synthetic control arm in single-arm trials or to augment control arms of RCTs has been proposed and implemented (44). For example, the Medical Device Innovation Consortium (MDIC) published an External Evidence Methods (EEM) Framework, which highlights the potential for incorporating data external to a clinical trial into the analysis of a medical device (45). The Drug Information Association Adaptive Design Scientific Working Group (DIA-ADSWG) provided a practical roadmap from design to analysis of a clinical trial to address the selection and inclusion of historical controls while maintaining scientific validity (46).

1.3.1 RWD/RWE Case Studies

The DAPA-MI trial is a pioneering registry-based PCT that combines elements of an RCT with innovative real-world trial elements. This study is among the first indication-seeking pragmatic trials and will evaluate the effect of dapagliflozin versus placebo on heart failure hospitalizations and cardiovascular death in patients without diagnosed diabetes who have an acute myocardial. This trial is unique in that it is sponsored by industry for the purpose of registration, while it is double blinded and placebo controlled. The DAPA-MI pragmatic trial enrolled patients from two high-quality national registries: SWEDEHEART in Sweden and MINAP in the UK. Routine follow-up data is captured automatically, resulting in a substantial reduction of the burden on both patients and investigators. Other pragmatic elements include the use of mobile phone applications to query patients about clinical events and "CleverCap Lite" bottle caps, which record the number of pills dispensed from the container by the patient and allow real-time tracking of adherence to medication. The unique design features led to a higher recruitment rate and lower overall costs in comparison to conventional clinical trials.

RWE has been used to provide critical evidence for drug approval (47). FDA recently approved Prograf (tacrolimus) in combination with other immunosuppressant drugs for preventing organ rejection in adult and pediatric patients receiving lung transplantation. The approval demonstrates that a well-designed, noninterventional (observational) study with reliable and relevant RWD can be considered adequate for regulatory approval. Specifically, the noninterventional study supporting approval for this new indication used RWD from the US Scientific Registry of Transplant Recipients (SRTR), supported by the Department of Health and Human Services. The data were collected on all lung transplants in the United States and were supplemented by information from the Social Security Administration's Death Master File as a trusted repository of mortality data. A dramatic improvement in outcomes was observed among lung transplant patients receiving Prograf as part of their immunosuppression medications compared to the well-documented natural history of lung transplant with no or minimal immunosuppressive therapy.

As more drugs are approved by regulatory authorities either through the FDA orphan drug and breakthrough therapy designations or EMA Conditional Approval, using RWE to supplement the findings in RCTs helps avoid costly postmarketing trials and ensures early access. For example, blinatumomab received accelerated approval for the treatment of Philadelphia chromosome-negative relapsed or refractory B-cell precursor ALL based on a single-arm trial of 189 adult patients (47). Historical control data for 694 patients were extracted from European national study groups and large individual sites from Europe and the United States. Two analytical approaches were used. The first was a weighted analysis, whereby outcomes from the historical data set were weighted according to the frequency distribution of predetermined prognostic baseline factors in the blinatumomab clinical trial population. The second was a propensity score analysis, which created a better balance between historical and blinatumomab-treated patients with respect to important baseline factors and enabled the quantification of differences in outcomes between the two groups. Both methods demonstrated significant benefits for patients receiving blinatumomab compared to historical controls.

1.4 Artificial Intelligence and Machine Learning

The role of artificial intelligence (AI) and machine learning (ML) has grown alongside RWD/RWE and the volume of data now available. These analytical methods are suited to large and complex datasets such as those from EHRs, medical images, genomic data, and continuous monitoring from wearable health sensors (4). These tools are used to find patterns in large datasets. They learn from previous data to gradually improve the ability to accomplish particular tasks such as diagnosing, predicting treatment outcomes for therapeutic decision making, or predicting a patient's individual risk for a future event (44). AI/ML technologies have been integrated into clinical development and are now becoming a cornerstone of successful modern clinical trials. AI/ML has been applied to virtually all stages of drug R&D (48). For example, ML has been used to predict the pharmaceutical properties of molecular compounds and targets for drug discovery. Pattern recognition and segmentation techniques on medical images, e.g., retinal scans, pathology slides and body surfaces, bones and internal organs, can enable faster diagnoses and tracking of disease progression; generative algorithms can be used for computational augmentation of existing clinical and imaging data sets; and deep-learning techniques on multimodal data sources such as combining genomic and clinical data are developed to detect new predictive models (49).

By matching patient characteristics from linked databases to clinical trial eligibility criteria, AI/ML tools can be used to identify, recruit, and monitor patients within clinical trials (50). It has been shown that AI-based clinical trial matching resulted in an increase in the enrollment of a lung cancer trial by 58.4%. Deep learning has exhibited remarkable success in identifying potential new drug candidates and improving the prediction of their properties and the possible safety risks (51). AI can improve the efficiency in searching for correlation between indications and biomarkers and help in selecting lead compounds that could have a higher chance of success during clinical development (50).

AI techniques, in combination with wearable technology, are valuable in efficient, real-time, and personalized monitoring of patients automatically and continuously during the trial. This can improve compliance with protocol requirements and the reliability of the assessment of endpoints. DL models, by analyzing data from wearable sensors and video monitoring, can generate patient-specific disease diaries adapted to behavioral changes and disease expression. Such dynamic disease diaries facilitate efficient and reliable collection of compliance and endpoints. ML technologies, approved for the detection of medical images, would play an important role in image-based endpoint detection (50). ML-based algorithms have been tried to determine the smallest and fewest doses required to shrink brain tumors while reducing chemotherapy adverse effects, in simulated trials. This could reduce the risk of dropouts due to safety issues (50).

1.4.1 AI/ML Case Study

AI/ML technology has been crucial in speeding up the development process for the COVID-19 vaccine (52): starting from drug discovery to clinical trials, to supply chain management, to, finally, distribution to people. The development of the Pfizer-BioNTech COVID-19 vaccine is a successful example of using AI/ML technologies (53). First, ML algorithms helped the company predict yields during the manufacturing stage before tens of thousands of volunteers from six countries were recruited for testing. AI systems were used to analyze any discrepancies in the participants' symptoms. Both AI and ML were used to predict product temperatures and enable preventative maintenance for the more than 3000 freezers that store vaccine doses. In addition, Internet of Things (IoT) and sensors were utilized to monitor and track vaccine shipments and temperatures at close to 100% accuracy.

1.5 Decentralization and Diversity

Two key barriers to conducting a clinical trial are cost and difficulty in recruiting and retaining trial participants (54). The largest portion of a trial's total cost is attributable to clinical procedures, administrative staff, and site monitoring (54). Major opportunities to reduce costs include in-home testing and mobile technologies, where these strategies have the potential to reduce the cost of a phase III trial by 17% and 12%, respectively (54). A decentralized clinical trial is a clinical trial where participants may not always be required to visit the study site for the study procedures, but rather all or a portion of the trial activities are conducted remotely, at the participants' home, or at local health care facilities (6). Examples of decentralization include the shipping of study drug directly to participants' homes to self-administer, telemedicine or at-home healthcare visits, and data collection conducted through websites, mobile applications, or wearable devices (6,55).

Decentralization directly addresses some of the major costs of conducting a clinical trial, but these strategies also offer benefits in terms of participant recruitment and retention. Many of these features reduce the burden of clinical trial participation because the clinical trial activities are more integrated into daily living with fewer requirements to travel and spend time at the study site (6,55). This has been shown to enhance recruitment, decrease dropout, and increase compliance (5,6,55). However, decentralization may not be appropriate in every clinical trial setting. Clinical trials conducted in indications that require intensive care, where the safety profile of the drug is not well understood, or where the drug cannot be self-administered, such as intravenous routes, may be more limited in their ability to decentralize (6,55). However, low-risk and chronic diseases that are often somewhat self-managed may be viable candidates for decentralization (55). Additionally, rare disease indications might particularly benefit from decentralization because the ability to enroll would be less hindered by geography and access to a study site. Other concerns over decentralization include protecting the safety of the participants, particularly in terms of providing appropriate care and oversite to detect adverse events but also in terms of protecting their personal health information. Data quality is also a key area of consideration with possible issues related to data collection procedures, novel endpoints, and digital outcomes that may generate large datasets (55).

Clinical trial results provide the critical evidence base for evaluating the safety and efficacy of new medicines and medical products. Efficacy and safety may differ among population subgroups depending on intrinsic/extrinsic factors, including sex, age, race, ethnicity, lifestyle, and genetic background. A systematic evaluation of trial eligibility criteria on oncology trials showed that many patients who were excluded from the original trials could potentially benefit from the treatments (60). Racial and ethnic minorities continue to be underrepresented in many clinical trials (57). Besides the benefit of promoting social justice and health equity, clinical studies with diverse patient populations enjoy improved replicability and generalizability (58,59). The major barriers to more diverse clinical trials include lack of information and comfort with the clinical trials; time and resource constraints associated with clinical trial participation; and lack of awareness about the existence and importance of clinical trials (56).

Although barriers to diversity in trials are well recognized, sustainable solutions for overcoming them have proved elusive. Regulatory agencies, scientific communities, and health industries have all long recognized the importance of inclusion and diversity in clinical trials. *The New England Journal of Medicine* encouraged more diverse study populations for trials and required research studies to provide information on the selection and representativeness of study participants (61). The US Food and Drug Administration (FDA) has issued final guidance for addressing the diversity of individuals participating in clinical trials of new drugs or biologics. The aim is to increase enrollment for underrepresented groups to ensure a broader understanding of these products' risks and benefits (62). Health industries started to build the knowledge base of clinical trial diversity (63,64).

1.4.2 Case Studies in Decentralization and Diversity

The CHIEF-HF (Canagliflozin: Impact on Health Status, Quality of Life and Functional Status in Heart Failure) study was a randomized, double-blind, placebo-controlled trial designed to determine the superiority of canagliflozin in a broad heart failure population. The primary endpoint was the 12-week change in the Kansas City Cardiomyopathy Questionnaire (KCCQ), which is a patient-reported quality-of-life measurement. CHIEF-HF was designed to be completely decentralized. Patients were enrolled through a study website with electronic informed consent, study medication was shipped directly to the patient's home, and the KCCQ was completed with a mobile application. Other data collected in the trial included activity monitoring using a Fitbit and adverse events and other clinical events collected through patient self-reports and an all-payer claims database (65). CHIEF-HF was successfully launched and conducted during the COVID-19 pandemic, enrolling 448 participants and demonstrating the superiority of canagliflozin on the primary endpoint (66).

Two cancer drugs, surufatinib and sintilimab, were rejected by FDA because of lack of patient representativeness. Per the complete response letter, a multiregional clinical trial that includes patients representative of the US population and medical practice consistent with current US standards will be required for FDA approval (67). A clear message was delivered by the regulatory agency that racial and ethnic diversity in clinical trials cannot be an afterthought and a prospective plan to address the inclusion of representative numbers of patients from racial and ethnic subgroups in clinical trials is recommended.

1.5 Challenges and Opportunities

Breaking new ground in the design and conduct of clinical trials is challenging work. Many features of what would be considered a gold-standard clinical trial were set decades ago. For example, the threshold for statistical success, $p < 0.05$, was a matter of convenience precomputers and is now a matter of tradition more than it is always an appropriate reflection of scientific principles (68). However, these traditions have served us well because it is rare for an ineffective or unsafe therapy to receive FDA approval (68). The suitability for innovating in clinical trials must be judged relative to the context of the scientific questions. The traditional paradigm works well when the science is asking a simple question that can readily be answered by a feasible sample size and a standard trial design. However, insisting on conventions when they no longer fit the science may mean doing worse science, slowing the ability to get effective drugs to patients, or even preventing the development of a therapy entirely. The Drug Information Association (DIA) identified challenges associated with implementing Bayesian methods into clinical trials, but many of these apply more broadly to clinical trial innovation generally (69). These include the lack of training and fully worked case examples to follow, the perception of regulatory acceptance, and having appropriate tools and internal support.

Various groups are actively addressing these challenges in different ways. Examples of training and education include the Innovative Clinical Trials Resource launched by the National Heart Lung and Blood Institute and the Clinical Trials Methodology Course available through the Neurologic Emergencies Treatment Trials Network (70,71). There are also numerous professional organizations that are devoted to different clinical trial topics and offer published materials, meetings, working groups, and webinars. This includes the Clinical Trial Transformation Initiative, EU-PEARL (Patient Centric Clinical Trial Platforms), the Society for Clinical Trials, and the Drug Information Association (DIA). Johns Hopkins University and the University of Washington are examples of two academic institutions that offer summer institutes consisting of intensive short courses including clinical trials topics.

In terms of regulatory acceptance, the FDA has guidance on many of the modern trends we see in clinical trials including adaptive designs, master protocols, surrogate endpoints, RWE, and decentralization (5). The FDA also initiated a Complex Innovate Design Pilot Program with the goal of advancing complex and novel clinical trial designs. The trials accepted into the pilot program are under the condition that the details will be made public and a set of case studies has become available (73). The FDA Oncology Center of Excellence has also launched Project Significant to engage various trial stakeholder groups to discuss topics related to the design and analysis of cancer clinical trials. Topics have included master protocols, diversity, and rare pediatric cancers (74). This all signals a regulatory openness to innovate to bring safe and effective drugs to patients. However, no approach has either universal regulatory acceptance or refusal. Rather, regulatory acceptance is contingent on the details of the proposal including the specifics of the clinical trial design, the therapy under investigation, the population being studied, and the phase of drug development.

There is very little written on how to foster the application of clinical trial innovations within organizations (69). A report done for the US Department of Health and Human Services noted the sponsor's own excessive risk aversion as a barrier in clinical trials (54). Certainly, risk aversion plays a role in the decision to innovate. However, there are examples of different organizations successfully investing in the resources to innovate.

Eli Lilly and Company created a dedicated group to develop clinical trial methods and user-friendly tools and provide internal education (69) and many other pharmaceutical companies have followed suit. Amgen established the Center for Design and Analysis to evaluate advanced trial designs along with initiatives to accelerate their adoption (75) and Amgen achieved participation in the FDA's CID pilot program and now uses adaptive designs in their pipeline (75).

Tools and implementation tend to go hand in hand, where challenges can be separated into those regarding trial design versus those regarding trial execution. On the trial design side, challenges center on the ability to assess complex statistical methods and the advantages they may bring. Often extensive simulations are required to characterize the expected performance of different approaches. Software for many complex statistical methods is commercially available (76,77) or publicly available (78,79). However, challenges frequently remain when custom trial designs are not accommodated within existing software tools and bespoke programming is required. The ability to create, conduct, and communicate the results of extensive simulation studies may require dedicated and experienced personnel, computing resources, and additional training and education. These new trial designs must then be implemented, executed, and reported. The challenges related to implementation will vary depending on the innovative aspects. For example, a trial with adaptive randomization or arm dropping does not have a set drug supply, including a novel digital health device may require new databases, and the use of decentralized trial elements may require additional service providers and contracting. Within an organization, creativity and flexibility is required in policies and procedures to create or modify the necessary systems along with corresponding quality monitoring and validation procedures (80,81).

The final challenge is the communication of the trial design and results. Innovative clinical trials will often involve specialized expertise in the innovation being applied. The methods being proposed and their benefits and risks versus other viable alternatives may not be transparent to all trial stakeholder groups. Furthermore, the innovation could be approached with skepticism by some due to their experiences with what has worked well in the past. Getting past this challenge requires continuing education and transparent and open dialogue (69,80,82).

While the challenges associated with innovating in clinical trials should not be underestimated, the literature has examples where these challenges have been overcome and innovations have been put into practice (80,81). Given the activities surrounding education and training, the channels of dialogue that are open with regulatory bodies, and the growing set of case studies, the future opportunities for growing and applying the novel approaches described in this chapter are boundless.

References

1. Lamberti M.J., Getz K. Profiles of new approaches to improving the efficiency and performance of pharmaceutical drug development. *Tufts Center for the Study of Drug Development* White Paper. May 2015. https://f.hubspotusercontent10.net/hubfs/9468915/TuftsCSDD_June2021/pdf/PROFILES+OF+NEW+APPROACHES+TO+IMPROVING+THE+EFFICIENCY+AND+PERFORMANCE+OF+PHARMACEUTICAL+DRUG+DEVELOPMENT+.pdf
2. Anderson R.M., Hadjichrysanthou C., Evans S., Wong M.M. Why do so many clinical trials of therapies for Alzheimer's disease fail? *The Lancet*. Nov 25: 390(10110): 2327–9. 2017.

3. Biankin A.V., Piantadosi S., Hollingsworth S.J. Patient-centric trials for therapeutic development in precision oncology. *Nature*. Oct: 526(7573): 361–70. 2015.
4. Rajkomar A., Dean J., Kohane I. Machine learning in medicine. *The New England Journal of Medicine*. Apr 4: 380(14): 1347–58. 2019.
5. Dhaliwal A. Council post: Four trends in the clinical research industry propelled by the pandemic. *Forbes*. Mar 23. www.forbes.com/sites/forbesbusinesscouncil/2021/08/16/four-trends-in-the-clinical-research-industry-propelled-by-the-pandemic/. 2022.
6. Apostolaros M., Babaian D., Corneli A., Forrest A., Hamre G., Hewett J., et al. Legal, regulatory, and practical issues to consider when adopting decentralized clinical trials: recommendations from the clinical trials transformation initiative. *Therapeutic Innovation & Regulatory Science*. Jul 1: 54(4): 779–87. 2020.
7. Bhatt A. Evolution of clinical research: a history before and beyond James Lind. *Perspectives in Clinical Research*. 1(1): 6–10. 2010.
8. Pocock S. Group sequential methods in the design and analysis of clinical trials. *Biometrika*. 64(2): 191–9. 1977.
9. Biswas S., Liu D.D., Lee J.J., Berry D.A. Bayesian clinical trials at the University of Texas M. D. Anderson Cancer Center. *Clinical Trials*. Jun 1: 6(3): 205–16. 2009.
10. Bothwell L.E., Avorn J., Khan N.F., Kesselheim A.S. Adaptive design clinical trials: a review of the literature and ClinicalTrials.gov. *BMJ Open*. Feb 10: 8(2):e018320. 2018.
11. Berry D.A. Bayesian clinical trials. *Nature Reviews Drug Discovery*. Jan: 5(1): 27–36. 2006.
12. Ryan E.G., Bruce J., Metcalfe A.J., Stallard N., Lamb S.E., Viele K., et al. Using Bayesian adaptive designs to improve phase III trials: a respiratory care example. *BMC Medical Research Methodology*. May 14: 19(1): 99. 2019.
13. Luce B.R., Connor J.T., Broglio K.R., Mullins C.D., Ishak K.J., Saunders E., et al. Using Bayesian adaptive trial designs for comparative effectiveness research: a virtual trial execution. *Annals of Internal Medicine*. Sep 20: 165(6): 431–8. 2016.
14. Broglio K., Meurer W.J., Durkalski V., Pauls Q., Connor J., Berry D., et al. Prospective comparison of Bayesian and frequentist adaptive clinical trials: the SHADOW – SHINE project. *medRxiv*. Mar 23. p. 2021.06.02.21257838. 2021. www.medrxiv.org/content/10.1101/2021.06.02.21257838v1
15. Nogueira R.G., Jadhav A.P., Haussen, D.C., Bonafe A., Budzik R., Bhuva, P. et al. Thrombectomy 6 to 24 hours after stroke with a mismatch between deficit and infarct. *New England Journal of Medicine*. Jan 4. 2018. www.nejm.org/doi/full/10.1056/nejmoa1706442
16. Woodcock J., LaVange L.M. Master protocols to study multiple therapies, multiple diseases, or both. *New England Journal of Medicine*. Jul 6: 377(1): 62–70. 2017.
17. Cunanan K.M., Gonen M., Shen R., Hyman D.M., Riely G.J., Begg C.B., et al. Basket trials in oncology: a trade-off between complexity and efficiency. *Journal of Clinical Oncology*. Jan 20: 35(3): 271–3. 2017.
18. Saville B.R., Berry S.M. Efficiencies of platform clinical trials: a vision of the future. *Clinical Trials*. Jun: 13(3): 358–66. 2016.
19. Lesser N., Naaz B. Master protocols. *Deloitte Insights*. Sept 17. 2018. www2.deloitte.com/content/www/us/en/insights/industry/life-sciences/master-protocol-clinical-trial-drug-development-process.html
20. Society for Clinical Trials. Mar 23. 2022. Available from: www.sctweb.org/toty.cfm
21. Lu C.C., Li X.N., Broglio K., Bycott P., Jiang Q., Li X., et al. Practical considerations and recommendations for master protocol framework: basket, umbrella and platform trials. *Therapeutic Innovation & Regulatory Science*. Nov: 55(6): 1145–54. 2021.
22. Sridhara R., Marchenko O., Jiang Q., Pazdur R., Posch M., Berry S., et al. Use of nonconcurrent common control in master protocols in oncology trials: report of an American Statistical Association Biopharmaceutical Section Open Forum Discussion. *Statistics in Biopharmaceutical Research*. Jun 3: 14(3): 353–7. 2021.
23. Subbiah V., Bang Y.J., Lassen U.N., Wainberg Z.A., Soria J.C., Wen P.Y., et al. ROAR: a phase 2, open-label study in patients (pts) with BRAF V600E–mutated rare cancers to investigate the efficacy and safety of dabrafenib (D) and trametinib (T) combination therapy. *JCO*. May 20: 34(15_suppl): TPS2604–TPS2604. 2016.

24. Subbiah V., Kreitman R.J., Wainberg Z.A., Cho J.Y., Schellens J.H.M., Soria J.C. et al. Dabrafenib plus trametinib in patients with BRAF V600E-mutant anaplastic thyroid cancer: updated analysis from the phase II ROAR basket study. *Annals of Oncology*. April: 33(4): 406–15. 2022. www.sciencedirect.com/science/article/pii/S0923753422000059

25. Mullard A. RECOVERY 1 year on: a rare success in the COVID-19 clinical trial landscape. *Nature Reviews Drug Discovery*. Apr 16: 20(5): 336–7. 2021.

26. FDA-NIH Biomarker Working Group. BEST (Biomarkers, EndpointS, and other Tools) Resource. Silver Spring (MD): Food and Drug Administration (US). May 9. 2016 www.ncbi.nlm.nih.gov/books/NBK326791/

27. Fleming T.R., DeMets D.L. Surrogate end points in clinical trials: are we being misled? *Annals of Internal Medicine*. Oct: 125(7): 605–13. 1996.

28. U.S. Food & Drug Administration. Surrogate endpoint resources for drug and biologic development. FDA. Jan 29. 2021. www.fda.gov/drugs/development-resources/surrogate-endpoint-resources-drug-and-biologic-development

29. Paganoni S., Berry J.D., Quintana M., Macklin E., Saville B.R., Detry M.A., et al. Adaptive platform trials to transform amyotrophic lateral sclerosis therapy development. *Annals of Neurology*. Feb: 91(2): 165–75. 2022.

30. Servais L., Yen K., Guridi M., Lukawy J., Vissière D., Strijbos P. Stride velocity 95th centile: insights into gaining regulatory qualification of the first wearable-derived digital endpoint for use in Duchenne muscular dystrophy trials. *Journal of Neuromuscular Diseases*. 9(2): 335–46. 2022.

31. Skrivanek Z., Berry S., Berry D., Chien J., Geiger M.J., Anderson J.H., et al. Application of adaptive design methodology in development of a long-acting glucagon-like peptide-1 analog (Dulaglutide): statistical design and simulations. *Journal of Diabetes Science and Technology*. Nov 1: 6(6): 1305–18. 2012.

32. Novack V., Beitler J.R., Yitshak-Sade M., Thompson B.T., Schoenfeld D.A., Rubenfeld G., et al. Alive and ventilator-free: a hierarchical, composite outcome for clinical trials in the acute respiratory distress syndrome. *Critical Care Medicine*. Feb: 48(2): 158–66. 2020.

33. Gajewski B.J., Meinzer C., Berry S.M., Rockswold G.L., Barsan W.G., Korley F.K., et al. Bayesian hierarchical EMAX model for dose-response in early phase efficacy clinical trials. *Stat Med*. 38(17): 3123–38. 2019.

34. Lake S.L., Quintana M.A., Broglio K., Panagoulias J., Berry S.M., Panzara M.A. Bayesian adaptive design for clinical trials in Duchenne muscular dystrophy. *Stat Med*. Aug 30: 40(19): 4167–84. 2021.

35. Wang G., Berry S., Xiong C., Hassenstab J., Quintana M., McDade E.M., et al. A novel cognitive disease progression model for clinical trials in autosomal-dominant Alzheimer's disease. *Stat Med*. Sep 20: 37(21): 3047–55. 2018.

36. Quintana M., Shrader J., Slota C., Joe G., McKew J.C., Fitzgerald M., et al. Bayesian model of disease progression in GNE myopathy. *Stat Med*. Apr 15: 38(8): 1459–74. 2019.

37. Carrillo N., Malicdan M.C., Leoyklang P., Shrader J.A., Joe G., Slota C., et al. Safety and efficacy of N-acetylmannosamine (ManNAc) in patients with GNE myopathy: an open-label phase 2 study. *Genetics in Medicine*. Nov: 23(11): 2067–75. 2021.

38. Administration UFD. Framework for FDA's real-world evidence program. D.o.H.a.H Services, Editor. 2018.

39. Kim H.S., Lee S., Kim J.H. Real-world evidence versus randomized controlled trial: clinical research based on electronic medical records. *Journal of Korean Medical Science*. Aug 20: 33(34): e213. 2018.

40. Barritt A.S., Gitlin N., Klein S., Lok A.S., Loomba R., Malahias L., et al. Design and rationale for a real-world observational cohort of patients with nonalcoholic fatty liver disease: the TARGET-NASH study. *Contemporary Clinical Trials*. Oct: 61: 33–8. 2017.

41. Hernán M.A., Robins J.M. Using big data to emulate a target trial when a randomized trial is not available. American Journal of Epidemiology. Apr 15: 183(8): 758–64. 2016.

42. Usman M.S, Van Spall H.G.C., Greene S.J., Pandey A., McGuire D.K., Ali Z.A., et al. The need for increased pragmatism in cardiovascular clinical trials. *Nature Reviews Cardiology*. May 17: 1–14. 2022.

43. Jahanshahi M., Gregg K., Davis G., Ndu A., Miller V., Vockley J., et al. The use of external controls in FDA regulatory decision making. *Therapeutic Innovation & Regulatory Science*. Sep: 55(5): 1019–35. 2021.

44. Ho M., van der Laan M., Lee H., Chen J., Lee K., Fang Y., et al. The current landscape in biostatistics of real-world data and evidence: causal inference frameworks for study design and analysis. *Statistics in Biopharmaceutical Research*. Feb 1: 15(1): 43–56. 2021.

45. Timbie J.W., Kim A.Y., Concannon T.W. Use of real-world evidence for regulatory approval and coverage of medical devices: a landscape assessment. *Value Health*. Dec: 24(12): 1792–8. 2021.

46. Ghadessi M., Tang R., Zhou J., Liu R., Wang C., Toyoizumi K., et al. A roadmap to using historical controls in clinical trials – by Drug Information Association Adaptive Design Scientific Working Group (DIA-ADSWG). *Orphanet Journal of Rare Diseases*. Mar 12: 15(1): 69. 2020.

47. Gökbuget N., Kelsh M., Chia V., Advani A., Bassan R., Dombret H., et al. Blinatumomab vs historical standard therapy of adult relapsed/refractory acute lymphoblastic leukemia. *Blood Cancer Journal*. Sep 23: 6(9): e473. 2016.

48. Bhatt A. Artificial intelligence in managing clinical trial design and conduct: man and machine still on the learning curve? *Perspectives in Clinical Research*. Jan 1: 12(1): 1. 2021.

49. Shah P., Kendall F., Khozin S., Goosen R., Hu J., Laramie J., et al. Artificial intelligence and machine learning in clinical development: a translational perspective. *NPJ Digit Medicine*. Jul 26: 2(1): 1–5. 2019.

50. Harrer S., Shah P., Antony B., Hu J. Artificial intelligence for clinical trial design. *Trends in Pharmacological Science*. Aug 1: 40(8): 577–91. 2019.

51. Mak K.K., Pichika M.R. Artificial intelligence in drug development: present status and future prospects. *Drug Discovery Today*. 24(3): 773–80. 2019. https://onwork.edu.au/bibi tem/2019-Mak,Kit-Kay-Pichika,Mallikarjuna+Rao-Artificial+intelligence+in+drug+developm ent+present+status+and+future+prospects/

52. Kolluri S., Lin J., Liu R., Zhang Y., Zhang W.. Machine learning and artificial intelligence in pharmaceutical research and development: a review. *AAPS Journal*. Jan 4: 24(1): 19. 2022.

53. Quach K. Pfizer used AI and big iron to design its COVID-19 vaccine. *The Register*. Mar 22. 2022. www.theregister.com/2022/03/22/pfizer_nvidia_ai/

54. Examination of clinical trial costs and barriers for drug development. ASPE. Jul 24. 2014. https://aspe.hhs.gov/reports/examination-clinical-trial-costs-barriers-drug-deve lopment-0

55. de Jong A.J., van Rijssel T.I., Zuidgeest M.G.P., van Thiel G.J.M.W., Askin S., Fons-Martínez J., et al. Opportunities and challenges for decentralized clinical trials: European regulators' perspective. *Clinical Pharmacology & Therapeutics*. April 30. 2022. https://onlinelibrary.wiley. com/doi/abs/10.1002/cpt.2628

56. Clark L.T., Watkins L., Piña I.L., Elmer M., Akinboboye O., Gorham M., et al. Increasing diversity in clinical trials: overcoming critical barriers. *Current Problems in Cardiolog*. May: 44(5): 148–72. 2019.

57. Loree J.M., Anand S., Dasari A., Unger J.M., Gothwal A., Ellis L.M., et al. Disparity of race reporting and representation in clinical trials leading to cancer drug approvals from 2008 to 2018. *JAMA Oncology*. Oct 10: 5(10): e191870. 2019.

58. Kennedy-Martin T., Curtis S., Faries D., Robinson S., Johnston J. A literature review on the representativeness of randomized controlled trial samples and implications for the external validity of trial results. *Trials*. Nov 3: 16: 495. 2015.

59. Usui T., Macleod M.R., McCann S.K., Senior A.M., Nakagawa S. Meta-analysis of variation suggests that embracing variability improves both replicability and generalizability in preclinical research. *PLOS Biology*. May 19. 2021. https://journals.plos.org/plosbiology/arti cle?id=10.1371/journal.pbio.3001009

60. Liu R., Rizzo S., Whipple S., Pal N., Pineda A.L., Lu M., et al. Evaluating eligibility criteria of oncology trials using real-world data and AI. *Nature.* Apr: 592(7855): 629–33. 2021.
61. Striving for diversity in research studies. *New England Journal of Medicine.* Oct 7: 385(15): 1429–30. 2021.
62. U.S. Food & Drug Administration. Enhancing the diversity of clinical trial populations – eligibility criteria, enrollment practices, and trial designs guidance for industry. Nov. 2020. www.fda.gov/regulatory-information/search-fda-guidance-documents/enhancing-diversity-clinical-trial-populations-eligibility-criteria-enrollment-practices-and-trial
63. Liu H., Chi Y., Butler A., Sun Y., Weng C. A knowledge base of clinical trial eligibility criteria. *Journal of Biomedical Informatics.* May: 117: 103771. 2021.
64. Rottas M., Thadeio P., Simons R., Houck R., Gruben D., Keller D., et al. Demographic diversity of participants in Pfizer sponsored clinical trials in the United States. *Contemporary Clinical Trials.* July: 106: 106421. www.sciencedirect.com/science/article/pii/S1551714421001579
65. Spertus J.A., Birmingham M.C., Butler J., Lingvay I., Lanfear D.E., Abbate A., et al. Novel trial design: CHIEF-HF. *Circulation: Heart Failure.* Mar: 14(3): e007767. 2021.
66. Spertus J.A., Birmingham M.C., Nassif M., Damaraju C.V., Abbate A., Butler J., et al. The SGLT2 inhibitor canagliflozin in heart failure: the CHIEF-HF remote, patient-centered randomized trial. *Nature Medicine.* Apr: 28(4): 809–13. 2022.
67. FDA's new diversity plan guidance, and what it means for sponsors developing cancer drugs. *Applied Clinical Trials Online.* June 9. 2022. www.appliedclinicaltrialsonline.com/view/fda-s-new-diversity-plan-guidance-and-what-it-means-for-sponsors-developing-cancer-drugs
68. Ruberg S.J., Harrell F.E., Gamalo-Siebers M., LaVange L., Jack Lee J., Price K., et al. Inference and decision making for 21st-century drug development and approval. *The American Statistician.* Mar 29: 73(sup1): 319–27. 2019
69. Natanegara F., Neuenschwander B., Seaman Jr. J.W., Kinnersley N., Heilmann C.R., Ohlssen D., et al. The current state of Bayesian methods in medical product development: survey results and recommendations from the DIA Bayesian Scientific Working Group. *Pharmaceutical Statistics.* 13(1): 3–12. 2014.
70. ICTR – Innovative Clinical Trial Resource. Cited Jul 20, 2022. https://innovativeclinicaltrial.org/
71. CTMC. NETT. Cited Jul 20, 2022. https://nett.umich.edu/training/ctmc
72. Office of the Commissioner. Clinical Trials Guidance Documents. FDA. Dec 23. 2021. www.fda.gov/regulatory-information/search-fda-guidance-documents/clinical-trials-guidance-documents
73. U.S. Food & Drug Administration. Complex innovative trial design pilot meeting program. FDA. Feb 8. 2022. www.fda.gov/drugs/development-resources/complex-innovative-trial-design-pilot-meeting-program
74. U.S. Food & Drug Administration. Project significant: statistics in cancer trials. FDA. Jun 15. 2022. www.fda.gov/about-fda/oncology-center-excellence/project-significant-statistics-cancer-trials
75. A strategy for making clinical trials more successful. Cited July 20. 2022. www.amgen.com/stories/2018/10/a-strategy-for-making-clinical-trials-more-successful
76. East Bayes. enhanced access to innovative bayesian clinical trial designs. Cited Jul 20. 2022. www.cytel.com/software/east-bayes/
77. Software – Berry Consultants. Cited Jul 20. 2022. www.berryconsultants.com/software/
78. Biostatistics Software Downloadable or Online. Cited Jul 20. 2022. https://biostatistics.mdanderson.org/softwaredownload/
79. R Core Team. R: a language and environment for statistical computing. Vienna, Austria: R Foundation for Statistical Computing. 2020. www.R-project.org/
80. Blagden S.P., Billingham L., Brown L.C., Buckland S.W., Cooper A.M., Ellis S., et al. Effective delivery of Complex Innovative Design (CID) cancer trials – a consensus statement. *British Journal of Cancer.* Feb: 122(4): 473–82. 2020.

81. Pallmann P., Bedding A.W., Choodari-Oskooei B., Dimairo M., Flight L., Hampson L.V., et al. Adaptive designs in clinical trials: why use them, and how to run and report them. *BMC Medicine*. Feb 28: 16(1): 29. 2018.

82. Guetterman T.C., Fetters M.D., Legocki L.J., Mawocha S., Barsan W.G., Lewis R.J., et al. Reflections on the adaptive designs accelerating promising trials into treatments (ADAPT-IT) process – findings from a qualitative study. *Clinical Research and Regulatory Affairs*. Oct 2: 32(4):119–28. 2015.

2

ANBL1531: The Children's Oncology Group (COG) Experience Using a Bayesian Approach

Arlene Naranjo, Rochelle Bagatell, Emily G. Greengard, and Steven G. DuBois

2.1 Background

ANBL1531 is a COG multiarm umbrella-type phase III clinical trial in children with newly diagnosed high-risk neuroblastoma. ANBL1531 is designed to simultaneously address multiple scientific questions about the benefits of adding ^{131}I-metaiodobenzylguanidine (MIBG) or a targeted inhibitor of signaling via the anaplastic lymphoma kinase (*ALK*) pathway to improve outcomes. ANBL1531 has five treatment arms. Two arms are nonrandom treatment assignments for patients who either have *ALK*-aberrant or MIBG non-avid disease. This chapter focuses on the remaining three arms, which are randomized treatment assignments for patients with MIBG-avid and *ALK* wild-type disease.

The current COG standard of care regimen for high-risk neuroblastoma includes induction chemotherapy, resection of the primary tumor, and consolidation therapy with tandem stem cell transplant and external beam radiation followed by post-consolidation immunotherapy. For patients with MIBG-avid and *ALK* wild-type disease, ANBL1531 was designed to elucidate the role of MIBG therapy added to the induction phase of therapy. However, there were also important questions about the consolidation phase of therapy. While the standard of care for consolidation in the United States is tandem stem cell transplants, other parts of the world use a different conditioning regimen, busulfan/melphalan (Bu/Mel), and perform a single stem cell transplant. Therefore, ANBL1531 included three randomized treatment arms for patients with MIBG-avid and *ALK* wild-type disease. Arm A is considered the control arm and is the current COG regimen for high-risk neuroblastoma. Arm B adds a block of MIBG therapy after the third induction cycle to current COG high-risk therapy. Arm C also adds a block of MIBG therapy after the third induction cycle to current COG high-risk therapy but substitutes Bu/Mel single stem cell transplant in place of tandem transplant during consolidation. The challenges of conducting clinical trials in pediatric oncology and the desire to address multiple different clinical questions within a single trial as efficiently as possible motivated the use of a Bayesian approach to the statistical design of this trial. However, this approach resulted in substantial challenges and delays during the review process, and multiple design revisions were required.

DOI: 10.1201/9781003288640-2

2.2 Trial Design Overview

The schema for ANBL1531 is shown in Figure 2.1. This study uses a delayed randomization. After enrollment, patients receive one cycle of induction chemotherapy while awaiting centralized determination of MIBG avidity and *ALK* status. Patients with MIBG non-avid, *ALK* wild-type disease are nonrandomly assigned to receive standard COG high-risk therapy (Arm D). Patients with *ALK* aberrant tumors are nonrandomly assigned to receive an ALK inhibitor added to standard COG high-risk therapy (Arm E). Patients with MIBG-avid and *ALK* wild-type disease are randomized to one of three arms (Arms A, B, and C) as described above. The primary endpoint is event-free survival (EFS), defined as the time from randomization to the first episode of disease relapse, progression, second malignancy, or death. Two comparisons of interest were defined across the three randomized arms. The primary objective was to compare the MIBG+tandem transplant arm (Arm B) to tandem transplant alone (Arm A) to determine the superiority of adding MIBG therapy during induction. A secondary objective was to compare MIBG+Bu/Mel (Arm C) to MIBG+tandem transplant (Arm B) to determine the noninferiority of the modified consolidation regimen. The target is to randomize 500 patients and the expected accrual rate is approximately 13 patients/month. The trial's final analysis was planned to take place after an additional 3 years of follow-up after accrual was complete.

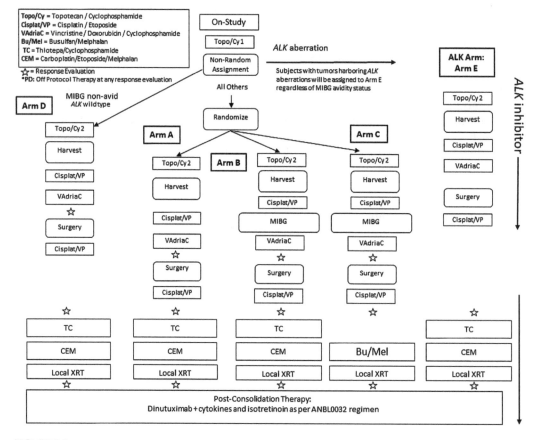

FIGURE 2.1
Study schema.

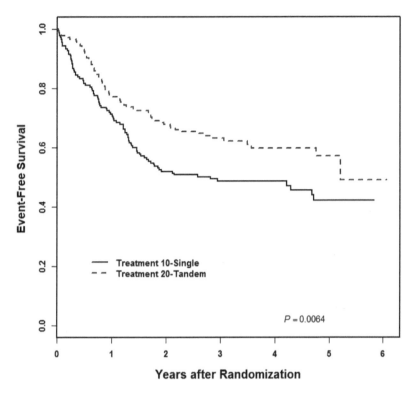

FIGURE 2.2
ANBL0532 initial results.

2.2.1 Bayesian Predictive Probabilities

The adaptive features of ANBL1531 are based on Bayesian predictive probabilities. A gamma-exponential model of EFS was defined to calculate these quantities. A previous COG trial, ANBL0532 (Park et al., 2019), evaluated single versus tandem stem cell transplant in the consolidation phase of treatment and showed the superiority of tandem transplant. Initial data from the 176 patients enrolled in the tandem transplant arm were used as the expected survival distribution for the standard-of-care COG treatment regimen (Arm A) for ANBL1531 (Figure 2.2). In ANBL0532, EFS was found to be 68% at 2 years, 60% at 4 years, and 49% at 6 years, when timed from randomization at the end of the induction phase of therapy. For ANBL1531, EFS was modeled as a piecewise exponential based on what was observed for the tandem transplant arm on ANBL0532. Pieces were defined at 0–2 years and 2+ years. Independent noninformative gamma prior distributions were assumed for each piece and the same priors were used for all arms. The prior distributions were centered on the expected survival for the tandem transplant arm.

The prior for the monthly hazard of the first 2 years is a gamma (shape parameter = 0.117, scale parameter = 0.1) distribution with a median of 0.016, which corresponds to an expected EFS rate on the tandem transplant arm of 68% at 2 years. Similarly, the prior for the second piece, the monthly hazard after 2 years, is a gamma (0.102, 0.1) distribution with a median of 0.0077. Taken with the first piece, this corresponds to the expectation that the EFS at 6 years from randomization on ANBL1531 will be 49%. This survival distribution, as well as those that would correspond to a benefit of the MIBG arms, is shown in Figure 2.3.

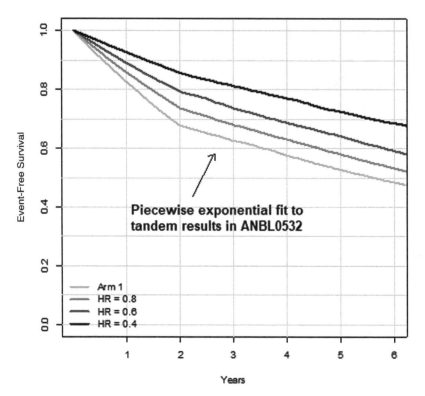

FIGURE 2.3
Hypothetical improvements on ANBL1531 over ANBL0532.

2.2.2 Original Bayesian Adaptive Design Features

The first trial design proposed included adaptive randomization, arm dropping, and early stopping as adaptive design features. Interim analyses were timed according to the number of patients randomized, starting when 250 patients were randomized and after every additional 50 patients were randomized. The adaptive decisions were to be evaluated at every interim and were based on the Bayesian predictive probabilities of success of each of the two comparisons of interest. The rationale for the accrual timed interims as well as each of the adaptive features was to make the most efficient use of the limited sample size available across the three randomized treatment arms. By taking frequent interim analyses during accrual to the trial, the trial would have the ability to move patients away from comparisons that were sufficiently addressed according to the accumulating data and redistribute patients to the questions where greater uncertainty remained.

Patients were to be initially randomized 1:1:½ to the tandem transplant:MIBG+tandem transplant:MIBG+Bu/Mel arms. The adaptive randomization scheme proposed to update the randomization ratio to the MIBG+Bu/Mel arm proportional to the probability of success for the primary comparison between MIBG+tandem transplant and tandem transplant. As the probability of success for the primary comparison increased, the sample size for this comparison could be reduced and more patients could be allocated to secondary comparison. In addition, the randomization ratio to the MIBG+Bu/Mel arm was limited in that it was scaled to be between ½ and 1 so that, at most, there would be equal allocation across the arms.

The superiority comparison between MIBG+tandem transplant and tandem transplant alone was monitored for both early futility and early success (Broglio et al. 2014). If the predictive probability of success for this primary comparison at the planned final analysis was low, below 5%, the entire randomized portion of the trial would stop early for futility. Alternatively, if the predictive probability of success for this primary comparison with the currently enrolled patients was high, greater than 90%, then accrual to the tandem transplant arm could be stopped early based on the expected success of the MIBG+tandem transplant arm. Follow-up of patients would continue to the planned final analysis, but the remaining patients to be randomized to the maximum sample size would be equally randomized between the two MIBG-containing arms. The secondary comparison, the noninferiority comparison between the MIBG+tandem transplant and MIBG+Bul/Mel arms, was monitored for early futility only. The MIBG+Bul/Mel arm could be dropped for predicted inferiority as compared to the MIBG+tandem transplant arm based on the predictive probability of observing a favorable hazard ratio (HR) between the arms. In this case, the trial would continue with patients randomized equally between the two primary comparison arms only.

While the interim analyses of the trial used Bayesian quantities, the planned final analyses were to be conducted according to standard frequentist statistical approaches. If the trial is not stopped early for futility, the final efficacy analysis for the primary comparison is an intent-to-treat log-rank test comparing EFS between the two treatment arms. The overall one-sided Type I error rate evaluated by simulation to control for the multiple interim analyses was less than 0.025. If the MIBG+Bu/Mel arm was not dropped early for futility, the MIBG+Bu/Mel arm would be deemed worthy of further consideration if the upper bound of the 90% confidence interval for the hazard ratio from a Cox proportional hazards model was less than 1.3.

2.2.3 Final Design

As a result of input from multiple review bodies (see next section), the final design of ANBL1531 reflected a change in the stated objective for the MIBG+Bu/Mel arm, a fixed randomization scheme, and a change in the timing of when the planned interim analyses could start by requiring a minimum number of events in each comparison before arm dropping was allowed. The final trial design had 81% power to determine the superiority of MIBG+tandem transplant over tandem transplant, assuming a hazard ratio of 0.63. The final test would be conducted at an alpha level of 0.0222 to account for the multiple interim analyses and the opportunity to stop early for predicted success.

2.3 Review Process and Revision of the Initial Trial Design

ANBL1531 was subject to review by multiple governing and regulatory bodies. Each of these groups had concerns about using a Bayesian approach for the statistical design. One review body expressed doubt that using Bayesian probabilities rather than the standard frequentist approaches to perform the interim analyses contributed positively to the trial and noted that the approach would likely complicate the interpretation of the final results. In this section, we describe the multiple changes to the trial design that were made in response to reviewer concerns.

2.3.1 Adaptive Randomization

Adaptive randomization was the first element of the original trial design that was discarded based on reviewer concerns. Reviewers commented that this feature draws patients away from the primary comparison and would reduce the power to determine the superiority of MIBG+tandem transplant over tandem transplant. Reviewers also expressed concerns that if the prognosis of patients enrolling in the trial changes over time, there is the potential for introducing bias into the treatment comparison due to temporal imbalance. Hence, a fixed randomization ratio of 1:1:½ was adopted, unless an arm was dropped.

2.3.2 Arm Dropping and Early Stopping

The first review of the trial design required that, in addition to having at least 250 patients randomized, interim analyses would not begin until at least 40% of the total number of expected events were observed to assure confidence in the results. Therefore, the design was changed such that 40% of the total information across all three arms was required before any arms could be dropped for either futility or predicted success. However, a subsequent meeting with a different review body required that a minimum of 50% of expected events be observed before any arm dropping would be allowed. Finally, a third review body indicated that the MIBG+Bu/Mel should be stopped earlier than 40% information if there were early evidence of insufficient efficacy. Therefore, the interim monitoring was revised such that the final arm dropping rules are:

1. When at least 50% of the total number of events expected for the primary comparison have been observed, enrollment to the tandem transplant arm may be stopped early for the predicted superiority of MIBG+tandem transplant if there is at least a 90% Bayesian predictive probability of success of MIBG+tandem transplant over tandem transplant alone with the currently enrolled patients.
2. When at least 40% of the total number of events expected for the primary comparison have been observed, the randomized portion of the trial may be stopped early for futility if there is less than a 5% Bayesian predictive probability that the primary comparison will be successful at the final analysis.
3. The MIBG+Bu/Mel may be dropped early for expected inferiority compared to MIBG+tandem transplant after at least 30% of the total number of events expected for the primary comparison have been observed. The MIBG+Bu/Mel arm will be dropped if there is less than a 10% predictive probability that the point estimate of the hazard ratio from a Cox proportional hazards model comparing MIBG+Bu/Mel to MIBG+tandem transplant is less than 1.1 should the trial continue to completion.

2.3.3 Secondary Comparison

During the review process, concerns regarding the inclusion of the MIBG+Bu/Mel arm were expressed. It appeared to reviewers that the design would not provide a clear answer to a Bu/Mel question and had the additional downside that it enrolled patients that could otherwise increase the power for the primary question. The reviewers recommended omitting the MIBG+Bu/Mel arm from the trial entirely. However, it was important to the COG neuroblastoma committee to retain this aim given the role of Bu/Mel as a transplant conditioning regimen in other parts of the world. Moreover, it was thought that a single Bu/Mel transplant could potentially result in lower rates of toxicity compared to two autologous stem cell transplants. Ultimately, the study committee was able to satisfy the reviewers and retain the arm by changing the objective from "comparing" the EFS of the MIBG+Bu/Mel versus MIBG+tandem transplant arms to the "estimation" of EFS for patients assigned to the MIBG+Bu/Mel arm.

2.3.4 Trial Conduct

While the prespecified rules for the arm dropping within the trial design are all based on Bayesian predictive probabilities, the Data Safety Monitoring Committee (DSMC) requested the calculation of more conventional statistical measures to help quantify evidence for stopping versus continuing the study. In addition, the DSMC required the estimated hazard ratios between the arms with two-sided 95% confidence intervals to be presented along with these other quantities to facilitate their decisions to drop arms for demonstrated futility or efficacy.

2.3.5 Impact on Operating Characteristics

The change from adaptive randomization to fixed randomization had little impact on the trial's operating characteristics. Ultimately, this adaptive feature did not add substantially to the goals of the adaptive design to redistribute patients to the different study questions over and above the arm dropping rules. Eliminating this feature addressed reviewer concerns, reduced the complexity of the trial, and retained the goals of the study.

However, the requirements imposed for a minimum number of events to be observed before arms could be stopped did make it more difficult for the trial to adapt during the accrual phase. Because the timing of arm dropping is later in accrual, the ability of the design to redistribute patients to other arms is limited, and this pushes the trial's expected sample size closer to a fixed sample size.

Operating characteristics for the primary comparison are shown in Table 2.1. Each row in the table has a top result (design with adaptive randomization), a middle result (design with fixed randomization), and a bottom result (final design with fixed randomization and imposed minimum number of events before arms can be dropped). In the original design, under the null hypothesis scenario, when the MIBG+tandem transplant arm is equivalent in EFS to tandem transplant alone, there is a 74% probability of stopping the trial early for futility with an average sample size savings of 110 patients. As the HR between the two arms decreases, the probability of futility stopping decreases, while the probability of stopping the tandem transplant arm for predicted success increases. At an HR of 0.60, there is a 77% probability of stopping the tandem transplant arm early. The operating characteristics also show that as the HR decreases, the total number of patients allocated to the tandem transplant only arm decreases while the total number of patients allocated to the two MIBG arms increases. In the final design, the probability of early futility under the null is reduced and the probability of early success under more optimistic HRs is reduced. The sample size distribution across the arms is close to 200:200:100, which would be the sample size of a fixed trial with no interims. Table 2.1 does show that, correspondingly, the power for the primary comparison is increased in the final design as compared to the original design. However, because the tandem transplant arm is less likely to stop early for success, the sample size on the MIBG+Bu/Mel arm is reduced, which ultimately reduces the information available for the additional question of interest between the two MIBG arms (results not shown).

TABLE 2.1

Operating Characteristics for Primary Comparison between Adaptive (top row), Fixed Randomization (middle row), and Final Design (bottom row) Probabilities.

True HR Arm B vs. Arm A	Mean Sample Size				Arm Dropping	Primary Comparison	
	Total	Arm A	Arm B	Arm C	Drop Arm A Predicted Success	Pr (Stop Early Futility)	Pr (Success)
1.0	393	155	155	82	1.0	74.2	2.2
	392	159	159	75	1.6	74.3	2.1
	435	176	176	83	0.9	64.2	2.2
0.8	440	170	174	97	8.4	40.3	24.0
	442	176	180	86	8.5	38.9	25.1
	475	191	192	92	6.6	27.3	30.0
0.7	459	173	181	105	18.6	23.6	51.6
	461	180	188	93	18.2	21.7	53.4
	487	195	197	95	11.8	13.7	59.7
0.6	470	168	186	117	36.5	10.9	77.4
	470	176	193	101	36.2	10.4	78.6
	495	197	200	98	17.1	4.2	86.8
0.5	474	158	190	127	57.9	4.4	93.0
	473	165	196	111	60.1	3.8	93.7
	498	198	201	99	15.2	0.7	98.0

HR: hazard ratio; Pr: probability.

The DSMC is tasked with protecting the safety of trial participants and the integrity of the study and should have access to any supplementary information they require to fulfill these duties. However, the decisions of the DSMC are not quantifiable. Should the DSMC overrule the prespecified adaptive design rules, there would be further impact on the trial's operating characteristics.

2.4 Discussion

Standard frequentist methods have historically been the preferred means to analyze randomized clinical trial data, but in rare diseases such as neuroblastoma, such methods may not be as efficient as other approaches. To advance treatment in pediatric cancers and other rare malignancies, Bayesian methods and other innovative statistical study design approaches are needed. COG conducts most of the childhood cancer clinical trials in the United States and houses a rich source of historical data that can help in designing future trials. Regulatory experience with Bayesian trials in pediatric oncology was minimal at the time ANBL1531 was designed and as such, additional time was needed during the design stage to obtain full approval from all review bodies tasked with oversight of this trial. Many of the requested design revisions were based on conventions surrounding interim analysis timings that come from traditional group-sequential trial design paradigms. While it is true that early interim analyses based on sparse data may lead to incorrect decisions based on spurious results, the Bayesian predictive probability does consider both the uncertainty of the current data and the uncertainty of the data yet to come (Saville et al. 2014). This is in contrast to the conditional power method that assumes a single, fixed-point estimate and considers only the uncertainty in the data yet to come. Additionally, case studies have demonstrated that Bayesian adaptive designs have the potential to be more efficient than traditional group sequential trial designs. However, Bayesian designs do rely heavily on simulations and sensitivity analyses, and acceptance of such methods as sufficient evidence to specify the study design characteristics is crucial for these methods to gain more widespread use.

During the approval process, conflicting requests were received from the various review bodies, and these had to be negotiated. Whenever a change was made to address a request from a review body, those changes then had to be submitted to agencies that had already approved the protocol to review and approve the modified design. This considerably slowed the ultimate regulatory approval and opening of ANBL1531 to patient accrual. It is possible that additional pre-meetings with these regulatory bodies may have facilitated review and ultimate approval. A more efficient model may be to form one committee comprised of members representing each of the regulatory bodies to review and provide approval for study protocols in a single comprehensive review. Coordinated review of this type would not only save time during the development of each individual trial but could also facilitate innovation in the design of clinical trials for patients with rare malignancies.

References

Broglio K.R., Connor J.T., Berry S.M. Not Too Big, Not Too Small: A Goldilocks Approach to Sample Size Selection. *J Biopharm Stat.* 24(3): 685–705. 2014.

Park J.R., Kreissman S.G., London W.B., Naranjo A., Cohn S.L., Hogarty M.D., et al. Effect of Tandem Autologous Stem Cell Transplantation vs. Single Transplantation on Event-Free Survival in Patients with High-Risk Neuroblastoma: A Randomized Clinical Trial. *J Am Med Assoc.* 322(8): 746–55. 2019.

Saville B.R., Connor J.T., Ayers G.D., Alvarez J. The Utility of Bayesian Predictive Probabilities for Interim Monitoring of Clinical Trials. *Clin Trials.* Aug; 11(4): 485–93. 2014.

3

Being SMART about Behavioral Intervention Trials for the Management of Chronic Conditions: Lessons Learned Using Sequential Multiple Assignment Randomized Trials (SMARTs)

Sylvie D. Lambert, Lydia Ould Brahim, and Erica E.M. Moodie

Introduction

In this chapter, lessons learned on the use of Sequential Multiple Assignment Randomized Trials (SMARTs) to optimize behavioral interventions for the management of chronic conditions are shared. Behavioral interventions usually aim to affect how individuals act, manage, and/or cope with a chronic condition (Cutler 2004). This is often achieved by combining psychoeducation and behavior change techniques such as goal setting and action planning to support individuals' learning and integration of new behaviors in daily life (Cutler 2004). Examples include making lifestyle changes and learning chronic disease self-management skills.

Behavioral interventions have positive effects on a wide range of health and clinical outcomes, and this across physical and mental health conditions (Allegrante et al., 2019, Bricca et al. 2022, Li et al. 2021, Peytremann-Bridevaux et al., 2015). Most of this evidence-base is derived from standard randomized controlled trials (RCTs), whereby a group of individuals given a fixed behavioral intervention is compared to a control group. The intervention is fixed because all participants in that group typically receive the same intervention for the entire duration of the trial, regardless of how they benefit or not from it (Collins, Murphy, and Bierman 2004).

However, managing a chronic condition is anything but fixed. Effective clinical care for chronic conditions typically requires a series of behavioral interventions, each tried for a certain period, with clinicians deciding to change or adapt the intervention based on how individuals respond (Almirall et al. 2014). For instance, to increase individuals' physical activity levels as part of diabetes management, clinicians may first suggest a home-based physical activity program. After using this intervention for several months, some individuals will have increased their physical activity levels and are referred to as responders. However, others will not and are referred to as nonresponders. Nonresponders to behavioral interventions may need more time, or they may require a different intervention entirely. The recognition of differential responses to interventions has prompted a growing interest in moving away from fixed, "one size fits all" interventions and toward developing adaptive interventions (Almirall et al. 2012).

DOI: 10.1201/9781003288640-3

3.1 Adaptive Interventions

Adaptive interventions are sequential interventions that are altered over time based on individuals' response (or nonresponse) (Nahum-Shani et al. 2012). Adaptive interventions are also known as adaptive treatment algorithms or strategies (Yan et al. 2021); dynamic treatment regimes (or regimens) or strategies (Chakraborty and Moodie 2013); multistage or multicourse treatment strategies (Thall, Sung, and Estey 2002); or treatment policies (Wahed and Tsiatis 2004).

Adaptive interventions are particularly well suited when there is a high level of heterogeneity in intervention response (Almirall et al. 2014), typical for behavioral interventions. They are also well suited when intervention goals change over time, such as when transitioning from an initial "active" intervention to maintenance or when the intervention benefits need to be balanced with its potential risks, such as participant burden (Almirall et al. 2012).

3.1.1 Components of an Adaptive Intervention

There are four key components to an adaptive intervention:

1. **Critical decision points**, which mark when changes to the intervention are considered. At least one decision point is included, and it may be based on the time since the intervention was initiated or a clinical marker, such as disease remission.
2. **Tailoring variables** are used to determine whether a change in the intervention is warranted at the decision point (Almirall et al. 2012, Kidwell and Hyde 2016). The success of an adaptive intervention particularly relies on which tailoring variable is used. Tailoring variables can include baseline, proximal, and/or distal variables (Almirall et al. 2014). Baseline variables are those obtained prior to the first decision point such as demographic information or clinical characteristics (Almirall and Chronis-Tuscano 2016). Proximal variables often lie on the causal pathway(s) of the intervention and capture its hypothesized mechanisms of action (Almirall et al., 2014). Distal outcomes include early measurements of the key clinical outcomes such as improvement in symptoms (Hong et al. 2019).
3. **Intervention options at each critical decision point** include maintaining or changing all or some aspects of the intervention (Lei et al. 2012, Murphy, Lynch, et al. 2007). The intervention options available at each decision point must take into account the intervention format and intensity as well as the ordered sequence and timing of the available options (Murphy, Lynch, et al. 2007).
4. **Decision rules** link the previous three components. These rules recommend when (critical decision point), based on what (tailoring variables) and how (intervention options) the intervention should be adapted (Lei et al. 2012, Yan et al. 2021).

As shown in Figure 3.1 below, for each component, several methodological questions need to be considered and SMART designs can answer these important questions (Almirall et al. 2014, Collins, Murphy, and Strecher 2007).

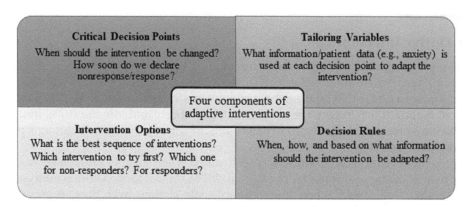

FIGURE 3.1
Questions to consider in developing an adaptive intervention.

3.2 Sequential Multiple Assignment Randomized Trials (SMARTs)

SMARTs accelerate the development and refinement of adaptive interventions by providing the evidence needed to identify which intervention is most effective for whom and when (Almirall et al. 2012, Collins, Nahum-Shani, and Almirall 2014). Initially, all participants are randomized to one of the intervention options. A tailoring variable is assessed at the first critical decision point, and participants are categorized as responders or nonresponders. Based on this categorization, some or all participants are rerandomized to other interventions (Collins, Nahum-Shani, and Almirall 2014, Murphy and Almirall 2009). Figure 3.2 illustrates a typical SMART design with two intervention stages. SMARTs are increasingly extending to behavioral interventions, including for weight loss (Jacques-Tiura et al. 2019, Naar et al. 2019, Sherwood et al. 2022), substance dependence (McKay et al. 2015, Petry et al. 2018, Morgenstern et al. 2021, Patrick et al. 2021), anxiety or depression (Karp et al. 2019, Sauer-Zavala et al. 2022), suicidal behavior (Czyz et al. 2021, Pistorello et al. 2017), stress management (Lambert, Grover, et al. 2022), symptom management in cancer (Wyatt et al. 2021), and physical activity (Gonze et al. 2020).

Several alternative primary analyses may be targeted in a SMART, but the two most common ones driving sample size calculations are to detect statistically significant differences (1) between initial interventions (at the decision point or final measure, averaging both intervention stages) or (2) between two intervention strategies with different initial interventions. Secondary or exploratory aims focused on identifying additional tailoring variables beyond responder status. Thus, statistical validity in terms of Type I error is preserved for the primary aim; however, additional aims require adjustments to guard against false discovery.

3.2.1 Advantages of SMARTs

One advantage of SMARTs is that heterogeneity in the sample is purposefully sought to ensure variability in response, which may improve the generalizability of the findings (Moodie, Karran, and Shortreed 2016, Rush et al. 2004). This contrasts with RCTs that typically target a very homogeneous patient population hypothesized to be most likely to respond to an intervention (limiting generalizability) (Kennedy-Martin et al. 2015, Kabisch et al. 2011).

SMARTs offer a transparent assessment of complex, multicomponent, behavioral interventions by comparing intervention options at each critical decision point (Lei et al. 2012). As each intervention option is sequentially added to form the adaptive intervention and then evaluated, its impact on outcomes, and cost-effectiveness, can be understood (Murphy, Lynch, et al. 2007). In addition, the potential synergistic effects of a sequence of interventions, that is, how an initial intervention magnifies or impedes subsequent ones, can also be explored (Lei et al. 2012). However, data analysis in SMARTs can become complex (Candlish et al. 2019) and a larger sample may be needed relative to a standard RCT, depending on the primary analysis goal. A SMART powered to detect a difference between first-stage interventions would require the same sample size as a traditional RCT, if conducted in the same population. However, as SMARTs are often conducted in more heterogeneous populations, a larger sample size is needed relative to the typically more homogenous population in which standard RCTs are conducted; this heterogeneity is accounted for in the design stage (sample size calculations and feasibility) of a SMART. Nevertheless, the sample size required in SMARTs to detect differences among adaptive interventions is still often smaller than what would be required for a series of independent RCTs, each addressing only one intervention option at a time (Kidwell 2014).

Other potential advantages of SMARTs include lower attrition and improved adherence. In a traditional RCT, nonresponders have no alternatives to the fixed intervention, which in turn may lead to high attrition or nonadherence (Almirall et al. 2012). In contrast, in SMARTs, nonresponders are often rerandomized to the next intervention option hypothesized to better meet their needs, potentially improving retention (Moodie, Karran, and Shortreed 2016). For responders, less burdensome step-down or maintenance intervention may be offered (Lei et al. 2012). Another factor associated with nonadherence is not knowing whether one is receiving an intervention or is in the control group in a double-blind RCT (Pettinati et al. 2000). Often in SMARTs, participants will receive an active intervention at some point over the course of the adaptive intervention, and this would be described in the consent form (Almirall et al. 2012), potentially then increasing engagement and retention. Table 3.1 summarizes the key advantages of SMARTs in comparison to RCTs.

Despite these advantages, some of the complexities of SMARTs remain underexplored. For example, there is no consensus on how to perform an intention-to-treat analysis when participants withdraw before the critical decision point since the "intended" second-stage intervention may not be known. In one of the best-known SMARTs, attrition and missing information was addressed via multiple imputation (Shortreed et al. 2014).

3.3 Overview of Two Behavioral Pilot SMART Studies

Given the advantages of SMARTs, this design was favored for two adaptive chronic disease self-management interventions developed by our team (Lambert et al. 2017, Lambert, Grover, et al. 2022). Despite the efficacy of self-management interventions across many chronic conditions (Allegrante, Wells, and Peterson 2019), their integration into clinical practice has been stalled mainly due to their high cost, as most are delivered face to face

TABLE 3.1

Summary of the main advantages of SMARTs in comparison to an RCT.

Limitations of RCTs	Advantages of SMARTs
Seek homogeneous sample	Seek heterogenous sample potentially leading to more generalizable findings
Multiple RCTs needed to differentiate among intervention components; only effect modifiers can be explored in a single RCT	Evaluate each component of complex behavioral interventions; detect a synergistic effect among these
Larger sample size across multiple RCTs	Sample size needed smaller than for multiple RCTs
Fix intervention provided regardless of response may lead to decreased adherence and increased attrition (especially for nonresponders)	Adaptive intervention may decrease nonadherence, reduce attrition, and reduce possible negative effects of inappropriate intervention or dose

Note.   Based on Almirall, Compton, Gunlicks-Soessel et al. 2012, Collins, 2014, Lavori and Dawson, 2008, Lei et al. 2012, Moodie et al. 2016, Murphy, Lynch, et al., 2007.

over multiple sessions by health care professionals often hired for the purpose of the study (Walters et al. 2012, Roberts et al. 2012). However, we know from clinical practice guidelines that this level of high-intensity support is only needed by 10–15% of patients; most individuals can benefit from self-directed or minimal-intensity interventions (Fitch 2015). Also, patients often prefer to attempt a self-directed intervention, before entering a more formal, intense program (Curry et al. 2002, Lambert, Kelly, et al. 2014). A SMART is ideal for developing adaptive self-management interventions tailored to the level of support individuals' need. This is also referred to as a stepped care approach (Van Straten et al. 2010).

In a stepped care approach, individuals begin with a low-intensity intervention. Response to this intervention is monitored, and nonresponders are "stepped up" to a higher intensity intervention that often involves more clinician contact (Van Straten et al. 2010). In this sense, stepped care ensures a sufficient intervention dose to meet each individual's needs while conserving finite health care resources for those who need them most and limiting the potential burden and cost of higher-intensity interventions for those who do not need them (Van Straten et al. 2010).

Both pilots were similar in their SMART design summarized in Table 3.2 and participant flow is illustrated in Figure 3.2. Both pilot SMARTs assessed the feasibility, acceptability, and clinical significance of an adaptive self-management intervention. In the first pilot, an adaptive web-based stress management intervention called My Health Checkup (https://myhealthcheckup.com) for patients with a cardiovascular disease (CVD) was evaluated (Lambert, Grover, et al. 2022). In this pilot, 59 patients with a CVD and moderate stress at eligibility screening (T0) were randomized (Stage 1) to My Health Checkup (self-directed) (n = 30) or the same intervention plus lay telephone-based guidance (minimally guided intervention, n = 29). Moderate stress was defined by a score of at least 16 on the Depression, Anxiety, and Stress Scale – Stress subscale (DASS) (Lovibond and Lovibond 1996). Stress was assessed with the same measure at baseline (T1, prior to randomization) and at 6 weeks postrandomization (T2 = decision point). Participants were categorized as responders if their stress (tailoring variable) score reduced by at least 50% between baseline (T1) and 6 weeks postrandomization (T2) or they reported a score of less than 16 at T2 on the DASS – Stress subscale (Lovibond and Lovibond 1996), irrespective of the baseline (T1) score. Nonresponders in either group were rerandomized to continue with their Stage

TABLE 3.2

Summary of CVD and Coping-Together Pilot SMARTs.

	CVD SMART	Coping-Together SMART
Sample	Adults with diagnosis of CVD and moderate baseline stress (≥16 stress subscale of the DASS)	Individuals with cancer + caregivers and moderate baseline distress (one member of the dyad ≥ 5 on the DT)
Decision Point	6 weeks postrandomization	6 weeks postrandomization
Tailoring Variable	Stress (DASS score) at 6 weeks	Distress level (DT) at 6 weeks
Primary Outcomes	Stress or quality of life	Anxiety and quality of life
Intervention Options	**Stage 1**, either Self-directed *My Health Checkup* OR *My Health Checkup* + lay guidance	**Stage 1**, either Self-directed Coping-Together OR Coping-Together + lay guidance
	Stage 2, continue with Stage 1 intervention OR *My Health Checkup* + MI	**Stage 2**, continue with Stage 1 intervention OR Coping-Together + MI
Decision Rules	If responder, then continue Stage 1 intervention for 6 weeks. If nonresponder, to the second stage programs for 6 weeks	

Notes: DASS = Depression, Anxiety, and Stress Scale; DT = Distress Thermometer; MI = motivational interviewing.

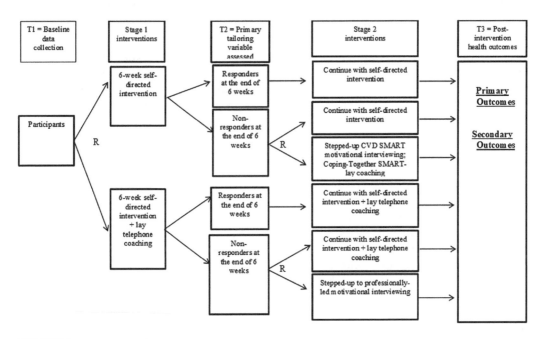

FIGURE 3.2
Design and participant flow for the CVD and Coping-Together SMARTs. *R* = randomization.

1 intervention or stepped up to professionally led motivational interviewing (MI). This pilot is herein referred to as CVD SMART.

In the second pilot, Coping-Together, a manual-based, self-directed coping skills training intervention for patients with cancer and their family caregivers was evaluated (Lambert et al. 2016, Lambert, Girgis, Turner, et al. 2013, Lambert, Girgis, McElduff, et al. 2013). In total, 48 patient-caregiver dyads with at least moderate distress at eligibility screening

(T0) were randomized (Stage 1) to Coping-Together (n = 25) or Coping-Together plus lay telephone-based guidance (n = 23). At 6 weeks postrandomization (T2), distress (tailoring variable) was assessed. Distress was measured by the Distress Thermometer (DT) (National Comprehensive Cancer Network 2020). Response was defined as a decrease of at least 1 point between screening (T0) at the decision point (T2) in both members of the dyad, or in only one member of the dyad, as long as the other member's score did not increase significantly from T0 to T2. Significant was defined as an increase of 2 if the DT (National Comprehensive Cancer Network 2020) score at T0 was below 5 or an increase of 1 if the DT score was 5 or above. Nonresponders to Coping-Together were rerandomized to either continue with Coping-Together or stepped up to receive lay telephone-based guidance. Nonresponders to Coping-Together plus lay telephone guidance were rerandomized to continue with this intervention or stepped up to MI. This pilot is referred to as Coping-Together SMART.

3.4 Lessons Learned: Key Methodological and Practical Decisions

This section focuses on the methodological and practical lessons learned in undertaking the CVD and Coping-Together SMARTs. Lessons learned are categorized according to the four components of adaptive interventions (see Figure 3.1). It should be noted that some of the lessons learned are not necessarily specific to SMARTs but are mostly due to the behavioral aspect of the interventions and associated self-administered measures commonly used in this field. Nonetheless, given the large sample needed and higher stakes of a SMART, it is pertinent to raise them here for consideration.

3.4.1 Critical Decision Points

The main lesson learned is to consider not only early response to Stage 1 interventions but potentially late response as well. In our examples, the decision point was 6 weeks postintervention (T2) to match the end of the interventions (i.e., early response). In hindsight, this time point could have been delayed, or potentially response could have been measured twice: at postintervention (i.e., early response), whereby responders are immediately rerandomized, but nonresponders could be reassessed 2–3 weeks later for any delayed response. In behavioral SMARTs, this delayed response has generally not been considered. Sherwood et al. (2022) conducted a SMART to optimize the identification of nonresponders to a behavioral weight loss treatment. Participants were randomized to assess response after 3 or 7 sessions (of 20). Nonresponders at either response time were offered the next intervention option. One suggestion from this SMART was that early responders may also need to be reassessed to ensure their improvements are sustained.

3.4.2 Tailoring Variables

The first lesson learned pertaining to the tailoring variable(s) relates to its selection and the remaining four to its measurement.

Leverage the interventions' mechanisms of action in selecting tailoring variables. In both SMART examples, the tailoring variables were distal outcomes focused on answering the question: Are the interventions resulting in a sufficient decrease in the targeted symptoms at this (early) point in time (Hong et al. 2019)? Alternatively, or in addition, we could have considered a proximal outcome answering the question: Are the mechanisms of action of the intervention working as expected? For instance, Coping-Together was designed based on Lazarus and Folkman's Stress and Coping Framework (Lazarus and Folkman 1984) and changes in coping and appraisal are proximal tailoring variable(s) that could be assessed in future SMARTs. A note of caution: some proximal variables in behavioral science are known to suffer from ceiling effects (e.g., self-efficacy) (Carey and Forsyth 2009) or are inconsistently correlated with outcomes (e.g., intervention adherence) (Donkin et al. 2011). Given this, a recommendation for future behavioral SMARTs would be to triangulate several tailoring variables, potentially using a combination of proximal and distal outcomes. For instance, in the CVD SMART, response could be defined as lower stress (distal outcome) as well as learning and applying at least one stress management strategy (proximal outcomes).

Beware of false-positive responders due to the Hawthorne effect and/or individual-level measurement error(s). In the CVD SMART, a subgroup of participants who reported moderate stress at eligibility screening (T0) were already below the stress threshold for response by baseline (T1) and remained below this threshold at the first decision point (T2). This might simply point to natural variations in health outcomes. Another explanation might be the Hawthorne effect, that is, attention given during screening or the mere promise of a stress reduction intervention might have led to improved stress (Bowling 2014). We tried to address these "false-positive responders" by raising the cut-point on the DASS from 16 to 18 at T0, but this did not resolve the issue. Even under this more stringent eligibility criterion, some participants' stress had sufficiently resolved by baseline (T1). Another explanation is that the false-positive responders may reflect measurement errors.

In RCTs, using large samples to establish intervention efficacy provides precision in score estimation and random measurement errors "cancel out" across the sample (King, Dueck, and Revicki 2019). However, in SMARTs, response (at the critical decision point) is determined at the individual level (N = 1) and measurement errors are not "cancelled out" (King, Dueck, and Revicki 2019). Nonetheless, a decision will be made to change the intervention at that point, which might lead to a cascade effect in the subsequent intervention stage(s). While one can expect that, with randomization, the proportion of false-positive responders in each arm might equal out in Stage 1, the impact of potentially assigning the wrong Stage 2 intervention to individuals is less likely to be equally distributed across all intervention sequences (or at least there is uncertainty around this). This lesson learned further supports the previous recommendation of triangulating tailoring variables to ensure better certainty in determining response. Furthermore, the measures chosen for the tailoring variable should be appropriate for individual-level measurement (internal consistency) for the set response timeframe (responsiveness and test-retest). Higher internal consistency is needed for individual-level measurement than for group-level measurement (0.90 versus 0.70) (Hays et al. 2021).

Minimize testing effects as a threat to internal validity. Testing effects bias results due to repeatedly testing participants using the same measures (Nezu and Nezu 2008). In the CVD SMART, the DASS was administered four times within a short timeframe: T0 – screening, T1 – baseline, T2 – decision point, and T3 – postintervention. The screening might have given some indication to the participants of what was important to the researchers (Lavrakas 2008). By T3, some participants may have an improved score simply because of repeated exposure to the DASS. This was addressed in the Coping-Together SMART by using different measures for the tailoring variables versus the primary health outcomes. Testing effects could also be further addressed by relying on proximal tailoring variables.

Choose scales to assess the tailoring variable that mimics clinical practice. One of the main advantages of a SMART is that it mirrors the dynamic decision-making that unfolds in clinical care (Almirall et al. 2012). It follows from this that measurement of the tailoring variable needs to be reasonably done in *real-world* clinical settings. Some scales used in research are costly and burdensome for patients to complete and/or have complex scoring algorithms. This might preclude transferability to the *real-world,* where clinicians have limited time to determine response and apply the decision rule. However, any changes in the measurement of the tailoring variable from research to the *real-world* contexts will compromise the efficacy of the adaptive intervention. In both SMART pilots, short measures were purposefully used to determine response. For the Coping-Together SMART, the DT is the most widely used distress screening measure in oncology. It takes no more than 2 minutes to complete, and even less for clinicians to interpret (Ownby 2019). In addition, the most frequently implemented clinical cut-point of 5 was used to determine eligibility and response (Lambert et al. 2014).

Consider how the measures for the tailoring variables are administered. In the CVD SMART, Stage 1 response assessments were done over the telephone, allowing the research assistant to on-the-spot complete the Stage 2 randomization and inform the participant of their Stage 2 intervention. For the Coping-Together SMART, we initially planned to do the same. However, the approach quickly became more cumbersome, because of the dyadic nature of the study. It was not always feasible to assess the patient and caregiver at the same time, requiring the research assistant to delay Stage 2 randomization until both members of the dyad had completed their response assessment. Informing the dyad of the Stage 2 intervention was often done by email to ensure that both were sent the information at the same time. Study participants asked if the responsiveness assessment could be completed online, as this would allow them to complete the measures when it was more convenient to them. Based on this recommendation, the Stage 2 assessment was shifted online. Pilot data indicate that this method was more feasible and acceptable and led to a Stage 2 assignment within days.

3.4.3 Intervention Options

Three lessons learned pertain to intervention options.

Recognize that while intensity is an important intervention component, adapting timing and/or format might also be appropriate. When planning to adapt both self-management interventions, intensity was the only component set to vary over time through lay guidance and/or professionally led MI. No other intervention component was considered. However, we noticed in the Coping-Together SMART that even the lay guidance was too intense for some dyads (even if the guidance was minimal), which seems to have resulted in greater attrition and fewer responders in the minimally guided group than in the self-directed one. This was not noted in the CVD SMART potentially because much support was needed to navigate the website (less of an issue for Coping-Together). Of note, not all groups in a SMART need to receive an active intervention in Stage 1. In future Coping-Together SMARTs, we suggest a period of active monitoring or watchful waiting.

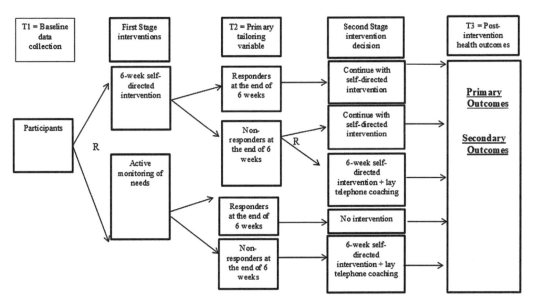

FIGURE 3.3
Sequential Multiple Assignment Randomization Trial (SMART) design with consideration of varying timing and intensity. *R* = randomization.

Figure 3.3 illustrates how the design in Figure 3.2 could be changed to reflect intervention adaptation based on both intensity and timing. This period of active monitoring might also help identify false responders due to the Hawthorne effect noted above.

Changes in intervention intensity meant changes in intervention provider. In the CVD SMART, stepping up from lay guidance to professionally led MI meant changing the intervention provider. This subgroup of participants reported low satisfaction scores, which was attributed to the disruption in the patient-interventionist therapeutic relationship (Karyotaki et al. 2018). Similarly, another SMART study reported high attrition rates (41.7%) among nonresponders who switched intervention providers from Stages 1 to 2 (Day, McGrath, and Wojtowicz 2013). To overcome this, in the Coping-Together SMART, a handover meeting among the Stages 1 and 2 intervention providers was scheduled and successfully facilitated the transition.

Sustain engagement for twice as long. In an RCT, intervention efficacy is typically measured postintervention. When there is a "long-term" follow-up (e.g., 12 months), there are often no expectations regarding individuals' "active" use of the intervention. The long-term follow-up is done more to document the potential lasting effects of the intervention. In SMARTs, participants remain actively engaged across intervention stages. In our pilots, this meant that engagement was 12 weeks, instead of the intervention's length of 6 weeks. Those who stepped up also needed to learn to use new intervention components. Whereas, for those who remained with the Stage 1 intervention, the challenge then became to sustain their adherence through maintenance. In our SMART pilots, those receiving lay guidance in Stage 1 who continued with this intervention in Stage 2 received booster calls from the lay guide, which were less frequent than in Stage 1 to minimize burden. However, those continuing in a self-directed manner in Stage 2 did not receive additional support.

In the CVD SMART, the highest attrition was among this group, i.e., nonresponders in the self-directed group rerandomized to this group in Stage 2 (Lambert, Grover, et al. 2022). In the future, information at the outset of Stage 2 will be provided to responders and nonresponders on the continued use of the self-directed intervention in Stage 2 to motivate sustained adherence. This highlights the need for additional resources to develop, deliver, and maintain adaptive interventions.

3.4.4 Decision Rules

For this last component of adaptive interventions, the main lesson learned is to keep the decision rules simple. Complex decision rules might need to be adapted when implemented in *real-world* settings, compromising the efficacy of the adaptive intervention. In the CVD SMART, the decision rule was simple. However, in the Coping-Together SMART the decision rule became complex, as it took into consideration two individuals' responses as well as the magnitude of the increase in DT scores. For a larger SMART, the decision rule would need to be simplified, potentially defining response as both members of the dyads scoring below 5 on the DT.

3.5 Discussion

This chapter initially described adaptive interventions and how they can be developed and evaluated using SMARTs. Then, methodological and practical lessons learned based on two pilot SMARTs of behavioral interventions were shared. Given the methodological considerations of a SMART, the complexities inherent in the design, and where the evidence currently lies, a pilot is potentially even more critical than prior to traditional RCTs. Adaptive behavioral interventions remain new and carry several challenges that are best discovered and managed through a pilot to assure the success of a full-scale SMART.

Key changes made to the Coping-Together SMART based on the CVD SMART were: the time points and the measures used to assess the primary health outcomes and the tailoring variable as well as the inclusion of a "handover session" between Stage 1 and Stage 2 intervention providers. The critical lessons learned from Coping-Together SMART that will be considered before a full-scale SMART are: considering using more proximal tailoring variables or triangulating tailoring variables, including an active monitoring group in Stage 1, and including an explicit maintenance plan for responders in the self-directed group.

As key lessons learned were discussed in this chapter, innovations for future SMARTs were identified, including triangulating the tailoring variables and randomizing in Stage 1 based on early or delayed response. In future dyadic SMARTs, consideration needs to be given to whether the tailoring variable should or needs to be the same for both patients and their caregivers. Previous studies have shown that often patients and their caregivers benefit differently from interventions (Lambert, Duncan, et al. 2022, Northouse et al. 2014, Northouse et al. 2007), which suggests that more personalized tailoring variables may need to be included.

More specific to dyadic SMARTs, the spillover or interference effect might need further attention. Spillover is typically considered in cases where the intervention of one individual may influence the outcomes of another person who is, by some measure, socially connected to the first (Wittenberg et al. 2013). In a dyadic SMART, both members of the pair received the same intervention; however, it may be the case that both members did not engage with the intervention to the same degree. The engagement of one person may impact the outcomes of the other member. Disentangling such effects requires further innovations in statistical analysis.

Another potential consideration for future SMARTs is the inclusion of a preference-based component. Preference is the intervention that individuals desire or want to receive or choose when given choices (Stalmeier et al. 2007). Preferences are now recognized to impact intervention adherence, attrition, and satisfaction (Sidani 2014). Accounting for preferences can positively impact recruitment and attrition rates (Sidani 2014). Metaanalyses report greater improvement in outcomes for participants randomly allocated to their preferred versus nonpreferred intervention, albeit effect sizes remain small (Preference Collaborative Review Group 2008, Swift, Callahan, and Vollmer 2011). Preferences were somewhat considered in the STAR*D SMART (Gaynes et al. 2009, Rush et al. 2004), whereby nonresponders' subsequent treatments were determined by randomization; however, the options to which they were randomized depended on whether participants chose the "switch" (new treatment class) or "augment" (add another agent to the current treatment) path for their treatment. Preference could be considered in future SMARTs by, for example, asking participants whether they want to be stepped up or not. Similarly, responders could be given alternative maintenance options.

SMARTs offer unprecedented flexibility within an experimental design and an ability to detect treatment synergies and optimal intervention sequences tailored to evolving patient needs. This trial design offers opportunities to gather evidence for stepped care in the management of chronic conditions. Despite their novelty and some remaining challenges, SMARTs provide an exciting new approach to studying behavioral interventions.

References

Allegrante, J.P., M.T. Wells, M and J.C. Peterson. 2019. "Interventions to support behavioral self-management of chronic diseases." *Annual Review of Public Health* 40: 127–146. doi: 10.1146/annurev-publhealth-040218-044008.

Almirall, D., and A. Chronis-Tuscano. 2016. "Adaptive interventions in child and adolescent mental health." *J Clin Child Adolesc Psychol* 45 (4): 383–95. doi: 10.1080/15374416.2016.1152555.

Almirall, D., S.N. Compton, M. Gunlicks-Stoessel, N. Duan, and S.A. Murphy. 2012. "Designing a pilot sequential multiple assignment randomized trial for developing an adaptive treatment strategy." *Stat Med* 31 (17): 1887–902. doi: 10.1002/sim.4512.

Almirall, D., I. Nahum-Shani, N.E. Sherwood, and S.A. Murphy. 2014. "Introduction to SMART designs for the development of adaptive interventions: with application to weight loss research." *Translational Behavioral Medicine* 4 (3): 260–274. doi: 10.1007/s13142-014-0265-0.

Bowling, A. 2014. *Research Methods in Health: Investigating Health and Health Services.* Milton Keynes: Open University Press.

Bricca, A., M. Jäger, M. Johnston, G. Zangger, L.K. Harris, J. Midtgaard, and S.T. Skou. 2022. "Effect of in-person delivered behavioural interventions in people with multimorbidity: systematic review and meta-analysis." *International Journal of Behavioral Medicine.* doi: 10.1007/s12529-022-10092-8.

Candlish, J., M.D. Teare, J. Cohen, and T. Bywater. 2019. "Statistical design and analysis in trials of proportionate interventions: a systematic review." *Trials* 20 (1): 151. doi: 10.1186/s13063-019-3206-x.

Carey, M.P., and A.D. Forsyth. 2009. *Teaching Tip Sheet: Self-Efficacy.* American Psychological Association (APA).

Chakraborty, B., and E. Moodie. 2013. *Statistical Methods for Dynamic Treatment Regimes.* London: Springer.

Collins, L.M., S.A. Murphy, and K.L. Bierman. 2004. "A conceptual framework for adaptive preventive interventions." *Prevention Science: The Official Journal of the Society for Prevention Research* 5 (3): 185–196. doi: 10.1023/b:prev.0000037641.26017.00.

Collins, L.M., S.A. Murphy, and V. Strecher. 2007. "The multiphase optimization strategy (MOST) and the sequential multiple assignment randomized trial (SMART): new methods for more potent eHealth interventions." *Am J Prev Med* 32 (5 Suppl): S112–8. doi: 10.1016/j.amepre.2007.01.022.

Collins, L.M., I. Nahum-Shani, and D. Almirall. 2014. "Optimization of behavioral dynamic treatment regimens based on the sequential, multiple assignment, randomized trial (SMART)." *Clin Trials* 11 (4): 426–434. doi: 10.1177/1740774514536795.

Curry, C., T. Cossich, J.P. Matthews, J. Beresford, and S.A. McLachlan. 2002. "Uptake of psychosocial referrals in an outpatient cancer setting: improving service accessibility via the referral process." *Support Care Cancer* 10 (7): 549–55. doi: 10.1007/s00520-002-0371-2.

Cutler, D.M. 2004. "Behavioral health interventions: what works and why?" In *Critical Perspectives on Racial and Ethnic Differences in Health in Late Life,* edited by R.A. Bulatao, N.B. Anderson, and B. Cohen. 643–677. Washington (DC): National Academies Press.

Czyz, E.K., C.A. King, D. Prouty, V.J. Micol, M. Walton, and I. Nahum-Shani. 2021. "Adaptive intervention for prevention of adolescent suicidal behavior after hospitalization: a pilot sequential multiple assignment randomized trial." *J Child Psychol Psychiatry* 62 (8): 1019–1031. doi: 10.1111/jcpp.13383.

Day, V., P.J. McGrath, and M. Wojtowicz. 2013. "Internet-based guided self-help for university students with anxiety, depression and stress: a randomized controlled clinical trial." *Behaviour Research and Therapy* 51 (7): 344–351. doi: https://doi.org/10.1016/j.brat.2013.03.003.

Donkin, L., H. Christensen, S.L. Naismith, B. Neal, I.B. Hickie, and N. Glozier. 2011. "A systematic review of the impact of adherence on the effectiveness of e-therapies." *Journal of Medical Internet Research* 13 (3): e52–e52. doi: 10.2196/jmir.1772.

Fitch, M. 2015. "Supportive care framework." *Canadian Oncology Nursing Journal / Revue Canadienne de soins Infirmiers en Oncologie* 18 (1):9.

Gaynes, B.N., D. Warden, M.H. Trivedi, S.R. Wisniewski, M. Fava, and A. John Rush. 2009. "What did STAR*D teach us? Results from a large-scale, practical, clinical trial for patients with depression." *Psychiatric Services* 60 (11): 1439–1445. doi: 10.1176/ps.2009.60.11.1439.

Gonze, B.B., R.D.C. Padovani, M.D.S. Simoes, V. Lauria, N.L. Proença, E.F. Sperandio, Tlvdp Ostolin, G.A.O. Gomes, P.C. Castro, M. Romiti, A. Gagliardi, R.L. Arantes, and V.Z. Dourado. 2020. "Use of a smartphone app to increase physical activity levels in insufficiently active adults: feasibility Sequential Multiple Assignment Randomized Trial (SMART)." *JMIR Res Protoc* 9 (10): e14322. doi: 10.2196/14322.

Hays, R.D., D. Hubble, F. Jenkins, A. Fraser, and B. Carew. 2021. "Methodological and statistical considerations for the National Children's Study." *Frontiers in Pediatrics* 9: 595059–595059. doi: 10.3389/fped.2021.595059.

Hong, N., D. Cornacchio, J.W. Pettit, and J.S. Comer. 2019. "Coal-mine canaries in clinical psychology: getting better at identifying early signals of treatment nonresponse." *Clinical Psychological Science* 7 (6): 1207–1221. doi: 10.1177/2167702619858111.

Jacques-Tiura, A.J., D.A. Ellis, A. Idalski Carcone, S. Naar, K. Brogan Hartlieb, E.K. Towner, N. Templin T, and K.C. Jen. 2019. "African-American adolescents' weight loss skills utilization: effects on weight change in a sequential multiple assignment randomized trial." *J Adolesc Health* 64 (3): 355–361. doi: 10.1016/j.jadohealth.2018.09.003.

Kabisch, M., C. Ruckes, M. Seibert-Grafe, and M. Blettner. 2011. "Randomized controlled trials: part 17 of a series on evaluation of scientific publications." *Deutsches Arzteblatt International* 108 (39): 663–668. doi: 10.3238/arztebl.2011.0663.

Karp, J.F., J. Zhang, A.S. Wahed, S. Anderson, M.A. Dew, G.K. Fitzgerald, D.K. Weiner, S. Albert, A. Gildengers, M. Butters, and C.F. Reynolds, 3rd. 2019. "Improving patient reported outcomes and preventing depression and anxiety in older adults with knee osteoarthritis: results of a Sequenced Multiple Assignment Randomized Trial (SMART) Study." *Am J Geriatr Psychiatry* 27 (10): 1035–1045. doi: 10.1016/j.jagp.2019.03.011.

Karyotaki, E., D.D. Ebert, L. Donkin, H. Riper, J. Twisk, S. Burger, A. Rozental, et al. 2018. "Do guided internet-based interventions result in clinically relevant changes for patients with depression? An individual participant data meta-analysis." *Clinical Psychology Review* 63: 80–92. doi: https://doi.org/10.1016/j.cpr.2018.06.007.

Kennedy-Martin, T., Sarah Curtis, Douglas Faries, Susan Robinson, and Joseph Johnston. 2015. "A literature review on the representativeness of randomized controlled trial samples and implications for the external validity of trial results." *Trials* 16:495–495. doi: 10.1186/s13063-015-1023-4.

Kidwell, K.M. 2014. "SMART designs in cancer research: past, present, and future." *Clin Trials* 11 (4):445–456. doi: 10.1177/1740774514525691.

Kidwell, K.M., and L.W. Hyde. 2016. "Adaptive interventions and SMART designs: application to child behavior research in a community setting." *The American Journal of Evaluation* 37 (3): 344–363. doi: 10.1177/1098214015617013.

King, M.T., A.C. Dueck, and D.A. Revicki. 2019. "Can methods developed for interpreting group-level patient-reported outcome data be applied to individual patient management?" *Med Care* 57 (Suppl 5 1): S38–s45. doi: 10.1097/mlr.0000000000001111.

Lambert, S.D., A. Girgis, P. McElduff, J. Turner, J.V. Levesque, K. Kayser, C. Mihalopoulos, S.T. Shih, and D. Barker. 2013. "A parallel-group, randomised controlled trial of a multimedia, self-directed, coping skills training intervention for patients with cancer and their partners: design and rationale." *BMJ Open* 3 (7). doi: 10.1136/bmjopen-2013-003337.

Lambert, S.D., A. Girgis, J. Turner, T. Regan, H. Candler, B. Britton, S. Chambers, C. Lawsin, and K. Kayser. 2013. "You need something like this to give you guidelines on what to do": patients' and partners' use and perceptions of a self-directed coping skills training resource." *Supportive Care in Cancer* 21 (12): 3451–3460. doi: 10.1007/s00520-013-1914-4.

Lambert, S. D., J. F. Pallant, K. Clover, B. Britton, M. T. King, and G. Carter. 2014. "Using Rasch analysis to examine the distress thermometer's cut-off scores among a mixed group of patients with cancer." *Qual Life Res* 23 (8): 2257-65. https://doi.org/10.1007/s11136-014-0673-0.

Lambert, S.D., B. Kelly, A. Boyes, A. Cameron, C. Adams, A. Proietto, and A. Girgis. 2014. "Insights into preferences for psycho-oncology services among women with gynecologic cancer following distress screening." *Journal of the National Comprehensive Cancer Network J Natl Compr Canc Netw* 12 (6): 899–906. doi: 10.6004/jnccn.2014.0084.

Lambert, S.D., P. McElduff, A. Girgis, J.V. Levesque, T. Regan, W., J. Turner, H. Candler, C. Mihalopoulos, S.T.F. Shih, K. Kayser, and P. Chong. 2016. " A pilot, multisite, randomized controlled trial of a self-directed coping skills training intervention for couples facing prostate cancer: accrual, retention, and data collection issues." *Supportive Care in Cancer* 24 (2):711–722.

Lambert, S., J. McCusker, E. Moodie, D. Da Costa, T. Schuster, L. Pilote, S. Grover, A.M. Laizner, M. Vallis, and G. Ménard. 2017. Adaptive internet-based stress management among adults with a cardiovascular disease: a pilot Sequential Multiple Assignment Randomized Trial (SMART) design. Grant obtained from Canadian Institutes of Health Research.

Lambert, S.D., L.R. Duncan, S. Nicole Culos-Reed, L. Hallward, C.S. Higano, E. Loban, and A. Katz, et al. 2022. "Feasibility, acceptability, and clinical significance of a dyadic, web-based, psychosocial and physical activity self-management program (TEMPO) tailored to the needs of men with prostate cancer and their caregivers: a multi-center randomized pilot trial." *Current Oncology* 29 (2): 785–804.

Lambert, S.D., S. Grover, A.M. Laizner, J. McCusker, E. Belzile, E.E.M. Moodie, J.W. Kayser, et al. 2022. "Adaptive web-based stress management programs among adults with a cardiovascular disease: a pilot Sequential Multiple Assignment Randomized Trial (SMART)." *Patient Education and Counseling* 105 (6): 1587–1597. doi: https://doi.org/10.1016/j.pec.2021.10.020.

Lavori, P.W., and R. Dawson. 2008. "Adaptive treatment strategies in chronic disease." *Annual Review of Medicine* 59: 443–453. doi: 10.1146/annurev.med.59.062606.122232.

Lavrakas, P. 2008. *Encyclopedia of Survey Research Methods.* Sage Publications, Inc. doi: 10.4135/9781412963947.

Lazarus, R.S, and S. Folkman. 1984. *Stress, Appraisal, and Coping.* New York: Springer Publishing Company.

Lei, H., I. Nahum-Shani, K. Lynch, D. Oslin, and S.A. Murphy. 2012. "A "SMART" design for building individualized treatment sequences." *Annual Review of Clinical Psychology* 8: 21–48. doi: 10.1146/annurev-clinpsy-032511-143152.

Li, Y., N. Buys, Z. Li, Li Li, Q. Song, and J. Sun. 2021. "The efficacy of cognitive behavioral therapy-based interventions on patients with hypertension: a systematic review and meta-analysis." *Preventive Medicine Reports* 23: 101477–101477. doi: 10.1016/j.pmedr.2021.101477.

Lovibond, P.F., and S.H. Lovibond. 1996. *Manual for the Depression Anxiety & Stress Scales.* 2nd ed. Sydney, Australia: Psychology Foundation of Australia.

McKay, J.R., M.L. Drapkin, D.H. Van Horn, K.G. Lynch, D.W. Oslin, D. DePhilippis, M. Ivey, and J.S. Cacciola. 2015. "Effect of patient choice in an adaptive sequential randomization trial of treatment for alcohol and cocaine dependence." *J Consult Clin Psychol* 83 (6): 1021–32. doi: 10.1037/a0039534.

Moodie, E.E., J.C. Karran, and S.M. Shortreed. 2016. "A case study of SMART attributes: a qualitative assessment of generalizability, retention rate, and trial quality." *Trials* 17 (1):242. doi: 10.1186/s13063-016-1368-3.

Morgenstern, J., A. Kuerbis, S. Shao, H.T. Padovano, S. Levak, N.P. Vadhan, and K.G. Lynch. 2021. "An efficacy trial of adaptive interventions for alcohol use disorder." *Journal of Substance Abuse Treatment* 123:108264. doi: https://doi.org/10.1016/j.jsat.2020.108264.

Murphy, S.A., and D. Almirall. 2009. "Dynamic treatment regimens." In *Encyclopedia of Medical Decision Making* edited by M.W. Kattan, 419–422. Thousand Oaks, CA: Sage Publications, Inc.

Murphy, S.A., K.G. Lynch, D. Oslin, J.R. McKay, and T. TenHave. 2007. "Developing adaptive treatment strategies in substance abuse research." *Drug and Alcohol Dependence* 88 (Suppl 2): S24–S30. doi: 10.1016/j.drugalcdep.2006.09.008.

Naar, S., D. Ellis, A.I. Carcone, A.J. Jacques-Tiura, P. Cunningham, T. Templin, K. B. Hartlieb, and K.L. Cathy Jen. 2019. "Outcomes from a sequential multiple assignment randomized trial of weight loss strategies for African American adolescents with obesity." *Annals of Behavioral Medicine: A Publication of the Society of Behavioral Medicine* 53 (10): 928–938. doi: 10.1093/abm/kaz003.

Nahum-Shani, I., M. Qian, D. Almirall, W.E. Pelham, B. Gnagy, G.A. Fabiano, J.G. Waxmonsky, J. Yu, and S.A. Murphy. 2012. "Experimental design and primary data analysis methods for comparing adaptive interventions." *Psychological Methods* 17 (4): 457–477. doi: 10.1037/a0029372.

National Comprehensive Cancer Network. 2020. "NCCN Guidelines for Patients: Distress during cancer care." www.nccn.org/patients/guidelines/content/PDF/distress-patient.pdf.

Nezu, A.M., and C. Maguth Nezu. 2008. *Evidence-Based Outcome Research: A Practical Guide to Conducting Randomized Controlled Trials for Psychosocial Interventions.* Oxford: Oxford University Press.

Northouse, L.L., D.W. Mood, A. Schafenacker, J.E. Montie, H.M. Sandler, J.D. Forman, M. Hussain, K.J. Pienta, D.C. Smith, and T. Kershaw. 2007. "Randomized clinical trial of a family intervention for prostate cancer patients and their spouses." *Cancer* 110 (12): 2809–18. doi: 10.1002/cncr.23114.

Northouse, L., A. Schafenacker, K.L.C. Barr, M. Katapodi, H. Yoon, K. Brittain, L. Song, D.L. Ronis, and L. An. 2014. "A tailored web-based psychoeducational intervention for cancer patients and their family caregivers." *Cancer Nursing* 37 (5): 321–330. doi: 10.1097/NCC.0000000000000159.

Ownby, K.K. 2019. "Use of the distress thermometer in clinical practice." *J Adv Pract Oncol* 10 (2): 175–179.

Patrick, M.E., G.R. Lyden, N. Morrell, C.J. Mehus, M. Gunlicks-Stoessel, C.M. Lee, C.A. King, E.E. Bonar, I. Nahum-Shani, D. Almirall, M.E. Larimer, and D.M. Vock. 2021. "Main outcomes of M-bridge: a sequential multiple assignment randomized trial (SMART) for developing an adaptive preventive intervention for college drinking." *J Consult Clin Psychol* 89 (7): 601–614. doi: 10.1037/ccp0000663.

Petry, N.M., S.M. Alessi, C.J. Rash, D. Barry, and K.M. Carroll. 2018. "A randomized trial of contingency management reinforcing attendance at treatment: Do duration and timing of reinforcement matter?" *Journal of Consulting and Clinical Psychology* 86 (10): 799–809. doi: 10.1037/ccp0000330.

Pettinati, H.M., J.R. Volpicelli, J.D. Pierce, Jr., and C.P. O'Brien. 2000. "Improving naltrexone response: an intervention for medical practitioners to enhance medication compliance in alcohol dependent patients." *J Addict Dis* 19 (1): 71–83. doi: 10.1300/J069v19n01_06.

Peytremann-Bridevaux, I., C. Arditi, G. Gex, P.O. Bridevaux, and B. Burnand. 2015. "Chronic disease management programmes for adults with asthma." *Cochrane Database Syst Rev* 5: Cd007988. doi: 10.1002/14651858.CD007988.pub2.

Pistorello, J., D.A. Jobes, S.N. Compton, N.S. Locey, J.C. Walloch, R. Gallop, J.S. Au, S.K. Noose, M. Young, J. Johnson, Y. Dickens, P. Chatham, T. Jeffcoat, G. Dalto, and S. Goswami. 2017. "Developing adaptive treatment strategies to address suicidal risk in college students: a pilot Sequential, Multiple Assignment, Randomized Trial (SMART)." *Arch Suicide Res* 22 (4): 644–664. doi: 10.1080/13811118.2017.1392915.

Preference Collaborative Review Group. 2008. "Patients' preferences within randomised trials: systematic review and patient level meta-analysis." *BMJ* 337 :a1864. doi: 10.1136/bmj.a1864.

Roberts, N.J., I. Younis, L. Kidd, and M.R. Partridge. 2012. "Barriers to the implementation of self management support in long term lung conditions." *London Journal of Primary Care* 5 (1): 35–47. doi: 10.1080/17571472.2013.11493370.

Rush, A.J., M. Fava, S.R. Wisniewski, P.W. Lavori, M.H. Trivedi, H.A. Sackeim, M.E. Thase, et al. 2004. "Sequenced treatment alternatives to relieve depression (STAR*D): rationale and design." *Controlled Clinical Trials* 25 (1): 119–142. doi: https://doi.org/10.1016/S0197-2456(03)00112-0.

Sauer-Zavala, S., M.W. Southward, N.E. Stumpp, S.A. Semcho, C.O. Hood, A. Garlock, and A. Urs. 2022. "A SMART approach to personalized care: preliminary data on how to select and sequence skills in transdiagnostic CBT." *Cogn Behav Ther*:1–21. doi: 10.1080/16506073.2022.2053571.

Sherwood, N.E., A.L. Crain, E.M. Seburg, M.L. Butryn, E.M. Forman, M.M. Crane, R.L. Levy, A.S. Kunin-Batson, and R.W. Jeffery. 2022. "BestFIT sequential multiple assignment randomized trial results: a smart approach to developing individualized weight loss treatment sequences." *Ann Behav Med* 56 (3): 291–304. doi: 10.1093/abm/kaab061.

Shortreed, S.M., E. Laber, T. Scott Stroup, J. Pineau, and S.A. Murphy. 2014. "A multiple imputation strategy for sequential multiple assignment randomized trials." *Stat Med* 33 (24): 4202–14. https://doi.org/10.1002/sim.6223.

Sidani, S. 2014. *Health Intervention Research: Understanding Research Design and Methods*. Los Angeles, CA: Sage.

Stalmeier, P.F.M., J.J. van Tol-Geerdink, E.N.J.Th. van Lin, E. Schimmel, H. Huizenga, W.A.J. van Daal, and J.-W. Leer. 2007. "Doctors' and patients' preferences for participation and treatment in curative prostate cancer radiotherapy." *Journal of Clinical Oncology* 25 (21): 3096–3100. doi: 10.1200/jco.2006.07.4955.

Swift, J.K., J.L. Callahan, and B.M. Vollmer. 2011. "Preferences." *Journal of Clinical Psychology* 67 (2): 155–165. doi: https://doi.org/10.1002/jclp.20759.

Thall, P.F., H.-G. Sung, and E.H Estey. 2002. "Selecting therapeutic strategies based on efficacy and death in multicourse clinical trials." *Journal of the American Statistical Association* 97 (457): 29–39.

Van Straten, A., W. Seekles, N. J.V. Veer-Tazelaar, A.T.F. Beekman, and P. Cuijpers. 2010. "Stepped care for depression in primary care: what should be offered and how?" *Medical Journal of Australia* 192 (S11):S36–S39. doi: https://doi.org/10.5694/j.1326-5377.2010.tb03691.x.

Wahed, A.S., and A.A. Tsiatis. 2004. "Optimal estimator for the survival distribution and related quantities for treatment policies in two-stage randomization designs in clinical trials." *Biometrics* 60 (1):124–33. doi: 10.1111/j.0006-341X.2004.00160.x.

Walters, J.A.E., H. Courtney-Pratt, H. Cameron-Tucker, M. Nelson, A. Robinson, J. Scott, P. Turner, E.H. Walters, and R. Wood-Baker. 2012. "Engaging general practice nurses in chronic disease self-management support in Australia: insights from a controlled trial in chronic obstructive pulmonary disease." *Australian Journal of Primary Health* 18 (1): 74–79. doi: https://doi.org/10.1071/PY10072.

Wittenberg, E., G.A. Ritter, and L.A. Prosser. 2013. "Evidence of spillover of illness among household members:EQ-5D scores from a US sample." *Medical Decision Making* 33 (2): 235–243. https://doi.org/10.1177/0272989x12464434.

Wyatt, G., R. Lehto, P. Guha-Niyogi, S. Brewer, D. Victorson, T. Pace, T. Badger, and A. Sikorskii. 2021. "Reflexology and meditative practices for symptom management among people with cancer: results from a sequential multiple assignment randomized trial." *Research in Nursing & Health* 44 (5): 796–810. doi: https://doi.org/10.1002/nur.22169.

Yan, X., D.B. Matchar, N. Sivapragasam, J.P. Ansah, A. Goel, and B. Chakraborty. 2021. "Sequential Multiple Assignment Randomized Trial (SMART) to identify optimal sequences of telemedicine interventions for improving initiation of insulin therapy: a simulation study." *BMC Medical Research Methodology* 21 (1): 200. doi: 10.1186/s12874-021-01395-7.

4

Adapting the Primary Endpoint of TULIP 2 – A Hybrid Bayesian-Frequentist Framework to Incorporate Relevant Information from Prior Studies in Confirmatory Trials in SLE Patients

Fredrik Öhrn, Anna Berglind, and Micki Hultquist

Introduction and overview of technical area

Traditionally, clinical trials have been designed and analyzed following the frequentist paradigm, as extensively discussed in Senn (2008) and Pocock (2013). The power to demonstrate the superiority of a new therapy versus control is calculated for some fixed effect size $\theta = \delta$, for a prespecified hypotheses test at level α, which is typically set at a one-sided 2.5% level (two-sided 5%) for confirmatory studies. The concept of assurance is described in O'Hagan, Stevens, and Campbell (2005) and seeks to extend traditional power calculations to account for uncertainty about the true treatment effect θ. To calculate assurance for a single study, we would integrate over the uncertainty in the treatment effect, represented by a prior distribution for θ. The prior distribution may typically be derived from historical data for the same or similar compounds, from the elicitation of expert knowledge, or a combination of the two. Refer to Holzhauer et al. (2022) for the use of elicitation in a case study in asthma and Grieve (2022) for a recent book on hybrid frequentist/Bayesian approaches to planning clinical trials.

4.1 Anifrolumab case study

Anifrolumab is a fully human monoclonal antibody that binds to the interferon receptor. All type I interferon signaling is mediated by the interferon receptor and anifrolumab prevents binding of type I interferons; hence it has the potential to block the biological effects of all type I interferons. In 2021, anifrolumab was approved by the Food and Drug Administration to treat patients with moderate to severe systemic lupus erythematosus (SLE). SLE is a disease with a high unmet medical need and anifrolumab was only the second new molecular entity approved to treat SLE in a decade. When the monoclonal antibody belimumab was first approved, 10 years earlier in 2011, it was the first new medicine to treat SLE patients for more than 50 years.

DOI: 10.1201/9781003288640-4

SLE is a complex autoimmune disease that can affect almost every organ in the body. The heterogeneity and complexity of the disease make it difficult to evaluate the efficacy of experimental drugs for SLE treatment, and composite endpoints are often used to evaluate disease activity across multiple organ systems. Two composite binary responder endpoints that have been widely incorporated in clinical trials are BICLA (BILAG-based composite lupus assessment) and SRI-k (k points improvement on the SLEDAI (SLE disease activity index) where k = 4 has often been applied. These are both regulatory-accepted endpoints in SLE that capture the change in disease activity across organ systems, but they do so in slightly different ways. Endpoints based on SLEDAI require full resolution of a symptom to result in an improvement in score, while partial improvement/worsening of existing symptoms has no effect on the score. SLEDAI-based endpoints also assign more weight to some organ systems than others. Endpoints based on BILAG, in contrast, capture partial improvement and weighs all organ systems equally. To be a BICLA responder, improvement in all organ systems of the BILAG with moderate-to-severe baseline activity is required.

The anifrolumab phase III studies TULIP 1 (Furie et al. 2019; NCT02446912) and TULIP 2 (Morand et al. 2020; NCT02446899) were designed as twin studies. There were only some minor differences between the studies with respect to geographic regions and the inclusion of one lower dose arm in TULIP 1. Both were initiated following the positive readout of the phase II study MUSE (Furie et al. 2017; NCT01438489). At the design stage, the assumption was that two positive studies would be required for regulatory approval. That said, it was recognized that any final decision would be based on the totality of evidence and the overall benefit-risk profile. All three studies (TULIP 1, TULIP 2, and MUSE) were randomized, double-blind, 1-year-long studies evaluating the efficacy and safety of anifrolumab versus placebo on top of standard of care (SOC). An overview of the studies is provided in Table 4.1 below. Additional dose arms were included in MUSE (1000 mg) and TULIP 1 (150 mg) but are not described here.

Another important design feature in the anifrolumab program was the handling of oral corticosteroids (OCSs), which is part of the SOC for the treatment of SLE. OCS is an effective treatment to reduce disease activity but is unfortunately accompanied by severe side effects. One of the treatment goals of SLE is to reduce the use of high-dose

TABLE 4.1

Overview of relevant studies in the anifrolumab development program.

Anifrolumab clinical studies in moderate to severe SLE patients (IV formulation)	Phase	N Randomized		Preplanned Primary endpoint
		Anifrolumab 300 mg	Placebo	
MUSE	II	102	99	SRI-4+OCS tapering
TULIP 1	III	180	184	SRI-4
TULIP 2	III	182	180	SRI-4 (adapted to BICLA)

SRI-4 was prespecified as the primary endpoint in the TULIP studies, based on both the regulatory precedence as it was used as the primary endpoint in the belimumab phase III program (Furie et al. 2011) and the reassuring SRI-4 results in MUSE. It is worth noting that BICLA was a prespecified efficacy endpoint in all three studies.

MUSE had dual primary hypotheses, evaluating the effect on SRI-4+OCS tapering in both the All-Comers and IFN-high population.

OCS. Therefore, tapering of the OCS dose was incorporated into the design. The studies were designed prior to the finalization of the ICH E9 R1, so the intercurrent event terminology was not available at the time of design. However, the intercurrent events that were incorporated in the analysis were: use of restricted medications/rescue, discontinuation of investigational product (IP), and lack of successful OCS tapering. The composite strategy was used for the use of restricted medications and discontinuations of IP in all three studies, as both these events were considered unfavorable events and hence led to nonresponse. For the intercurrent event connected to OCS tapering, the composite strategy (incorporating OCS tapering into the responder definition) was used for the primary analysis of MUSE. However, the treatment policy strategy was chosen when designing the TULIP studies, hence not requiring successful OCS tapering to be a responder for the prospectively defined primary endpoint.

Despite the promising phase II data, TULIP 1 did not meet its primary objective of achieving a statistically significant reduction in disease activity, as measured by SRI-4 at 52 weeks. However, other endpoints, including BICLA and measurements of organ-specific disease manifestations, suggested there was a clinically meaningful response to anifrolumab. A decision was made to leverage all available information, from both MUSE and TULIP 1, to optimize a potential redesign of TULIP 2. At the time of redesigning TULIP 2 the study was fully blinded, no interim analyses had been conducted, and the study had not yet been reported. In addition, all patients had completed 52 weeks of follow-up, so there was no potential for impact on study conduct that could affect the primary outcome. These conditions were important to protect the integrity of TULIP 2, making sure that no within-trial data were used to inform the potential adaptation.

The redesign of TULIP 2 included a choice of primary endpoint and a choice of the primary analysis population. Apart from the differences between SRI-4 and BICLA, there was also uncertainty about to what extent anifrolumab would be more efficacious in patients who had a high interferon gene signature at baseline versus those with a low gene signature (e.g., a prespecified biomarker defined subgroup motivated by the mechanism of action). This interferon subgroup had already been included in the testing strategy in TULIP 1 (Furie et al. 2019), so prespecified testing in the IFN-high subgroup was a natural option to consider. Furthermore, since reduction of high-dose OCS use is one of the treatment goals in SLE, the composite strategy for the intercurrent event connected to OCS tapering was explored where one had to be a responder for the SRI-4/BICLA and successfully taper OCS (BICLA+OCS tapering/SRI-4+OCS tapering), instead of using the treatment policy approach. There were thus seven possible redesign options, across primary endpoint and population choices, for the redesign of TULIP 2 as presented in Table 2.

TABLE 4.2

Design options for TULIP 2 redesign.

Design Option	Endpoint	Population
Current	SRI-4	All-Comers
1	SRI-4	IFN-high
2	BICLA	All-Comers
3	BICLA	IFN-high
4	SRI-4+OCS tapering	All-Comers
5	SRI-4+OCS tapering	IFN-high
6	BICLA+OCS tapering	All-Comers
7	BICLA+OCS tapering	IFN-high

The problem at hand can be viewed as an operationally seamless adaptive design, where we may adapt the primary endpoint and/or analysis population based on external information. We shall focus on quantitative methods to support this decision but certainly would recognize that clinical and regulatory aspects, as well as protecting the integrity of the ongoing trial, must also be considered. Finally, we should bear in mind that the overarching goal of clinical research must always be to benefit patients. The quantitative methods presented should be seen as supportive of the overall decision framework, not as defining a mathematical decision rule for the primary hypothesis selection.

To characterize the treatment effects for BICLA and SRI-4, we sampled with replacement from the patient level data, separately for 300 mg arm and placebo, in TULIP 1 and MUSE. In each bootstrap sample, we calculated the difference between BICLA and SRI-4 on the placebo-corrected treatment effect. As shown in Figure 4.1, there was only a minor difference between the placebo-corrected effect on the two endpoints in MUSE but a considerable difference in TULIP 1. Extensive exploratory modeling was conducted, without identifying obvious reasons for the discrepancy.

It was decided that a reasonable quantitative framework for comparing different redesign options would be to calculate the corresponding assurance for a given prior distribution derived from TULIP 1 and MUSE. This raises the question of how to combine the data from the two prior studies. We decided to use a straightforward approach where a weight w, $0 \leq w \leq 1$, decided the relative weight put on MUSE and TULIP 1, respectively. Setting $w = 1$ would correspond to only considering TULIP 1, while $w = 0$ would put all weight on MUSE. Since TULIP 1 had more observations than MUSE, it would in general seem reasonable to put more weight on TULIP 1. In many of the illustrations in this chapter we have chosen to display a full range of weights, while the weight derived from the relative sample size in the two studies is displayed with a dashed vertical line.

The primary method used to estimate the distribution of the treatment effect for the assurance calculation for a given design option in TULIP 2 was to bootstrap from patient-level data. For each arm shown in Table 4.1 with n patients, n patients were sampled

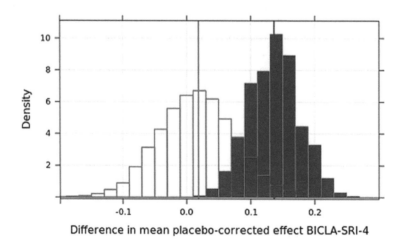

Difference in mean placebo-corrected effect BICLA-SRI-4

FIGURE 4.1

Difference in placebo-corrected treatment effects between BICLA and SRI-4. Histograms show this difference calculated for each bootstrap sample, separately for MUSE (white) and TULIP 2 (dark).

with replacement. For each of the 10,000 bootstrap samples, the treatment difference for anifrolumab versus placebo was calculated, for both TULIP 1 and MUSE. For a given weight w on the TULIP 1 treatment effect, it is then straightforward to calculate the power for a given number of observations per arm in TULIP 2. Finally, assurance was calculated as the average power across the bootstrap samples. This approach has been used in this chapter, unless otherwise stated. As a supportive analysis we assumed that success rates in each arm followed a beta distribution and applied the resulting prior to calculating the assurance, giving results virtually identical to those obtained from the bootstrap analysis.

The assurance for the seven possible redesign options in Table 4.2, as well as that for the current design using SRI-4 in the full population as the primary hypothesis, can be seen in Figure 4.2. The weighting of two studies is displayed on the x-axis, where the dashed line denotes weighting according to the actual respective sample sizes of the previous studies. The full weighting scheme was shown to facilitate reaching a consensus within the project team. Key stakeholders were also likely to agree with a given recommendation in case the corresponding redesign option would provide uniformly higher assurance regardless of how the studies were weighted.

It is evident from Figure 4.2 that BICLA would increase assurance over SRI-4 in both the full population and the IFN-high subgroup, for any w, $0 \le w \le 1$. This is because based on MUSE there is only a minor difference between the treatment effect measured by SRI-4 and BICLA, while for TULIP 1 the difference is substantial. Adding the OCS tapering requirement to BICLA increases the assurance slightly. Even if there is reason to prefer one of the two studies, the fact that BICLA would provide a uniformly higher assurance makes it easier to reach a consensus about the choice of endpoint from a quantitative perspective.

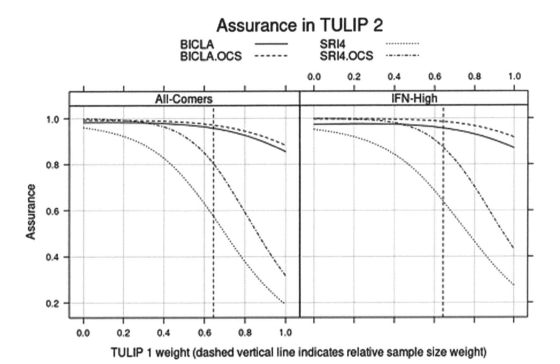

FIGURE 4.2
Assurance by endpoint and population.

Given that there was less precedent with a BICLA endpoint incorporating tapering, it was not felt that the increase in assurance motivated switching to BICLA+OCS as opposed to BICLA alone.

While the recommendation to change the primary endpoint holds regardless of study weighting, the choice of population is less obvious. Figure 4.3 shows the same assurance calculations as shown in Figure 4.2. While Figure 4.2 facilitates endpoint comparison, Figure 4.3 enables a direct comparison of the assurance for each population across each possible endpoint.

As described, there was special interest in the IFN-High subgroup due to the mechanism of action of anifrolumab. One way of approaching the choice of population (All-Comers vs. IFN-High) is to use a weighted assurance. In this approach, we consider the expected number of patients we could treat in the All-Comers population report a weighted assurance for the IFN-High subgroup, where a win in the subgroup is discounted by a factor equal to the proportion of patients in the subgroup. If we also account for the fact that additional patients could benefit from an approval in the All-Comers population, then as shown in Figure 4.4 the weighted assurance tends to be higher for tests in the All-Comers population. It would then appear reasonable to recommend testing BICLA in the All-Comers population, as opposed to the IFN-High subgroup only. While weighted assurance provides a clear recommendation for the full population as opposed to the subgroup, there was also a preference to keep the same broad primary analysis population as in TULIP 1, making it possible to include all the patients recruited in the primary analysis. In addition, it is worth pointing out that while the treatment effect in the IFN-High subgroup was more pronounced than IFN-Low, patients in the IFN-Low subgroup also

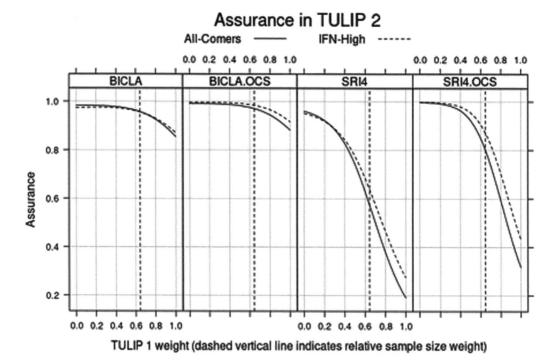

FIGURE 4.3
Assurance by population and endpoint.

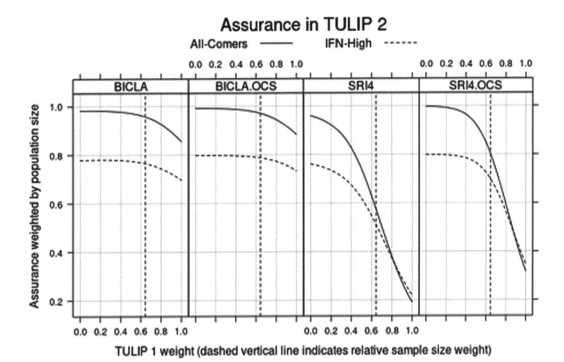

FIGURE 4.4

Weighted assurance, accounting for the size of the patient population where superiority vs placebo is demonstrated, by population and endpoint.

appeared to benefit in TULIP 1 and MUSE, as was later confirmed in TULIP 2 (Morand et al. 2020).

The TULIP 2 study stands on its own with no inflation of the within-study familywise type I error probability since an appropriate multiple test procedure was used. Neither will there be bias in estimation due to the adaptation because no data used to inform the adaptation were included in the final analysis. There was nevertheless a sponsor's risk of overestimating the likelihood of success due to the data-driven choice of primary endpoint and population. To this end, additional adjustments to prior distributions were also considered.

We shall now describe how one supportive analysis was conducted to achieve an adjusted estimate of the assurance. To approximate the bias introduced by taking the maximum over eight possible primary populations/endpoints, we simulated from the correlation matrix estimated from the prior data. The mean treatment effect for the selected endpoint/population across the simulations can be compared to keeping the original population/endpoint, in a scenario where all the true treatment effects are the same. The corresponding bias in mean treatment effect is then subtracted when calculating the assurance for the preferred redesign option (BICLA in the All-Comers population). This sensitivity analysis may in fact overestimate the bias because, in practice, other factors would also be considered when deciding the primary hypothesis. Nevertheless, we consider it to be a useful illustration of the bias introduced.

The adjusted and unadjusted assurance for BICLA in the All-Comers population is compared with keeping the original primary hypothesis, which it can be argued was not in

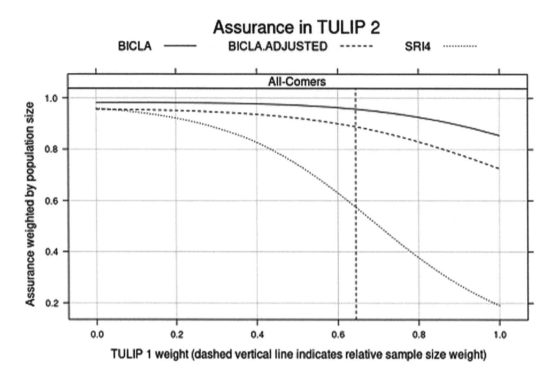

FIGURE 4.5
Adjusted assurance for BICLA versus unadjusted assurance for BICLA and SRI-4.

the same way selected in a data-driven way. As shown in Figure 4.5, the adjusted assurance for BICLA is still considerably higher than the unadjusted assurance for SRI-4, across the full range of weights. One reason for the adjustment not being more pronounced is that all the underlying treatment effects for all the candidate designs are strongly correlated.

This chapter would not be complete without providing the TULIP 2 results, which are reported in Morand et al. (2020). TULIP 2 demonstrated a positive treatment difference for anifrolumab compared with placebo for BICLA in the All-Comers population. Overall, the results for BICLA were consistent across studies, while the SRI-4 results were more variable. Looking at the pooled SRI-4 results across the two TULIP studies, the treatment effect was lower than in MUSE, which is not uncommon when moving compounds from phase II to phase III. The positive read-out in TULIP 2 (Morand et al. 2020), combined with the results for BICLA in TULIP 1 (Furie et al. 2019) and MUSE (Furie et al. 2017) as supportive information, formed the body of evidence which was the basis for approval across multiple regions and jurisdictions.

4.2 Lessons learned

It is worth having a general discussion about conducting a single trial versus requiring two positive trials. As discussed in Senn (2008), conducting a single trial requiring a two-sided p value of less than 2×0.025^2 would generally be more efficient from a power perspective than requiring superiority from two independent trials, each with a two-sided alpha level of 0.05. While it is possible to conduct a retrospective evaluation of strategies for the two trials, we must acknowledge that any such evaluation will be post hoc. A strength of the redesign described in the case study is that it was prospective in nature with an independent evaluation of TULIP 2, from which no data internal to the trial was used to inform the design change.

We shall now discuss the extent to which the results for BICLA would have met even more stringent thresholds than two-sided 0.05, focusing on nominal two-sided p-values either for the pooled TULIP data or for TULIP 2 alone. The pooled data from the two TULIP trials were assessed in Vital et al. (2022). The two-sided nominal p value for BICLA in this pooled analysis was reported to be < 0.001, so hence, $< 2 \times 0.025^2$. In fact, the two-sided nominal p-value was equal to $0.001 < 2 \times 0.025^2$ also based on TULIP 2 alone (Morand et al. 2020). Hence, there is no doubt that the efficacy of BICLA has been confirmed in an independent trial. We might also have considered dual primary hypotheses for the pooled trial. Using a classical unweighted Holm procedure (Holm, 1979), testing each endpoint at two-sided $2 \times 0.025^2 / 2$ in the first step, we can retrospectively evaluate the pooled results. We note that the corresponding two-sided nominal p-value for BICLA is indeed below $2 \times 0.025^2 / 2 = 0.025^2$ (data on file); i.e., based on the pooled data BICLA would have been rejected in the first step of such a test procedure.

Finally, we might view the two TULIP trials as an adaptive design, where a combination test for choice of endpoint is applied at two-sided $\alpha = 2 \times 0.025^2$. We would then select the endpoint after TULIP 1, where the stage 1 p-value would have to be adjusted for multiplicity, while for stage 2 we would apply the nominal p-value for the selected endpoint in TULIP 2. In the last step, we could apply, for example, the weighted inverse normal method (Lehmacher and Wassmer, 1999). If applied retrospectively, the combination test p-value would be significant by a wide margin. A related, albeit different, approach to endpoint selection in SLE was recently highlighted by FDA in their complex innovative designs (CID) pilot program. An adaptive choice of endpoint was proposed based on interim data (FDA 2022), allowing for an optimized primary endpoint at week 52.

A final possibility not considered in this case study would be a fully Bayesian analysis, borrowing on the treatment effect scale from previous trials. In such a scenario, we would recommend discussing with regulators and seeking agreement about the amount of borrowing before the read-out of the TULIP 2 study. This approach of more formally incorporating the prior data in the primary analysis is appealing but would undoubtedly have type I error implications.

Decisions about trial designs can be made both before and during the conduct of a trial. Trial integrity and consideration of patients are always critical aspects, but even more so when adaptations are done during the trial. No data from TULIP 2 was used to inform the adaptation, ensuring that the recommendation based on data from TULIP 1 and MUSE could be independently verified in TULIP 2. In addition, no unblinded interim analysis for efficacy had been conducted and all patients were included in the primary analysis.

When adapting to external information it is typically due to new data that it is hard to ignore, and hence, it is natural to update our assumptions. Adaptation may provide an opportunity to increase the probability of success, but honest assessment may be complex given the challenges of exactly modeling the bias introduced via the decision-making process. The independent analysis of the confirmatory trial, TULIP 2 in our case study, is, however, more straightforward and no α adjustment is needed when the adaptation is external. Adaptive designs based on within-trial information provide opportunities for further efficiency gains, but adaptations are then likely to be based on uncertain estimates, if done based on interim data for the primary endpoint. More data may, however, be available through external information.

There are potential power gains in applying a one-trial rule as opposed to conducting two independent trials, as discussed in the previous paragraph. Moreover, we may prefer to have a single decision point that is provided with a one-trial rule, for example, conducting a pooled analysis vs two-sided $\alpha = 2 \times 0.025^2$. One phase III trial backed up by prior evidence, or a multiple test procedure with dual primary endpoints, is a robust option as having more data from the two trials may compensate for any α loss. For midcourse adaptation of the primary endpoint, we would then have more data to inform the adaptation than when considering a single trial only. The recent CID pilot, or a more traditional combination test approach, are reasonable suggestions for how such midcourse adaptation of an endpoint can be conducted.

References

Food and Drug Administration. 2022. "CID case study: a study in patients with systemic lupus erythematosus," www.fda.gov/media/155404/download.

Furie, Richard, Munther Khamashta, Joan T Merrill, Victoria P Werth, Kenneth Kalunian, Philip Brohawn, Gabor G Illei, et al. 2017. "Anifrolumab, an anti-interferon-± receptor monoclonal antibody, in moderate-to-severe systemic lupus erythematosus." *Arthritis & Rheumatology* 69 (2): 376–86.

Furie, Richard, Eric Morand, Ian Bruce, Susan Manzi, Kenneth Kalunian, Edward Vital, Theresa Lawrence Ford, et al. 2019. "Type I interferon inhibitor anifrolumab in active systemic lupus erythematosus (TULIP-1): a randomised, controlled, phase 3 trial." *The Lancet Rheumatology* 1 (4): e208–19.

Furie, Richard, Michelle Petri, Omid Zamani, Ricard Cervera, Daniel J Wallace, Dana Tegzová, Jorge Sanchez-Guerrero, et al. 2011. "A phase III, randomized, placebo-controlled study of belimumab, a monoclonal antibody that inhibits B lymphocyte stimulator, in patients with systemic lupus erythematosus." *Arthritis & Rheumatism* 63 (12): 3918–3930.

Grieve, Andrew P. 2022. *Hybrid Frequentist/Bayesian Power and Bayesian Power in Planning Clinical Trials.* CRC Press.

Holm, Sture, 1979, "A simple sequentially rejective multiple test procedure." *Scandinavian Journal of Statistics*: 65–70.

Holzhauer, Björn, Lisa V Hampson, John Paul Gosling, Björn Bornkamp, Joseph Kahn, Markus R Lange, Wen-Lin Luo, et al. 2022. "Eliciting judgements about dependent quantities of interest: the sheffield elicitation framework extension and copula methods illustrated using an asthma case study." *Pharmaceutical Statistics*, 21 (5): 1005–1021.

ICH E9 (R1) addendum on estimands and sensitivity analysis in clinical trials to the guideline on statistical principles for clinical trials. European Medicines Agency. 2020. www.ema.europa.eu/en/documents/scientific-guideline/ich-e9-r1-addendum-estimands-sensitivity-analysis-clinical-trials-guideline-statistical-principles_en.pdf.

Lehmacher, Walter, and Gernot Wassmer. 1999. "Adaptive sample size calculations in group sequential trials." *Biometrics* 55(4): 1286–1290.

Morand, Eric F, Richard Furie, Yoshiya Tanaka, Ian N Bruce, Anca D Askanase, Christophe Richez, Sang-Cheol Bae, et al. 2020. "Trial of Anifrolumab in active systemic lupus erythematosus." *New England Journal of Medicine* 382 (3): 211–21.

O'Hagan, Anthony, John W Stevens, and Michael J Campbell. 2005. "Assurance in clinical trial design." *Pharmaceutical Statistics: The Journal of Applied Statistics in the Pharmaceutical Industry* 4 (3): 187–201.

Pocock, Stuart J. 2013. *Clinical Trials: A Practical Approach.* John Wiley & Sons.

Senn, Stephen S. 2008. *Statistical Issues in Drug Development.* Vol. 69. John Wiley & Sons.

Vital, EM, JT Merrill, EF Morand, et al. 2022. "Anifrolumab efficacy and safety by Type I interferon gene signature and clinical subgroups in patients with SLE: post hoc analysis of pooled data from two phase III trials", *Annals of the Rheumatic Diseases* 81: 951–961.

5

Unblinded Sample Size Reestimation: A Case Study

Silke Jörgens and Vladimir Dragalin

Introduction

Unblinded sample size reestimation (SSR) based on conditional power has become one of the most popular adaptive design features in clinical trials. At the planning stage of a given trial the target treatment effect to be detected is used to calculate the required number of subjects to achieve a desired power. This target treatment effect is usually determined based on many considerations including information from previous studies investigating the compound, the competitive landscape, compound differentiation at the time of approval, etc. However, this target effect is based on many assumptions and may be different from the true treatment effect. The SSR design allows the opportunity to revisit these assumptions during the study and adjust the final sample size, in light of new data on the treatment effect and its variability in the trial population.

Several methods have been developed for SSR designs under the frequentist statistical paradigm that provide analytical control of the Type I error rate. A commonly employed class of SSR designs utilizes the fact that the standard test statistics can be used if the sample size is increased only when a minimum conditional power is reached. Conditional power is defined as the power for the final analysis given the interim result and assuming the observed interim treatment effect is the true treatment effect for the remainder of the trial. This is commonly known as the "promising zone" approach (Mehta and Pocock (2011)). Further enhancement of the promising zone approach was suggested by relaxing the requirement to use the standard test statistics at the final analysis (Hsiao et al. (2018)). However, the FDA guidance on adaptive designs highlights approaches that combine p-values from the different stages using preplanned weights (Lehmacher and Wassmer (1999), Cui et al. (1999), Brannath and Bauer (2004)). The respective advantages of these methods have been discussed (e.g., Jennison and Turnbull (2015), Emerson et al. (2011), Glimm (2012)). For a comprehensive comparison, see a recent publication by Mehta et al. (2022).

The example we present in this chapter is modeled after a completed phase 3 trial that had an unblinded SSR design based on combining p-values from two stages. Due to confidentiality reasons, the study will not be identified, and data are altered. We use this example to illustrate the issues related to setting up and implementing such trials. In the first two sections we introduce the design of the study and provide statistical considerations and details of the SSR design. We then describe the conduct of the study including the interim results and the Independent Data Monitoring Committee (IDMC) recommendations,

DOI: 10.1201/9781003288640-5

implementation issues, and a description and discussion of the final analysis results. We close with a discussion on lessons learned and what could have been done differently.

5.1 Outline of the Study Design

The example study was a randomized, double-blind, active-controlled, multicenter study with a preplanned maximum sample size of 348 male and female adult subjects. Its primary objective was to evaluate the efficacy of two doses of experimental treatment against a control, as assessed by the change in a continuous primary outcome from day 1 prerandomization to the end of a 4-week double-blind treatment phase.

The study consisted of three parts: (1) 4-week screening, (2) 4-week double-blind treatment, and (3) up to 24 weeks of follow-up or roll-over into a long-term extension study. A diagram of the study design is provided below in Figure 5.1. Here, we consider the 4-week double-blind treatment period only.

5.2 Statistical Considerations

The primary efficacy endpoint, the change in a continuous outcome from baseline (day 1) to day 28, was analyzed using a mixed-effects repeated measures model (MMRM). The model included an adjustment for baseline, a patient-level random intercept, and fixed effects for treatment assignment, region, type of concomitant medication, study day, and a study day-by-treatment assignment interaction. The changes from baseline for all postbaseline outcome measurements (days 2, 8, 15, 22, and 28) were included in the model as the repeated measures.

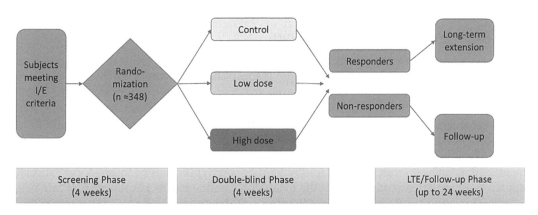

FIGURE 5.1
Study Design.
Abbreviations: I/E – Inclusion/exclusion; LTE – long-term extension.

Multiple testing arises from the two doses of the experimental treatment to be tested against control, and from key secondary endpoints included in the confirmatory testing stream. While the details for key secondary endpoints are not of interest here, it is important to note that the multiplicity across the two doses of experimental treatment was tested in a modified fixed sequence. The high dose was tested first at full one-sided alpha of 0.025, and upon a positive result, a one-sided alpha of 0.02125 was allocated to the primary endpoint for the low dose group.

Phase 2 study results led to a sample size of 86 subjects per treatment group, providing 90% power at a one-sided significance level of 0.0125. The actual number of subjects to be randomized in the study was adjusted to account for the assumed drop-out rate of 25%. The maximum number of subjects to be randomized was therefore 116 subjects per treatment group for a total of 348 subjects.

However, based on other previous studies, it was possible that a larger treatment effect may be observed, which would require a smaller sample size of only 78 subjects per arm for a total of 234 subjects. As the assumptions of the expected treatment effect and variability may or may not be upheld, an interim analysis was planned with the purpose of stopping the study due to futility or reestimating the sample size. The sample size may be adjusted to achieve the desired conditional power while maintaining control of the overall Type I error rate. Early efficacy stopping was not an option. Simulations were performed to assess the operating characteristics of this design. Such simulation studies are needed to demonstrate that type I error control is maintained. Further, they allow for assessing whether operating characteristics are acceptable. Desirable operating characteristics are a high probability of a futility stop in the case of no treatment effect, and vice versa, a low probability of a futility stop if the true treatment effect is worthwhile. Additionally, the introduction of a futility option impacts the global power of a study. Regarding sample size reassessment, simulations ensure that the planned procedure is suitable to accommodate necessary changes based on interim results. Assessing different interim analysis timepoints in simulations can help find a timepoint where, on the one hand, sufficient information is available to ensure a meaningful interim analysis and, on the other hand, recruitment is not so far advanced as to preclude the required changes to the sample size.

5.3 Sample Size Reassessment Design

The target sample size per group for the SSR procedure was 78 subjects, corresponding to the sample size based on more optimistic assumptions. The timing of interim analyses was planned when 50% of this target sample size had complete primary endpoint information, i.e., 4 weeks after the first 120 subjects were randomized (40 per arm). An adaptive two-stage design was implemented based on the inverse normal p-value combination method with equal weights prespecified for both stages (Lehmacher and Wassmer, 1999). SSR at the interim analysis was based on the unblinded estimation of treatment effect measured as change from baseline to day 28. For the hypotheses of interest, conditional power was calculated assuming that the estimated treatment effect at the interim analysis was the true effect for the remainder of the study. SSR was performed in a discretized way. Guidance for the new sample size was provided to the IDMC based on outcomes of the conditional power for each treatment group, as shown in Table 5.1. Possible values were the 234 subjects required under the optimistic treatment effect, the 348 subjects required

TABLE 5.1

Sample Size Reestimation Based on Conditional Power for Each Treatment Comparison.

Scenario	Conditional Power (%)		Reestimated Total Sample Size
	Comparison 2: Low dose vs. control	Comparison 1: High dose vs. control	
1	$CP_2 < 10$	$CP_1 < 10$	Stop study
2a	$10 \leq CP_2 \leq 30$	$CP_1 < 10$	234
2b	$CP_2 < 10$	$10 \leq CP_1 \leq 30$	234
2c	$10 \leq CP_2 \leq 30$	$10 \leq CP_1 \leq 30$	234
3a	$30 < CP_2 < 50$	$CP_1 \leq 30$	348
3b	$CP_2 \leq 30$	$30 < CP_1 < 50$	348
3c	$30 < CP_2 < 50$	$30 < CP_1 < 50$	348
4a	$50 \leq CP_2 < 80$	$CP_1 \leq 30$	291
4b	$CP_2 \leq 30$	$50 \leq CP_1 < 80$	291
4c	$50 \leq CP_2 < 80$	$50 \leq CP_1 < 80$	291
5a	$CP_2 \geq 80$	$CP_1 \leq 30$	234
5b	$CP_2 \leq 30$	$CP_1 \geq 80$	234
5c	$CP_2 \geq 80$	$CP_1 \geq 80$	234
6a	$50 \leq CP_2$	$30 < CP_1 < 50$	348
6b	$30 < CP_2 < 50$	$50 \leq CP_1$	348
7a	$CP_2 \geq 80$	$50 \leq CP_1 < 80$	291
7b	$50 \leq CP_2 < 80$	$CP_1 \geq 80$	291

under the smallest expected treatment effect, and an intermediate sample size of 291 total subjects. Generally, the SSR scheme recommended that if either the conditional power was quite low for both doses or the conditional power for at least one dose was quite high, the recommended sample size was the smaller 234 subjects due to expected futility or expected success, respectively. More moderate conditional powers resulted in one of the two larger possible sample sizes.

As usual with adaptive designs, the statistical validity of the procedure needs to be ascertained. Wang (2010) showed that if the sample size is increased proportionately in all treatment groups, then the regular (unconditional) distributions of the combination test statistics used for the final analysis, both for the primary and the secondary endpoints, are the same as the distribution of these test statistics in a fixed design without an adaptive sample size adjustment. As a result, the distributional assumptions used in the serial gatekeeping procedure proposed for this study are met and strong control of the overall Type I error rate is not compromised.

5.4 Logistics and Operational Considerations

Following FDA (2019) Guidance, procedures were put in place to ensure that the results of the interim analysis do not influence the conduct of the study, investigators, or subjects. In order to minimize operational bias that may occur if the study continued to enroll beyond the minimum sample size, only the maximum sample size of 348 subjects was mentioned in the study protocol. A rigorous interim statistical analysis plan (SAP) and IDMC charter were developed detailing the algorithm for a sample size reestimation based on the interim data and how the analysis was to be executed. An independent, external statistician was contracted to perform the interim analysis and make recommendations to the IDMC for any sample size adjustment based on the rules defined in the interim SAP. Any changes to the sample size were communicated by the independent, external statistician to the IWRS vendor to ensure that the appropriate number of subjects was enrolled in the trial. None of the study team members or staff members at the investigational sites conducting the clinical trials were informed of the specific sample size adjustment resulting from this interim analysis.

5.5 Outcome of Interim Analysis

The prespecified interim analysis was performed 4 weeks after randomizing 121 subjects. Recruitment was not paused between data cut-off for the interim analysis and time of IDMC recommendation. This approach ensures that the timepoint of the interim analysis does not become known to the investigators, which is a further piece contributing to operational integrity of the study. On the other hand, this practice may lead to overenrollment. In this example, approximately 60 subjects were randomized between randomization of the 121st subject and the communication of the IDMC recommendation to the IWRS vendor. While this allowed accommodating all possible changes in sample size, overrun would have been substantial in the event of an early futility stop.

Results on the primary endpoint are presented in Table 5.2 below.

Conditional power for the high dose group was rather low at 0.0059%. Figure 5.2 shows that the high dose group shows an effect close to control (difference in LS means: 0.52 points). The low-dose group appears to perform somewhat better, with a one-sided p-value of 0.115 and a conditional power of 19%.

According to the prespecified guideline for the sample size reestimation (see Table 5.1), the IDMC recommended continuing the study with the final sample size of 234 patients. Figure 5.3 shows how the reduction from the original randomization cap of 348 subjects to the SSR result of 234 subjects was communicated to the IWRS vendor.

The sponsor study team and study site staff were not informed of the adjusted sample size until it had been met to ensure no impact on study conduct. As an ethical obligation, the sponsor allowed patients in the screening phase or who had a screening visit already scheduled to continue participation in the study if all entry criteria were met. Despite the

TABLE 5.2

Change from Baseline to Day 28 of the Double-Blind Phase.

	Low dose	High dose	Control
Number of subjects enrolled	42	37	42
Number of subjects with day 28 data	39	31	37
Mean (SD)	-20.7 (15.86)	-18.6 (12.58)	-16.6 (15.46)
1-Sided p-value	0.115	0.436	
Difference of LS Means (SE)	-3.7 (3.07)	-0.52 (3.23)	
95% CI on difference	(-9.77; 2.37)	(-6.93; 5.88)	
Conditional power	0.1900	0.0059	

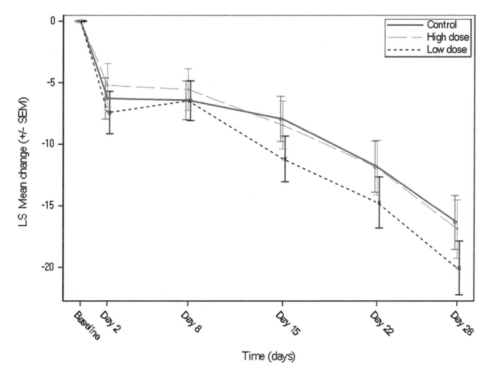

FIGURE 5.2
LS mean change and +/− SE over time for the data from stage 1.

Cap and Milestone update:

Event:	Type:	Current Value:			New Value:		
☒ Study-Wide Randomization Cap	☐ Soft Cap	3	4	8	2	3	4
☐ Live Project Data Review Milestone	☒ Hard Cap						
	☐ Milestone						

FIGURE 5.3
Operational change form for IWRS vendor.

IDMC recommending the sample size to be capped at the preplanned 234 patients, this obligation resulted in 346 patients being randomized.

5.6 Final Analysis

For the final analysis, the MMRM analysis was performed as planned, separately for both stages. Results were then combined according to the inverse normal combination test procedure.

Differences in the primary endpoint results were observed between the stages as shown in Figures 5.2 and 5.4, specifically a smaller improvement in the control group in Stage 2 leading to a larger treatment difference in the two experimental treatment arms in this stage. There are reasons for that including that experienced sites were added as the study progressed, additional training of sites was implemented, and an open label extension study became available.

Table 5.3 shows the results for the full dataset. While within-treatment group results are calculated on the pooled data over stages, results given for the comparisons to control combine the results from the stages according to the adaptive design. The p-value results from the inverse normal combination of the p-values from both stages, and the difference to control is the median unbiased estimate, which is a weighted combination of the LS means of the difference to control from the two stages.

According to the predefined testing sequence, the comparison between the high dose and control is the first in sequence. The one-sided p-value is 0.041, so the high dose was not superior to control at the predefined one-sided alpha level of 2.5%. Thus, the comparison of the low dose against control cannot be performed in a confirmatory fashion.

In addition to the p-value corresponding to the two-stage design, the overall p-value was calculated, disregarding the adaptive nature of the study. This overall p-value is 0.027 one-sided for the high dose, just shy of the boundary of being significant, in contrast to the 0.041 one-sided given in Table 5.3. This discrepancy is not a sign of methodological flaws in the adaptive design, but rather a direct result of the combination of stages with

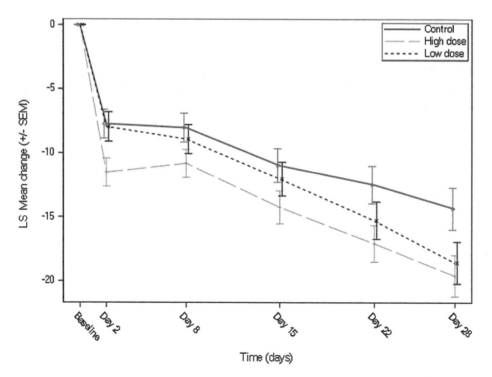

FIGURE 5.4
LS mean change and +/− SE over time for the data from stage 2.

TABLE 5.3

Change from Baseline to Day 28 of the Double-Blind Induction Phase.

	Low Dose	High Dose	Control
Number of patients enrolled	114	115	113
Number of patients with day 28 data	108	102	107
Mean (SD)	-19.1 (15.10)	-19.2 (13.20)	-15.2 (14.68)
1-Sided p-value	0.016	0.041	
Diff. of LS Means	-4.0	-2.9	
95% CI on difference	(-9.26; 1.33)	(-8.33; 2.55)	

TABLE 5.4

Final p-Values for Different Weighting Schemes.

Weights based on a total sample size of	Weight for Stage 1	Final p-Value	
		High Dose Arm	Low Dose Arm
234	120/234=0.5	0.0411	0.0158
291	120/291=0.41	0.0309	0.0146
348	120/348=0.34	0.0250	0.0141

the prespecified weights chosen for the study and the heterogeneity seen over stages. For the lower dose, the overall p-value is 0.013 one-sided, much closer to the inverse normal combination p-value given in Table 5.3.

5.7 Choice of Weights over the Two Stages

In such a type of design as we present here, the choice of weights for both stages can play a crucial role. On the one hand, the weights need to be prespecified if an adaptive design with a p-value combination test is pursued. On the other hand, the efficiency of the statistical test procedure is maximized if the weights are close to the actual stage size proportion.

In the example on hand, the weights were derived based on the minimum sample size allowed. Under the optimistic treatment effect assumption, 234 subjects were planned and the interim occurred after approximately half of these subjects had been followed for 4 weeks, 121 subjects. The weights were therefore chosen as 50% for each stage. However, the sample size maximum in the SSR plan was 348 subjects, in which case the 121 interim analysis subjects would correspond to a percentage of only 34%. This choice of weights does not benefit from the main advantage of the inverse normal p-value combination method that if no adaptations were made to the sample size, the final test statistic is optimal.

Table 5.4 shows the weights for each stage according to their size for the different possible maximum sample sizes, and the p-values that would correspond to each weighting scheme. A more appropriate target sample size in this case might have been 291 subjects with the option to either reduce it to 234 or increase it up to 348.

We can see in more detail here what has already been touched upon in the previous section, which is that the p-values derived for the high-dose group depend very much on the weights chosen. In particular, the prespecified weights in this case resulted in the most conservative results compared to other options in Table 5.4. The last row of the table, which closely mirrors a pooled result across the two stages, even results in a borderline statistically significant outcome. The reason is that, of the three options shown in Table 5.4, this places the least weight of all three options on the first stage data, in which there was no separation from control for the high-dose group. It also places a weight close to the true proportion on the patients in each stage. Thus, this adaptive p-value is very close to the overall p-value reported. However, this choice of weights should not be considered generally appropriate because it implicitly assumes that the study will be extended to the maximum sample size.

5.8 Discussion

Such a large discrepancy in study results for the different weighting schemes, due to differences seen over stages, is not a typical outcome for an adaptive design. Usually, a careful operational approach will ensure a higher degree of homogeneity over stages. In an ideal world, with identical p-values from both stages, the weighting scheme would have a much lower impact on the final p-value. The low-dose group is a good example of this.

It is important to note that in this approach, no weighting scheme is more or less correct than another. They are all valid choices. However, choosing the weight on the inter-mediate sample size, 291 subjects, limits the extent of possible deviation from the theor-etical optimal weighting corresponding to the true proportion of the sample size in each stage. While the interim analysis happens at the same timepoint, the setup of such a study would be different from the actual design. Instead of allowing a sample size increase if the optimistic assumptions about the treatment effect are not met, the trial is planned on a realistic assumption. A sample size correction in both directions, upward and downward, would then be allowed if a lower or higher effect size was observed in the interim ana-lysis. The inverse normal p-value combination method allows such flexible changes to the sample size in contrast to other methods which allow increases only, such as the original "promising zone" approach. In the past, health authorities have sometimes pushed back against a possible sample size decrease. This was based on results for blinded SSR, where it was shown by simulations that the type I error rate is controlled only if the sample size is allowed to be increased. However, the p-value combination method for unblinded SSR analytically controls the Type I error rate even if the sample size is allowed to be decreased. Nevertheless, as in all adaptive designs, it is advisable to gain health authority feedback before embarking on such a trial.

As noted above, the inverse normal method allows full flexibility in determining the sample size of subsequent stages. That also applies to the set of potential new sample sizes. Instead of a discrete set, as was done for this trial, a more granular recalculation is possible where all intermediate values would also be allowed. Additionally, the min-imum and maximum total sample size are not imposed by the statistical method but were rather a conscious choice made at the design stage and, perhaps, fine-tuned through intensive simulation to obtain acceptable performance. When choosing the actual set of recalculated sample sizes to be permitted, the following two aspects should be weighed against each other. First, a continuous sample size reassessment procedure may allow the best approximation to the target conditional power. However, it must not be forgotten that it is still an approximation because the method assumes that the true treatment effect in the second stage is what was observed in the first stage. This may create a false precision in the recalculated sample size. Second, the issue of back-calculating the observed treatment effect from a recalculated sample size has often been raised. This concern can at least be partly attenuated by introducing some fuzziness into the recalculation such as by discretizing the set of new possible sample sizes. When the set of new possible sample sizes is very small, such as in the current example, it may also be worthwhile to further use simulations for comparing the operational characteristics of the design against a group sequential design. This group sequential design would have the same maximum sample size and allow early efficacy stops at the possible recalculation outcomes of the adaptive design. In this case, the maximum sample size would have been 348 subjects with interim analysis after 234 subjects and after 291 subjects.

In addition to the above, two further details in the proposed conditional power table are worth reconsidering. The first one is specific to the multiplicity correction applied to testing two doses against control. The testing hierarchy precludes the test on the lower dose from having a confirmatory connotation if the higher dose cannot show statistical significance over control. In contrast to this, the conditional power table treats both treatment groups in a symmetric way, leading to a futility recommendation only if the conditional power is below 10% for both treatment groups. An alternative approach would be to base futility on the higher dose alone given that its future success is independent of the performance of the low-dose group, and conversely the lower dose cannot succeed if the higher dose does not. If the conditional power for the first test in hierarchy, the high-dose group, is sufficiently high, then it may be a reasonable decision not to increase the sample size and give up on the lower dose if its conditional power is low. If the conditional power for the high dose group is low but still above futility, it does not seem promising to stay at the minimum sample size even if the second dose group has a high conditional power. This is a general criticism often voiced regarding the promising zone approach. By design, there is a zone with relatively low conditional power where the sample size is kept as originally planned. Others have shown (see e.g., Jennison and Turnbull (2015) and Glimm (2012)) that trial efficiency can be significantly improved if this region is eliminated and possible decisions are to either stop for futility or increase the sample size if the conditional power is low, but above the futility boundary.

It is worth mentioning a couple of further options to consider when defining conditional power for sample size reassessment. They do not so much refer to the example at hand but are more generally applicable. Depending on the sample size reached at an interim analysis, the interim effect estimate will still be subject to a certain degree of volatility. There are several suggestions that have been proposed to deal with this (Wassmer and Brannath (2016), Kieser (2020)). Basically, they represent different degrees of incorporating planning assumptions.

- **Using the initially specified effect.** A very simple approach is to calculate the conditional power with the protocol planned treatment effect. This ignores any new information about the possible true treatment effect from the trial data and allows sample size changes only to make up for deviations from the protocol assumption seen in the first stage. A similar approach would be to use the minimal clinically relevant effect size. However, this may lead to overly high increases if the effect of the drug is actually much better than the minimal clinically relevant effect. Such a conditional power may be relatively large under the no-treatment effect situation or behave as uniformly distributed when the observed treatment effect is smaller than anticipated.
- **Using the interim effect estimate.** The most frequent approach is to use the interim estimate of the treatment effect in the calculation of conditional power, as was done

in the example at hand. However, this "double" use of the interim data (in plugging in the value of the effect estimate and conditioning on it for future data) can cause erratic behavior of the resulting conditional power and careful determination of the minimum and maximum sample size is required.

- **Using prior information and the interim effect estimate.** The effect size estimate to be plugged into the conditional power calculation can be chosen as the posterior mean after updating the prior distribution of the treatment effect using the data seen at the interim analysis. This allows for balancing prior belief and current information.
- **Using Bayesian Predictive Power.** Instead of using the conditional power, a further step in incorporating uncertainty is choosing the Bayesian predictive power defined as average of the conditional power with respect to the posterior distribution of the treatment effect after the interim analysis. One can expect the method of sample size reestimation using a required threshold on predictive power to be more robust; however, there are "perils" and potential misuse of predictive power (see Dallow and Fina (2011)). Specifically, the additional uncertainty taken into account with this approach can lead to much larger sample sizes than the conditional power approach and in some cases, even an increase in sample size does not correspond to an increase predictive power.

In this context, it is important to note that the adaptive design using the inverse normal combination test is not an automatic procedure in the sense that a predefined recalculation rule needs to be adhered to for ensuring the validity of the procedure. This means that it may be valuable to provide the IDMC with the outcomes of different recalculation procedures to allow them to issue an informed recommendation. In addition, it may also be of value to provide the conditional power under the planned sample size with the same options as described above for the choice of the treatment effect estimate. This gives the IDMC additional guidance as to whether a change in sample size should be recommended or if the preplanned sample size still provides reasonable power, thus ensuring that the patients are equally weighted in the final analysis. We emphasize again the need for thorough preparation together with the IDMC to make sure that recommendations are made according to the study team's intents.

Adaptive designs with sample size reassessment require careful planning to build the basis for a successful conduct of the trial. Apart from statistical considerations and properties, alignment with operational conduct is needed and can be complex. As mentioned above, simulations can be utilized to determine a suitable interim analysis timepoint. For this assessment, not only the projected time of data cut-off should be considered but also the time needed from this cut-off to when a change to the IWRS system can be made. If there is no alignment between these different pieces of the trial, then in the worst case a successful outcome of the trial may be put in jeopardy.

Acknowledgment

The authors would like to thank their colleagues Rosanne Lane, Rama Melkote, Yevgen Tymofyeyev, Bart Michiels, and Tobias Mielke for helpful comments and discussion.

References

Brannath W, Bauer P. (2004). Optimal conditional error functions for the control of conditional power. *Biometrics*. 60(3):715–723.

Cui L, Hung JH, Wang SJ. (1999). Modification of sample size in group sequential clinical trials. *Biometrics*. 55(3):853–857.

Dallow N, Fina P. (2011). The perils with the misuse of predictive power. *Pharm Stat*. 10(4):311–317.

Emerson SS, Levin GP, Emerson SC. (2011). Comments on "Adaptive increase in sample size when interim results are promising: a practical guide with examples". *Stat Med*. 30(28):3285–3301.

FDA (2019). *Adaptive Designs for Clinical Trials of Drugs and Biologics*. CDER/CBER. Rockville, MD.

Glimm E. (2012). Comments on "Adaptive increase in sample size when interim results are promising: a practical guide with examples". *Stat Med*. 31(1):98–99.

Hsiao ST, Liu L, Mehta CR. (2018). Optimal promising zone designs. *Biom Journal*. 61(5):1175–1186.

Jennison C, Turnbull B. (2015). Adaptive sample size modification in clinical trials: start small then ask for more? *Stat Med*. 34(29):3793–3810.

Kieser M. (2020). Methods and applications of sample size calculation and recalculation in clinical trials. *Springer Series in Pharmaceutical Statistics*. New York: Springer.

Lehmacher W, Wassmer G. (1999). Adaptive sample size calculations in group sequential trials. *Biometrics*. 55:1286–1290.

Mehta CR, Bhingare A, Liu L, Senchaudhuri P. (2022). Optimal adaptive promising zone designs. *Stat Med*. 41:1950–1970.

Mehta CR, Pocock SJ. (2011). Adaptive increase in sample size when interim results are promising: a practical guide with examples. *Stat Med*. 30(28):3267–3284.

Wang J. (2010). Many-to-one comparison after sample size reestimation for trials with multiple treatment arms and treatment selection. *J Biopharmaceutical Statistics*. 20:927–940.

Wassmer G, Brannath W. (2016). Group sequential and confirmatory adaptive designs in clinical trials. *Springer Series in Pharmaceutical Statistics*. New York: Springer.

6

Evaluation of a Method for Sample Size Reestimation for a Confirmatory Phase 3 Clinical Trial to Compare Two Test Treatments to Control

Elaine K. Kowalewski and Gary G. Koch

Introduction

Consider a confirmatory phase 3 clinical trial with two different regimens for a test treatment, such as a higher dose and a lower dose versus a placebo control. Suppose both doses of test treatment are expected to be effective, but there is uncertainty about the usefulness of the effect for one of the doses and the tolerability for the other, with the lower dose being the one that is possibly somewhat less effective and the higher dose being the one that might not be sufficiently tolerable. Both doses are being investigated to determine the benefit/risk and thus which dose is more appropriate for regulatory approval. An example of such a scenario is the suvorexant Phase 3 clinical trial to investigate the efficacy and safety of a higher and lower dose of suvorexant in the treatment of insomnia (Herring et al., 2016; Sun et al., 2018). Through safety analyses, it was determined that there is a potential for tolerability issues with the higher dose. Although the efficacy of the lower dose was not assessed with rigorous control of Type I error in the trials, FDA ultimately approved the lower dose. Another such example is the phase 3 pivotal study to investigate the efficacy and safety of a higher and lower dose of brexpiprazole in patients with major depression disorder (Ouyang et al., 2020).

The suvorexant development program was underpowered to assess the efficacy of the lower dose. Prior to conducting a clinical trial, the sample size is determined using statistical power calculations based on assumptions about the expected treatment difference and variability along with the desired Type I error level and power for the primary analysis (Mehta & Pocock, 2011). However, these assumptions are not always realistic due to estimates of treatment differences and corresponding variances being based on small previous trials, changes in medical practice over time, changes in patient populations, etc. (Gao et al., 2008). Trials can be unsuccessful due to insufficient sample size and therefore insufficient power, or the treatment differences may have been underestimated and resources have been committed that should not have been. Sample size reestimation in confirmatory phase 3 trials is a method to address these challenges by using unblinded interim results of the estimated treatment effect for the primary endpoint (Mehta & Pocock, 2011). However, a major challenge for sample size reestimation is controlling the overall Type I error rate at the final analysis, and methods have been proposed to address this challenge. Cui et al. (1999) proposed combining the test statistics from the two periods for before and after the

DOI: 10.1201/9781003288640-6

interim analysis using prespecified weights for the corresponding fractions of information. A possible issue with this approach is that it down-weights the contribution of patients after the interim analysis that led to an increase in sample size because the weights were prespecified without knowledge of the increase in sample size. This implies that not all patients are managed equally in the analysis. Chen et al. (2004) showed that if the sample size is increased only when interim results are promising, which they define to be when the conditional power based on the effect size at the interim analysis is greater than 50%, then the overall Type I error rate at the final analysis is not inflated and so a statistical adjustment is not necessary.

This chapter focuses on the promising zone method discussed by Mehta and Pocock (2011), which is implemented in the EAST software produced by Cytel. Mehta and Pocock's approach for sample size reestimation is to evaluate the conditional power for the effect size at the interim analysis and, based on this calculation, either maintain the sample size or increase the sample size by a prespecified amount. This conditional power at interim is the conditional probability of rejecting the null hypothesis at the final analysis given the observed results for the effect size at interim (Lan & Wittes, 1988). Mehta and Pocock (2011) propose maintaining the planned sample size if the conditional power is too low or too high and increasing the sample size up to a prespecified upper limit if the conditional power is in a *promising* zone. More specifically, the range of possible conditional power values is *a priori* partitioned into the *favorable*, *promising*, and *unfavorable* zones. Let $(1-\beta)$ denote the prespecified level of power for the study, let CP denote the observed conditional power for the study at interim (as expressed by (3) in Appendix Section 6.5.1), and let CP_2 denote the prespecified minimum conditional power value for the interim analysis results to be deemed favorable. Therefore, $CP_2 \leq CP \leq 1$ defines the *favorable* zone. If CP_2 is similar to $(1-\beta)$, the desired level of power at the interim analysis nearly applies for rejection of the null hypothesis at final analysis. Let CP_1 denote the prespecified minimum conditional power value for the interim analysis results to be deemed promising. Therefore, $CP_1 \leq CP \leq CP_2$ defines the *promising* zone, which implies that $0 \leq CP \leq CP_1$ defines the *unfavorable* zone. Sometimes this methodology also involves a futility zone, which is defined as $0 \leq CP \leq CP_0$, where $CP_0 \ll CP_1$ denotes the prespecified maximum conditional power value for the interim analysis to indicate futility. As indicated previously, Mehta and Pocock (2011) propose maintaining the originally planned sample size if the observed conditional power falls into either the *unfavorable* or *favorable* zones, since the interim results are either too disappointing or sufficiently favorable, respectively, and therefore do not imply a need to increase the sample size. On the other hand, when the observed conditional power falls into the *promising* zone, the interim results are not clearly disappointing but may also not be favorable enough to support the power desired at the final analysis, so the sample size is increased to attempt to recover the originally planned power.

The promising zone methods provided by Mehta and Pocock (2011) are for a clinical trial to compare a test treatment to a control treatment. This chapter applies the promising zone methodology to a confirmatory phase 3 clinical trial, with two potentially effective doses compared to a control treatment and where response to the treatment is evaluated by up to two endpoints. In this regard, the rationale of this methodology is avoidance of "borderline" results for a trial that could provide a confirmatory result for either the higher and/or lower dose with an appropriately larger sample size. Alternatively, for phase 2/3 trials for which dose finding is a major objective, there are many references that deal with sample size reestimation, including Bischoff and Miller (2009), Wang (2010), and Liu et al. (2021), but these references address a different topic than this chapter. The scope of the discussion in the chapter includes clinical trials with a single primary endpoint, clinical trials with two coprimary endpoints, clinical trials with two dual primary endpoints, and clinical trials with one primary endpoint and one key secondary endpoint. For all these paradigms, methods for multiple comparisons are presented for the control of Type I error.

6.1 Introduction to Suvorexant Development Program

Suvorexant is an orexin receptor antagonist developed for the treatment of insomnia (Herring et al., 2016). The suvorexant development program included two phase 3 clinical trials to evaluate the efficacy and safety of suvorexant (Sun et al., 2018). Both trials were randomized, double-blind, placebo-controlled, parallel-group, 3-month trials in nonelderly (18–64 years) and elderly (≥ 65 years) patients with insomnia. Two doses of suvorexant were evaluated, including 40/30 mg (nonelderly/elderly) and 20/15 mg (nonelderly/elderly), although the primary focus was for 40/30 mg. Each trial had a 2-week, single-blind placebo run-in period and a 3-month three-arm treatment phase. Patients were assessed for subjective sleep measures using an electronic sleep diary questionnaire (e-diary). Many patients (approximately 75%) also had objective sleep evaluation overnight by polysomnography (PSG) over 8 hours. In trial 1, patients were randomized in the treatment phase in a 3:2:3 ratio to suvorexant 40/30 mg, suvorexant 20/15 mg, or placebo. In trial 2, the randomization ratio was 1:1:1 for the Q-cohort, which included patients who received only the subjective assessment, and the randomization ratio was 2:1:2 for the PQ-cohort which included patients who had assessments for both the subjective and objective sleep measures (Herring et al., 2016).

Efficacy was assessed for the subjective and objective measures of sleep maintenance and sleep onset. The primary efficacy endpoints were change from baseline at months 1 and 3 for the subjective (e-diary) and the objective (PSG) measures of sleep maintenance and sleep onset for suvorexant 40/30 mg. Tests for these measures at 1 month preceded those for month 3 in the specified multiplicity method (Sun et al., 2018)). For sleep maintenance, subjective total sleep time in minutes (sTST) was the subjective measure and wakefulness after persistent sleep (WASO) was the objective measure. The subjective and objective measures for sleep onset were subjective time to sleep onset in minutes (sTSO) and latency to onset of persistent sleep (LPS), respectively. Secondary efficacy endpoints for suvorexant 40/30 mg were the subjective endpoints at week 1 and the objective endpoints at night 1. Also, all of these endpoints were assessed for the 20/15 mg dose as secondary (trial 1) or exploratory (trial 2) endpoints (Herring et al., 2016).

After their review, the FDA approved suvorexant in August 2014 at the lower doses of 5 mg, 10 mg, 15 mg, and 20 mg, although the efficacy of the 20/15 mg dose with respect to sleep onset and maintenance was not formally assessed in either of the two phase 3 studies with strong control of Type I error and/or adequately planned power (Sun et al., 2018). In this regard, endpoints for the 40/30 mg dose were primary, whereas those for the 20/15 mg dose were secondary or exploratory. Also, the 20/15 mg dose had less sample size than the 40/30 mg dose (254 versus 383 in trial 1 and 239 versus 387 in trial 2) (Herring et al., 2016). As noted by Herring et al. (2016), each trial was expected to have 91% power to declare all primary sleep maintenance endpoints significant for suvorexant 40/30 mg versus placebo and 62% power to declare all primary sleep onset endpoints significant for suvorexant 40/30 mg versus placebo. The trials had lower power for suvorexant 20/15 mg versus placebo due to smaller sample size.

For a future study like those for the suvorexant development program, information for its planning could be based on the effect sizes and covariance structure of the endpoints observed in the suvorexant trial 1 and trial 2. Accordingly, we show here how the methodology developed in this chapter can be used to improve the power for the formal assessment of the endpoints for both doses. For the illustration of the methods in this chapter for a future study like those for the suvorexant development program, we will only consider the measures of sleep maintenance as sTST and WASO, and we will refer to the 40/30 mg dose and the 20/15 mg dose as the high dose and the low dose, respectively. Appendix Section 6.5.3 provides details for how the treatment effects are estimated from the published results of the suvorexant development program. These treatment effect estimates are used in the simulations in Section 6.3 to compare the expected Type I error, mean sample size, and power for fixed sample size trials to trials with potential increase in sample size by promising zone methodology.

6.2 Methods

Let $h = 1, 2$ index the two periods in the trial that correspond to before and after the interim analysis to evaluate whether to increase the sample size. Let $i = 1, 2$ index the two endpoints, where $i = 1$ for sTST and $i = 2$ for WASO; and let $j = 0, 1, 2$ index the three treatment groups, where $j = 0$ corresponds to the placebo group, $j = 1$ corresponds to the lower dose, and $j = 2$ corresponds to the higher dose. Let r be the information fraction for the interim analysis, and it expresses the extent of study completion as a proportion of the initially planned sample size. Let N be the initially planned total sample size for the trial, and let $n_{ij} = s_i t_j N$ be the initially planned total sample size for the i-th endpoint and j-th treatment group, where t_j is the proportion of the sample size for the j-th treatment group and s_i is the proportion of the sample size for the i-th endpoint. Usually, $s_i = 1.0$, although for the suvorexant trials, only about 75% of patients were assessed for the WASO endpoint and so for WASO as the second endpoint $s_2 = 0.75$ and for sTST as the first endpoint, $s_1 = 1.0$. Let N_+ be the total potential sample size increase.

Let $\mu = \left(\mu_1', \mu_2' \right)' = \left(\mu_{10}, \mu_{11}, \mu_{12}, \mu_{20}, \mu_{21}, \mu_{22} \right)'$ be the true population means for each dose for each endpoint (e.g., μ_{10} for placebo for sTST, μ_{11} for the lower dose for sTST, and μ_{12} for the higher dose for sTST, and μ_2 is similar for WASO). Let Y_{hijk} denote the response of patient k in treatment group j for endpoint i during period h of the trial, where $k = 1, 2, \ldots, n_{hij}$ and n_{hij} is the initially planned number of patients in treatment group j in period h of the trial for endpoint i. With an information fraction of r, $n_{1ij} = r n_{ij}$, and with no increase in sample size after the interim analysis, $n_{2ij} = (1 - r) n_{ij}$ so that $n_{1ij} + n_{2ij} = n_{ij}$. For each treatment group, the patients are assumed to represent a corresponding population in a manner comparable to independent simple random samples for the two periods. The sample sizes for each treatment group for each endpoint during each period are assumed to be sufficiently large that sample means for a response variable of interest independently have approximately normal distributions with essentially known variances through consistent estimators.

The conditional power at interim CP_{Iij} for the i-th endpoint and j-th treatment comparison ($j = 1$ corresponds to the difference between the lower dose and placebo and $j = 2$ corresponds to the difference between the higher dose and placebo) is produced given the observed responses. For additional details, see Appendix Section 6.5.1 and expression (3). For trials with a single endpoint (i.e., $i = 1$ only), let $u_1 = I \left(CP_1 \leq CP_{I11} \leq CP_2 \right)$, $u_2 = I \left(CP_1 \leq CP_{I12} \leq CP_2 \right)$, and $u_0 = \max(u_1, u_2)$, where $I(\cdot)$ is the indicator function (which equals 1 when $(\cdot)$ applies and equals 0 otherwise). Then, u_0, u_1, u_2 determine whether there is a sample size increase in the second period of the trial in the manner described subsequently. For trials with more than one endpoint, there are various rules that can be applied to determine sample size increase at the interim analysis, and they depend on whether the two endpoints are coprimary, dual primary, or primary and key secondary. In any event, the determination to increase sample size is based on the treatment groups and so there cannot be a sample size increase for one endpoint and no sample size increase for another endpoint. Thus, u_0, u_1, u_2 can be interpreted as the final indicator variables for sample size increase after the two endpoints are considered. These rules are described in Section 6.3. For single endpoint trials, if $u_0 = 1$, then there is a sample size increase for the second period of the trial. With N_+ as the total potential sample size increase, the sample size for the second period of the trial for each treatment group, n_{2ij+} is given in (1).

$$n_{2ij+} = (1-r)n_{ij} + u_j s_i t_j N_+ = n_{2ij} + u_j s_i t_j N_+ \tag{1}$$

Therefore, the overall sample size for each treatment group, $n_{\ast ij+}$, is given in (2).

$$n_{\ast ij+} = n_{1ij} + n_{2ij+} = rn_{ij} + (1-r)n_{ij} + u_j s_i t_j N_+ = n_{ij} + u_j s_i t_j N_+ \tag{2}$$

The second period of the trial is then conducted, with an increase in sample size in certain scenarios. For combining the observed treatment differences from both periods (i.e., before interim and after interim), two different methods of weighting are considered.

Method 1: Information fraction weighting (Cui et al., 1999):

$$w_1 = w_2 = r$$

Method 2:

1. If $u_1 = 0, u_2 = 1$, meaning increase the sample size for the higher dose but not for the lower dose:

$$w_1 = r$$

$$w_2 = \frac{rN}{N + N_+}$$

2. If $u_1 = 1, u_2 = 0$, meaning increase the sample size for the lower dose but not for the higher dose:

$$w_1 = \frac{rN}{N + N_+}$$

$$w_2 = r$$

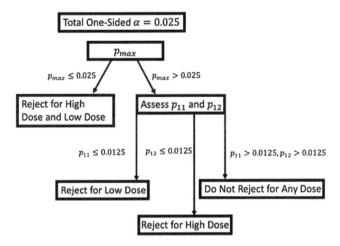

FIGURE 6.1
Hochberg's method with one-sided $\alpha = 0.025$ for a single endpoint with two doses.

3. If $u_1 = u_2 = 1$, meaning increase the sample size for both doses:

$$w_1 = \frac{rN}{N + N_+}$$

$$w_2 = \frac{rN}{N + N_+}$$

4. If $u_1 = u_2 = 0$, meaning do not increase the sample for either dose:

$$w_1 = w_2 = r$$

Given the treatment differences observed in each period, and the chosen weighting method, the test statistics and p-values are produced for each endpoint for each dose. See Appendix Section 6.5.1 for additional technical details. The p-values for the trial with a single endpoint and two doses, p_{11}, p_{12} with $p_{max} = \max(p_{11}, p_{12})$, are evaluated with strong control of Type I error at one-sided $\alpha = 0.025$ using Hochberg's (1988) method as shown in Figure 6.1. Multiplicity methods for trials with two endpoints will be discussed in Section 6.3.

6.3 Application of Methods to Suvorexant Trial Design – Simulations

6.3.1 Simulation Specifications

Simulations are used to assess power and Type I error under various specifications, as well as to evaluate mean sample sizes considering potential sample size increase. Table 6.1 includes the si mulation specifications for $t, N, r, N_+, \tilde{\Delta}_{12} = (\mu_{12} - \mu_{10}) / \sigma_1, \tilde{\Delta}_{22} = (\mu_{22} - \mu_{20}) / \sigma_2$, and

TABLE 6.1

Simulation specifications.

Parameter		Values
Randomization Ratios	t	$\left(\dfrac{1}{3},\dfrac{1}{3},\dfrac{1}{3}\right)'$
Total Sample Size	N	600
Information Fraction	r	0.5
Total Sample Size Increase	N_+	$0.5N$
Standardized Treatment Effect for High Dose on sTST	$\tilde{\Delta}_{12} = (\mu_{12} - \mu_{10})/\sigma_1$	$\dfrac{1}{3},\dfrac{2}{5}$
Treatment Effect for High Dose on WASO	$\tilde{\Delta}_{22} = (\mu_{22} - \mu_{20})/\sigma_2$	$\dfrac{1}{2}$
Proportion of High Dose Treatment Effect for Low Dose	$\delta = \dfrac{\mu_{11} - \mu_{10}}{\mu_{12} - \mu_{10}} = \dfrac{\mu_{21} - \mu_{20}}{\mu_{22} - \mu_{20}}$	0.7, 0.85

δ for the ratio of lower dose treatment effect versus higher dose treatment effect for both endpoints. For all simulations, we use one-sided $\alpha = 0.025$ as the overall Type I error. In addition to evaluating rules for increasing sample size for the period after the interim analysis (i.e., period 2) based on the results in period 1, the scope of the simulations includes the usual fixed trial with no sample size increase in period 2, regardless of interim results.

The subsequent sections describe four different types of trials as follows: a trial with a single primary endpoint, a trial with two coprimary endpoints, a trial with dual primary endpoints, and a trial with a primary endpoint and key secondary endpoint. For each type of trial, each endpoint has two treatment effects of interest, one for the higher dose of treatment and another for the lower dose of treatment. In the subsequent sections, we describe the rules for increasing sample size based on a promising zone specification of 0.30 to 0.80 for conditional power, and the methods for managing multiplicity based on the type of trial. Technical details for the simulations are in Appendix Section 6.5.2.

6.3.2 Single Primary Endpoint

First, we consider the trial for a single primary endpoint (i.e., sTST) for two doses.

Let $u_j = I\left(0.30 \leq CP_{I1j} \leq 0.80\right)$ for the sTST endpoint; and $u_0 = \max(u_1, u_2)$. Then, the sample size for period 2 of the trial for each treatment group for the sTST endpoint $(i = 1)$ based on the sample size increase due to the observed conditional power at interim with one-sided Type I error $\alpha = 0.0125$ is computed using (1). Let $p_{max} = \max(p_{11}, p_{12})$. The resulting p-values are evaluated using Hochberg's (1988) method as described in Figure 6.1.

6.3.3 Coprimary Endpoints

We next consider the trial with coprimary endpoints (i.e., sTST and WASO), each with two doses. For coprimary endpoints, the null hypotheses for both endpoints for a given dose need to be rejected to declare overall success for a dose. We evaluated two rules for how to increase sample size for coprimary endpoints:

TABLE 6.2

Criteria for increasing the sample size for a given dose based on conditional powers for sTST and WASO falling above, within, or below the promising zone.

sTST	WASO	Coprimary Rule 1	Coprimary Rule 2	Dual Primary	sTST Primary WASO Key Secondary
Above	Above	No	Possibly[1]	No	No
Above	Within	Yes	Probably[1]	No	Yes
Above	Below	No	No	No	No
Within	Above	Yes	Probably[1]	No	Yes
Within	Within	Yes	Possibly[1]	Yes	Yes
Within	Below	No	No	Yes	Yes
Below	Above	No	No	No	No
Below	Within	No	No	Yes	No
Below	Below	No	No	No	No

[1] Possibly and probably depend on the product of the conditional powers being in the promising zone.

Rule 1: The separate conditional power values for the two endpoints with one-sided Type I error $\alpha = 0.0125$ for the two doses provide the criteria for the promising zone. Let $q_{ij} = I\left(0.30 \le CP_{Iij} \le 0.80\right)$ and $r_{ij} = I(CP_{Iij} > 0.80)$. If $q_{1j} = 1$ and $q_{2j} = 1$, then there is sample size increase for the j-th dose (and placebo). Moreover, if $r_{1j} = 1$ and $q_{2j} = 1$, or if $r_{2j} = 1$ and $q_{1j} = 1$, then there is sample size increase for the j-th dose (and placebo). Let $u_j = \left(q_{1j} \cap q_{2j}\right) \cup \left(r_{1j} \cap q_{2j}\right) \cup \left(r_{2j} \cap q_{1j}\right)$ (where $\cup$ is the union operator and $\cap$ is the intersection operator), and let $u_0 = \max\left(u_1, u_2\right)$.

Rule 2: The product of the conditional power values for the two coprimary endpoints provides the criterion for the promising zone. Let $u_j = I\left(0.30 \le CP_{I1j}CP_{I2j} \le 0.80\right)$ and $u_0 = \max\left(u_1, u_2\right)$.

Then, the sample size for the second period of the trial for each treatment group and for each endpoint, as based on the sample size increase due to observed conditional power at interim, is computed using (1), where u_j is determined by Rules 1 and 2. A summary of the rules is provided in the columns labeled "Coprimary Rule 1" and "Coprimary Rule 2" in Table 6.2.

We use Hochberg's method (1988) to manage multiplicity for the coprimary endpoints as shown in Figure 6.2.

6.3.4 Dual Primary Endpoints

In this section, we consider the trial with dual primary endpoints for the comparisons of two doses to placebo. For dual primary endpoints, both endpoints are managed as "primary" for a dose, usually with equal alpha splitting for management of multiplicity. In this regard, unlike for coprimary endpoints as described in the previous section, there is success for the trial if either endpoint has success for either dose. For example, WASO could have success for the higher dose even if sTST did not have success for the higher dose. The main objective is to have at least one primary endpoint with success for at least one dose, and this objective is made more obvious in the rule for increasing sample size as described subsequently.

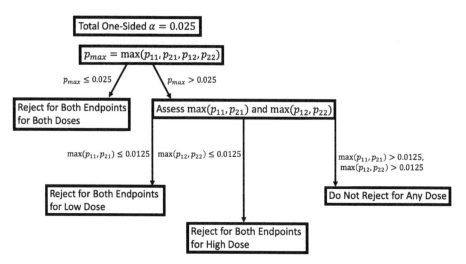

FIGURE 6.2

Hochberg's method with one-sided $\alpha = 0.025$ for coprimary endpoints with two doses.

For this type of trial, we compute CP_{lij} using (3) with one-sided $\alpha = 0.00625$, and in order to determine whether to increase sample size for the second period, we evaluate the following rule:

> **Rule:** Let $q_{ij} = I\left(0.30 \leq CP_{lij} \leq 0.80\right)$ and $r_{ij} = I\left(CP_{lij} < 0.30\right)$. If $q_{1j} = 1$ and $q_{2j} = 1$, then there is sample size increase for the jth dose (and placebo). Also, if $q_{1j} = 1$ and $r_{2j} = 1$, or if $q_{2j} = 1$ and $r_{1j} = 1$, then there is sample size increase for the jth dose (and placebo). In other words, let $u_j = \left(q_{1j} \cap q_{2j}\right) \cup \left(q_{1j} \cap r_{2j}\right) \cup \left(r_{1j} \cap q_{2j}\right)$ and $u_0 = \max\left(u_1, u_2\right)$.

Therefore, the sample size for the second period of the trial for each treatment group and for each endpoint based on the sample size increase due to observed conditional power at interim is given in (1), where u_j is determined by the previously stated Rule. A summary of this rule is provided in the column labeled "Dual Primary" in Table 6.2. For this type of trial, we manage multiplicity with the PA multiplicity strategy in Sun et al. (2018), also known as a parallel gatekeeper. In this regard, for each dose, the two endpoints are evaluated with the Hochberg procedure at one-sided $\alpha = 0.0125$. If both p-values for a given dose are < 0.0125 (one-sided), then one-sided $\alpha = 0.0125$ is recycled to the other dose. If one endpoint for a dose has one-sided $p < 0.00625$ while the other has one-sided $p > 0.0125$, then success can be declared for the dose for this endpoint with one-sided $p < 0.00625$, but one-sided $\alpha = 0.0125$ cannot be recycled to the other dose. The method is shown graphically in Figure 6.3.

6.3.5 Primary Endpoint and Key Secondary Endpoint

In this section, we consider the trial with a primary endpoint (i.e., sTST) and a key secondary endpoint (i.e., WASO), and with two doses. The main objective for such a trial is to have success for the primary endpoint, which is sTST, for at least one dose. The null hypotheses for the primary endpoint are evaluated first and success for at least one of them is a prerequisite for subsequent evaluation of the key secondary endpoint. Also, a

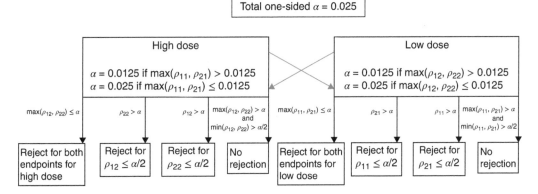

FIGURE 6.3
Parallel gatekeeper method with one-sided $\alpha = 0.025$ for dual primary endpoints with two doses.

secondary objective is success for the secondary endpoint for a dose with success for the primary endpoint. To determine when to increase sample size for the second period, we analyzed the following rule:

Rule: Let $q_{ij} = I\left(0.30 \leq CP_{Iij} \leq 0.80\right)$ and $r_{ij} = I\left(CP_{Iij} > 0.80\right)$. Let $u_j = q_{1j} \cup \left(r_{1j} \cap q_{2j}\right)$, and let $u_0 = \max\left(u_1, u_2\right)$. In other words, if the conditional power with one-sided Type I error $\alpha = 0.0125$ for the j-th dose falls into the promising zone for sTST, then there is sample size increase for the j-th dose (and placebo). Additionally, if the conditional power for the j-th dose falls into the promising zone for WASO and is above the promising zone for sTST, then there is also sample size increase for the j-th dose.

Therefore, the sample size for the second period of the trial for each endpoint for each treatment group, as based on the sample size increase due to observed conditional power at interim, is given in (1), where u_j is determined by the previously stated Rule. Table 6.2 includes the criteria for the decisions for increasing the sample size for the two endpoints for a given dose in the column labeled "sTST Primary WASO Key Secondary." In this regard, if either dose has sample size increase, then the placebo group has sample size increase.

   For the trial with the endpoints managed with sTST as the primary endpoint and WASO as the key secondary endpoint, we manage multiplicity with a version of the PA multiplicity strategy in Sun et al. (2018), also known as a parallel gatekeeper. In this regard, for each dose, the primary endpoint, sTST, is assessed at one-sided $\alpha = 0.0125$. If its one-sided p-value is < 0.0125, then the key secondary endpoint, WASO, for this dose is assessed at one-sided $\alpha = 0.0125$. If its one-sided p-value is< 0.0125, then the one-sided 0.0125 is recycled to the other dose. The method is shown graphically in Figure 6.4.

6.3.6 Simulation Results – Type I Error

6.3.6.1 Single Endpoint

The three methods for the trial with the single endpoint include the two weighting methods described in Section 6.2. We compare to a fixed trial where there is no increase in sample

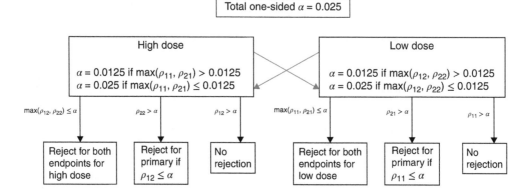

FIGURE 6.4

Parallel gatekeeper method with one-sided $\alpha = 0.025$ for primary endpoint and key secondary endpoint with two doses.

TABLE 6.3

Type I error for Single Endpoint Trial.

	Δ_{11}	Δ_{12}	Method 1	Method 2	Fixed Trial	Mean SS
P (Reject Any True Null Hypothesis)	0.000	0.000	0.0230	0.0227	0.0215	626.41
	0.000	0.333	0.0247	0.0222	0.0249	657.91
	0.000	0.400	0.0257	0.0230	0.0251	643.32

size regardless of interim results. For the fixed trial, information fraction weighting is used to weight results before and after interim. Table 6.3 provides the Type I error rates and mean sample sizes (SSs) for the single endpoint trial. For all null scenarios considered, both methods and the fixed trial have Type I error control to a reasonable extent with respect to the number of replications in the simulations. For an actual Type I error level of 0.025, we would expect that the observed one-sided Type I error level would fall within

$0.025 \pm 2 \times \sqrt{\dfrac{0.025 \times 0.975}{10000}} = (0.022, 0.028)$ due to sampling error based on the 10,000 replications of the simulations.

6.3.6.2 Coprimary Endpoints

The five methods for the coprimary endpoint paradigm include the fixed trial, as well as the four methods that correspond to the combinations of the two weighting methods with the two rules for increasing sample size based on interim results. Table 6.4 provides the Type I error rates and mean SS for both rules for the coprimary endpoints trial. The results in this table indicate that all methods have Type I error control for the null scenarios considered.

6.3.6.3 Dual Primary Endpoints

The three methods for the trial with dual primary endpoints include the two weighting methods described in Section 6.2 and the fixed trial. Table 6.5 provides the Type I error

TABLE 6.4

Type I error for Coprimary Endpoints Trial.

	Δ_{11}	Δ_{12}	Δ_{21}	Δ_{22}	Method 1 Rule 1	Method 1 Rule 2	Method 2 Rule 1	Method 2 Rule 2	Fixed Trial	Rule 1 Mean SS	Rule 2 Mean SS
P (Reject Any True Null Hypothesis for Both Endpoints)	0.000	0.000	0.000	0.000	0.0004	0.0002	0.0002	0.0001	0.0002	603.26	601.88
	0.000	0.000	0.000	0.500	0.0122	0.0125	0.0114	0.0115	0.0119	614.72	613.52
	0.000	0.000	0.350	0.500	0.0234	0.0239	0.0223	0.0223	0.0217	624.59	622.08
	0.000	0.000	0.425	0.500	0.0242	0.0250	0.0228	0.0234	0.0230	625.91	624.04
	0.000	0.333	0.000	0.000	0.0117	0.0119	0.0105	0.0105	0.0115	615.01	612.65
	0.000	0.400	0.000	0.000	0.0125	0.0127	0.0111	0.0113	0.0126	615.94	614.32
	0.000	0.400	0.000	0.500	0.0011	0.0011	0.0009	0.0009	0.0009	644.83	644.91
	0.233	0.333	0.000	0.000	0.0201	0.0206	0.0174	0.0175	0.0185	623.11	619.40
	0.280	0.400	0.000	0.000	0.0224	0.0232	0.0203	0.0205	0.0214	624.95	622.38
	0.283	0.333	0.000	0.000	0.0217	0.0223	0.0196	0.0196	0.0205	624.13	620.85
	0.340	0.400	0.000	0.000	0.0243	0.0247	0.0221	0.0223	0.0235	626.40	624.04

TABLE 6.5

Type I error for Dual Primary Endpoints Trial.

	Δ_{11}	Δ_{12}	Δ_{21}	Δ_{22}	Method 1	Method 2	Fixed Trial	Mean SS
P (Reject Any True	0.000	0.000	0.000	0.000	0.0238	0.0227	0.0236	637.68
Null Hypothesis)	0.000	0.000	0.000	0.500	0.0243	0.0244	0.0243	646.18
	0.000	0.000	0.350	0.500	0.0238	0.0250	0.0229	675.51
	0.000	0.000	0.425	0.500	0.0240	0.0245	0.0234	664.49
	0.000	0.333	0.000	0.000	0.0235	0.0239	0.0235	666.56
	0.000	0.400	0.000	0.000	0.0247	0.0247	0.0239	652.15
	0.000	0.400	0.000	0.500	0.0271	0.0254	0.0256	628.84
	0.233	0.333	0.000	0.000	0.0211	0.0232	0.0217	697.20
	0.280	0.400	0.000	0.000	0.0223	0.0239	0.0235	684.63
	0.283	0.333	0.000	0.000	0.0218	0.0236	0.0231	696.50
	0.340	0.400	0.000	0.000	0.0237	0.0242	0.0241	676.08

TABLE 6.6

Type I error for Primary Endpoint and Key Secondary Endpoint Trial.

	Δ_{11}	Δ_{12}	Δ_{21}	Δ_{22}	Method 1	Method 2	Fixed Trial	Mean SS
P (Reject Any True	0.000	0.000	0.000	0.000	0.0243	0.0245	0.0241	626.82
Null Hypothesis)	0.000	0.000	0.000	0.500	0.0239	0.0240	0.0241	627.08
	0.000	0.000	0.350	0.500	0.0244	0.0238	0.0241	627.63
	0.000	0.000	0.425	0.500	0.0234	0.0232	0.0241	627.52
	0.000	0.333	0.000	0.000	0.0279	0.0268	0.0271	664.70
	0.000	0.400	0.000	0.000	0.0294	0.0285	0.0285	652.45
	0.000	0.400	0.000	0.500	0.0268	0.0242	0.0251	657.64
	0.233	0.333	0.000	0.000	0.0229	0.0221	0.0211	702.96
	0.280	0.400	0.000	0.000	0.0256	0.0249	0.0242	691.07
	0.283	0.333	0.000	0.000	0.0246	0.0235	0.0228	701.45
	0.340	0.400	0.000	0.000	0.0274	0.0261	0.0259	682.71

rates and mean SS for the dual primary endpoints trial. The results in this table indicate that all methods have Type I error control for the null scenarios considered.

6.3.6.4 *Primary Endpoint and Key Secondary Endpoint*

The three methods for the trial with a primary endpoint and a key secondary endpoint include the two weighting methods described in Section 6.2 and the fixed trial. Table 6.6 provides the Type I error rates and mean SS for the primary endpoint and key secondary endpoint trial. The results in this table indicate that all methods have Type I error control to a reasonable extent for the null scenarios considered, except for the scenario where the high dose for the sTST (primary) endpoint was the only nonnull endpoint. For this scenario, all of the methods show slight Type I error inflation.

6.3.7 Simulation Results – Power

The following subsections will provide results for the simulations about powers to address nonnull alternatives for hypotheses.

TABLE 6.7

Power for Single Endpoint Trial.

	Δ_{11}	Δ_{12}	Method 1	Method 2	Fixed Trial	Mean SS
P (Reject Both Null Hypotheses)	0.233	0.333	0.6830	0.6762	0.6222	691.15
	0.280	0.400	0.8382	0.8342	0.7961	675.78
	0.283	0.333	0.8226	0.8178	0.7700	687.79
	0.340	0.400	0.9377	0.9364	0.9107	665.72
P (Reject Null Hypothesis for High Dose)	0.000	0.333	0.8956	0.8953	0.8590	657.91
	0.000	0.400	0.9716	0.9715	0.9592	643.32
	0.233	0.333	0.9179	0.9175	0.8813	691.15
	0.280	0.400	0.9809	0.9808	0.9690	675.78
	0.283	0.333	0.9287	0.9281	0.8937	687.79
	0.340	0.400	0.9851	0.9848	0.9739	665.72

6.3.7.1 Single Endpoint

For the trial with the single endpoint of sTST with two doses, the simulation results (Table 6.7) demonstrate that the power to reject the null hypothesis for both doses when both doses are nonnull is slightly higher for Method 1 than for Method 2 and for the fixed trial. Moreover, Method 1 and Method 2 have similar power to reject the null hypothesis for at least one dose when at least one dose is nonnull, and they provided higher power than the fixed trial.

6.3.7.2 Coprimary Endpoints

For the trial with coprimary endpoints, the probability of rejecting both endpoints for at least one dose and the probability of rejecting both endpoints for both doses are of interest. Part A of Table 6.8 provides the probability of rejecting both endpoints for at least one dose for scenarios in which both endpoints for at least one dose are nonnull. Part B of Table 6.8 provides the probability of rejecting both endpoints for both doses for scenarios in which both endpoints for both doses are nonnull. In both parts of Table 6.8, the powers are similarly higher for Methods 1 and 2 than for the fixed trial. Powers are slightly higher for Rule 1 compared to Rule 2 for each of them to a similar extent. For given Δ_{12} and Δ_{22} values, as δ increases for relatively larger treatment effects of the lower dose, all of the powers increase.

6.3.7.3 Dual Primary Endpoints

For trials with dual primary endpoints, the probability of rejecting the same endpoint for both doses, the probability of rejecting both endpoints for at least one dose, and the probability of rejecting both endpoints for both doses are of interest. Part A of Table 6.9 provides the probability of rejecting the same endpoint for both doses for scenarios in which both doses for at least one endpoint are nonnull. Part B of Table 6.9 provides the probability of rejecting both endpoints for at least one dose for scenarios in which both endpoints for at least one dose are nonnull. Part C of Table 6.9 provides the probability of rejecting both endpoints for both doses for scenarios in which both endpoints for both doses are nonnull. In all three parts of this table, the powers are similarly higher for Methods 1 and 2 than for the fixed trial. In Parts B and C of the table for given Δ_{12} and Δ_{22} values, as δ increases for relatively larger treatment effects of the lower dose, all of the powers increase.

6.3.7.4 Primary and Key Secondary Endpoints

For trials with primary and key secondary endpoints, the powers of interest are as follows:

i.   The probability of rejecting the primary endpoint for at least one dose (Part A of Table 6.10).
ii. The probability of rejecting the primary endpoint for both doses (Part B of Table 6.10).
iii. The probability of rejecting the primary and key secondary endpoint for at least one dose (Part C of Table 6.10).
iv. The probability of rejecting the primary and key secondary endpoint for both doses is of interest (Part D of Table 6.10).

In all four parts of this table, the powers are similarly higher for Methods 1 and 2 than for the fixed trial. For given Δ_{12} and Δ_{22} values as δ increases for relatively larger treatment effects of the lower dose, all of the powers increase as well.

6.4 Discussion and Conclusions

This chapter applies the *promising zone* methodology discussed by Mehta and Pocock (2011) to a confirmatory phase 3 clinical trial with up to two endpoints for two different regimens for a test treatment, such as a higher dose and a lower dose, compared to a control treatment. The objective is adequate power for the trial to assess the possibly somewhat smaller efficacy of the lower dose and control the overall Type I error rate at the final analysis. The methodology in this chapter can apply to two different regimens for a test treatment, such as two different schedules for administration of the same total dose. For convenience of explanation, the discussion is for the two regimens corresponding to a higher dose and a lower dose of test treatment, with the higher dose being more efficacious than the lower dose. Nevertheless, the methodology does not make any assumptions about which treatment regimen is more efficacious and thereby also applies to scenarios in which the higher dose might actually be less effective than the lower dose.

At the interim analysis, the conditional power (as the conditional probability of rejecting the null hypothesis at the final analysis given the results observed at interim) is computed for both the higher and lower doses (Lan & Wittes, 1988; Mehta & Pocock, 2011; Wiener et al., 2020). The conditional power values for both doses are evaluated for being in the *favorable, promising,* or *unfavorable zone.* For a single endpoint trial, if at least one conditional power value is in the prespecified *promising zone,* then this treatment group and the placebo group have the sample size increased by a prespecified amount. If both conditional power values are in the prespecified *promising zone,* then all treatment groups have the sample size increased subsequent to the interim analysis. For trials with two endpoints, various rules for increasing sample size for treatment groups were considered, depending on the relationship between the endpoints (i.e., coprimary, dual primary, and primary and key secondary). For coprimary endpoint trials, two different rules for using the conditional

TABLE 6.8

Power results for Coprimary Endpoints paradigm.

	Δ_{11}	Δ_{12}	Δ_{21}	Δ_{22}	δ	Method 1 and Rule: 1	Method 1 and Rule: 2	Method 2 and Rule: 1	Method 2 and Rule: 2	Fixed Trial	Rule 1 Mean SS	Rule 2 Mean SS
Part A:												
P (Reject Both Endpoints for At Least One Dose)	0.000	0.400	0.000	0.500	0.00	0.9604	0.9600	0.9605	0.9600	0.9426	644.83	644.91
	0.233	0.333	0.350	0.500	0.70	0.9171	0.9145	0.9171	0.9140	0.8793	704.64	700.66
	0.280	0.400	0.350	0.500	0.70	0.9762	0.9753	0.9759	0.9750	0.9595	699.45	696.69
	0.283	0.333	0.425	0.500	0.85	0.9420	0.9401	0.9415	0.9394	0.9150	707.26	705.73
	0.340	0.400	0.425	0.500	0.85	0.9868	0.9863	0.9868	0.9861	0.9762	696.04	696.55
Part B:												
P (Reject Both Endpoints for Both Doses)	0.233	0.333	0.350	0.500	0.70	0.6129	0.6054	0.6024	0.5952	0.5285	704.64	700.66
	0.280	0.400	0.350	0.500	0.70	0.7464	0.7400	0.7400	0.7334	0.6745	699.45	696.69
	0.283	0.333	0.425	0.500	0.85	0.7964	0.7943	0.7918	0.7899	0.7317	707.26	705.73
	0.340	0.400	0.425	0.500	0.85	0.9061	0.9044	0.9045	0.9027	0.8660	696.04	696.55

TABLE 6.9

Power results for Dual Primary Endpoints paradigm.

	Δ_{11}	Δ_{12}	Δ_{21}	Δ_{22}	δ	Method 1	Method 2	Fixed Trial	Mean SS
Part A									
P (Reject Same Endpoint for Both Doses)	0.000	0.000	0.350	0.500	0.70	0.7672	0.7700	0.7007	675.51
	0.233	0.333	0.000	0.000	0.70	0.4746	0.4781	0.4021	697.20
	0.233	0.333	0.350	0.500	0.70	0.9259	0.9287	0.8893	661.21
	0.280	0.400	0.000	0.000	0.70	0.6797	0.6837	0.5981	684.63
	0.280	0.400	0.350	0.500	0.70	0.9610	0.9615	0.9392	650.93
	0.000	0.000	0.425	0.500	0.85	0.9092	0.9096	0.8661	664.49
	0.283	0.333	0.000	0.000	0.85	0.6464	0.6501	0.5567	696.50
	0.283	0.333	0.425	0.500	0.85	0.9822	0.9827	0.9689	643.00
	0.340	0.400	0.000	0.000	0.85	0.8503	0.8515	0.7884	676.08
	0.340	0.400	0.425	0.500	0.85	0.9937	0.9938	0.9888	631.31
Part B:									
P (Reject Both Endpoints for at Least One Dose)	0.000	0.400	0.000	0.500	0.00	0.9552	0.9563	0.9471	628.84
	0.233	0.333	0.350	0.500	0.70	0.9013	0.9073	0.8729	661.21
	0.280	0.400	0.350	0.500	0.70	0.9712	0.9735	0.9584	650.93
	0.283	0.333	0.425	0.500	0.85	0.9270	0.9311	0.9068	643.00
	0.340	0.400	0.425	0.500	0.85	0.9828	0.9836	0.9753	631.31
Part C:									
P (Reject Both Endpoints for Both Doses)	0.233	0.333	0.350	0.500	0.70	0.5790	0.5930	0.5176	661.21
	0.280	0.400	0.350	0.500	0.70	0.7307	0.7409	0.6719	650.93
	0.283	0.333	0.425	0.500	0.85	0.7620	0.7698	0.7241	643.00
	0.340	0.400	0.425	0.500	0.85	0.8887	0.8915	0.8654	631.31

TABLE 6.10

Power results for Primary and Key Secondary Endpoint paradigm.

	Δ_{11}	Δ_{12}	Δ_{21}	Δ_{22}	δ	Method 1	Method 2	Fixed Trial	Mean SS
Part A: P (Reject Primary Endpoint for at Least One Dose)									
	0.000	0.333	0.000	0.000	0.00	0.8946	0.8948	0.8600	664.70
	0.000	0.400	0.000	0.000	0.00	0.9701	0.9703	0.9590	652.45
	0.000	0.400	0.000	0.500	0.00	0.9706	0.9707	0.9590	657.64
	0.233	0.333	0.000	0.000	0.70	0.9245	0.9245	0.8896	702.96
	0.233	0.333	0.350	0.500	0.70	0.9261	0.9257	0.8896	716.96
	0.280	0.400	0.000	0.000	0.70	0.9829	0.9827	0.9712	691.07
	0.280	0.400	0.350	0.500	0.70	0.9832	0.9826	0.9712	710.27
	0.283	0.333	0.000	0.000	0.85	0.9463	0.9465	0.9183	701.45
	0.283	0.333	0.425	0.500	0.85	0.9478	0.9474	0.9183	713.86
	0.340	0.400	0.000	0.000	0.85	0.9892	0.9892	0.9806	682.71
	0.340	0.400	0.425	0.500	0.85	0.9893	0.9892	0.9806	699.71
Part B: P (Reject Primary Endpoint for Both Doses)									
	0.233	0.333	0.000	0.000	0.70	0.5907	0.5884	0.5173	702.96
	0.233	0.333	0.350	0.500	0.70	0.6933	0.6822	0.6145	716.96
	0.280	0.400	0.000	0.000	0.70	0.7684	0.7672	0.7019	691.07
	0.280	0.400	0.350	0.500	0.70	0.8411	0.8359	0.7854	710.27
	0.283	0.333	0.000	0.000	0.85	0.7462	0.7452	0.6662	701.45
	0.283	0.333	0.425	0.500	0.85	0.8227	0.8185	0.7535	713.86
	0.340	0.400	0.000	0.000	0.85	0.8979	0.8972	0.8545	682.71
	0.340	0.400	0.425	0.500	0.85	0.9392	0.9376	0.9093	699.71
Part C: P (Reject Primary and Key Secondary Endpoints for at Least One Dose)									
	0.000	0.400	0.000	0.500	0.00	0.9591	0.9598	0.9416	657.64
	0.233	0.333	0.350	0.500	0.70	0.9163	0.9167	0.8699	716.96
	0.280	0.400	0.350	0.500	0.70	0.9755	0.9758	0.9556	710.27
	0.283	0.333	0.425	0.500	0.85	0.9414	0.9413	0.9051	713.86
	0.340	0.400	0.425	0.500	0.85	0.9844	0.9844	0.9710	699.71
Part D: P (Reject Primary and Key Secondary Endpoints for Both Doses)									
	0.233	0.333	0.350	0.500	0.70	0.6286	0.6222	0.5281	716.96
	0.280	0.400	0.350	0.500	0.70	0.7598	0.7603	0.6718	710.27
	0.283	0.333	0.425	0.500	0.85	0.8019	0.7991	0.7188	713.86
	0.340	0.400	0.425	0.500	0.85	0.9123	0.9118	0.8659	699.71

power at interim to determine sample size increase were considered, and the powers were found to be slightly higher for Rule 1 compared to Rule 2.

This chapter discusses two methods for weighting the test statistics of the results from both periods of the trial: (1) information fraction weighting (Cui et al., 1999) and (2) a mixture method. With respect to Type I error for single endpoint trials, both methods controlled Type I error at the specified one-sided $\alpha = 0.025$ level for the overall null hypothesis, the null hypothesis for the higher dose, and the null hypothesis for the lower dose. For two endpoint trials, Type I error was similarly controlled by the various methods. Another method to weight the two test statistics is inverse variance weighting. Exploration in the simulations indicated that the power of the inverse variance weighting method was similar to the powers for Method 1 and Method 2 for the situations that were evaluated, and so results for this method are not reported in this chapter.

For this chapter, results from the suvorexant clinical trials as published in both Herring et al. (2016) and Sun et al. (2018), enabled determination of standardized effect sizes to be used in the simulations. Accordingly, this chapter provides methodology to enable appropriate power for the design of a new study like the suvorexant clinical trials for which there may be two doses of a test treatment. Also, its scope includes two endpoints, with one possibly having planned measurement for fewer patients than the other.

The importance of the reported methodology is its potential for enabling the lower dose to have regulatory approval in situations where it may not be as efficacious as the higher dose, but its safety profile is preferable to the higher dose. In this regard, trials do not always have adequate power to assess the efficacy of the lower dose, and this chapter provides methodology for appropriate power for the lower dose through assessment of the corresponding conditional power at the interim analysis. Also, this capability applies to the higher dose if the true treatment difference for it is smaller than expected.

References

Bischoff, W., & Miller, F. (2009). A seamless phase II/III design with sample-size re-estimation. *J Biopharm Stat*, 19(4), 595–609. https://doi.org/10.1080/10543400902963193

Chen, Y. H., DeMets, D. L., & Lan, K. K. (2004). Increasing the sample size when the unblinded interim result is promising. *Stat Med*, 23(7), 1023–1038. https://doi.org/10.1002/sim.1688

Cui, L., Hung, H. M., & Wang, S. J. (1999). Modification of sample size in group sequential clinical trials. *Biometrics*, 55(3), 853–857. https://doi.org/10.1111/j.0006-341x.1999.00853.x

Gao, P., Ware, J. H., & Mehta, C. (2008). Sample size re-estimation for adaptive sequential design in clinical trials. *J Biopharm Stat*, 18(6), 1184–1196. https://doi.org/10.1080/10543400802369053

Herring, W. J., Connor, K. M., Ivgy-May, N., Snyder, E., Liu, K., Snavely, D. B., Krystal, A. D., Walsh, J. K., Benca, R. M., Rosenberg, R., Sangal, R. B., Budd, K., Hutzelmann, J., Leibensperger, H., Froman, S., Lines, C., Roth, T., & Michelson, D. (2016). Suvorexant in patients with insomnia: results from two 3-month randomized controlled clinical trials. *Biol Psychiatry*, 79(2), 136–148. https://doi.org/10.1016/j.biopsych.2014.10.003

Hochberg, Y. (1988). A sharper Bonferroni procedure for multiple tests of significance. *Biometrika*, 75(4), 800–802. https://doi.org/10.1093/biomet/75.4.800

Lan, K. K., & Wittes, J. (1988). The B-value: a tool for monitoring data. *Biometrics*, 44(2), 579–585.

Liu, Q., Hu, G., Ye, B., Wang, S., & Wu, Y. (2021). Sample size re-estimation design in phase II dose finding study with multiple dose groups: frequentist and Bayesian methods. *arXiv pre-print server* . https://doi.org/https://doi.org/10.48550/arXiv.2012.14589

Mehta, C. R., & Pocock, S. J. (2011). Adaptive increase in sample size when interim results are promising: a practical guide with examples. *Stat Med*, 30(28), 3267–3284. https://doi.org/https://doi.org/10.1002/sim.4102

Ouyang, J., Zhang, P., Carroll, K. J., Lee, J., & Koch, G. (2020). Comparisons of global tests on intersection hypotheses and their application in matched parallel gatekeeping procedures. *J Biopharm Stat*, 30(4), 593–606. https://doi.org/10.1080/10543406.2019.1696355

Sun, H., Snyder, E., & Koch, G. G. (2018). Statistical planning in confirmatory clinical trials with multiple treatment groups, multiple visits, and multiple endpoints. *J Biopharm Stat*, 28(1), 189–211. https://doi.org/10.1080/10543406.2017.1378664

Wang, J. (2010). Many-to-one comparison after sample size reestimation for trials with multiple treatment arms and treatment selection. *J Biopharm Stat*, 20(5), 927–940. https://doi.org/10.1080/10543401003618959

Wiener, L. E., Ivanova, A., & Koch, G. G. (2020). Methods for clarifying criteria for study continuation at interim analysis. *Pharm Stat*, 19(5), 720–732. https://doi.org/10.1002/pst.2027

6.5 Appendix

6.5.1 Technical Details for Methods

Let $\overline{Y}_{1ij} = \dfrac{1}{n_{1ij}} \sum_{k=1}^{n_{1ij}} Y_{1ijk}$ denote the sample mean of the responses Y_{1ijk} for patients in treatment group j in period 1 of the trial for endpoint i. By the assumptions in Section 6.2 and the central limit theorem, $\overline{Y}_{1ij}$ has an approximately $N\left(\mu_{ij}, \dfrac{\sigma_i^2}{n_{1ij}}\right)$ normal distribution. Let

$$\overline{Y}_1 = \left(\overline{Y}'_{11}, \overline{Y}'_{12}\right)' = \left(\overline{Y}_{110}, \overline{Y}_{111}, \overline{Y}_{112}, \overline{Y}_{120}, \overline{Y}_{121}, \overline{Y}_{122}\right)'$$ denote the vector of the sample means of the observed responses for the three treatment groups for the interim analysis for the first period of the trial for both endpoints ($\overline{Y}_{11}$ for sTST as the first endpoint and $\overline{Y}_{12}$ for WASO as the second endpoint). In this regard, $E\left[\overline{Y}_1\right] = \mu$. Let $B = \begin{pmatrix} -1 & 1 & 0 & 0 & 0 & 0 \\ -1 & 0 & 1 & 0 & 0 & 0 \\ 0 & 0 & 0 & -1 & 1 & 0 \\ 0 & 0 & 0 & -1 & 0 & 1 \end{pmatrix}$ such

that $d_1 = B\overline{Y}_1 = \left(d_{111}, d_{112}, d_{121}, d_{122}\right)'$. Given $\overline{Y}_1$, d_1 is computed, where $E\left[d_{1ij}\right] = \left(\mu_{ij} - \mu_{i0}\right)$

and $Var\left(d_{1ij}\right) = \sigma_i^2 \left(\dfrac{1}{n_{1i0}} + \dfrac{1}{n_{1ij}}\right)$. Let $f_{1ij} = \dfrac{d_{1ij}}{\sigma_i \sqrt{\dfrac{1}{n_{1i0}} + \dfrac{1}{n_{1ij}}}}$, where j indexes the two treatment

differences of interest ($j = 1$ corresponds to the difference between the lower dose and placebo and $j = 2$ corresponds to the difference between the higher dose and placebo). Then (3) provides the conditional power (relative to one-sided Type I error α) for the assessment of d_{1ij} (for each treatment difference of interest j for each endpoint i at interim) with information fraction r (as defined in Section 6.2) if there is no increase in sample size. In (3), $\Phi(\cdot)$ is the cumulative distribution function of the standard normal distribution and $Z_{(1-\alpha)}$ is the $(1-\alpha)$-th quantile of the standard normal distribution (Lan & Wittes, 1988; Mehta & Pocock, 2011; Wiener et al., 2020).

$$CP_{lij} = \Phi\left\{\left(\sqrt{\frac{r}{1-r}}+\sqrt{\frac{1-r}{r}}\right)f_{lij} - \frac{Z_{(1-\alpha)}}{\sqrt{1-r}}\right\}$$ (3)

The sample means from the second period of the trial, $\bar{Y}_{2ij}^{*}$, are defined as $\bar{Y}_{2ij}^{*}=\frac{1}{n_{2ij+}}\sum_{k=1}^{n_{2ij+}}Y_{2ijk}$ where

$k=1,2,\ldots,n_{2ij},\ldots,n_{2ij+}$. Let $\bar{\boldsymbol{Y}}_{2}^{*}=\left(\bar{\boldsymbol{Y}}_{21}^{*\prime},\bar{\boldsymbol{Y}}_{22}^{*\prime}\right)=\left(\bar{Y}_{210}^{*},\bar{Y}_{211}^{*},\bar{Y}_{212}^{*},\bar{Y}_{220}^{*},\bar{Y}_{221}^{*},\bar{Y}_{222}^{*}\right)^{\prime}$ denote the vector of the sample means of the observed responses for the three treatment groups for both endpoints in the second period of the trial. Since $E\left[\bar{\boldsymbol{Y}}_{2}^{*}\mid\boldsymbol{u}\right]=\boldsymbol{\mu}$, where $\boldsymbol{u}=\left(u_{0},u_{1},u_{2}\right)^{\prime}$ is determined from CP_{lij} as described in Section 6.2, it follows that $E\left[\bar{\boldsymbol{Y}}_{2}^{*}\right]=\boldsymbol{\mu}$. Let $\bar{\boldsymbol{Y}}^{*}=\left(\bar{\boldsymbol{Y}}_{1}^{\prime},\bar{\boldsymbol{Y}}_{2}^{*\prime}\right)^{\prime}$. Therefore, $E\left[\bar{\boldsymbol{Y}}^{*}\right]=\left(\boldsymbol{\mu}^{\prime},\boldsymbol{\mu}^{\prime}\right)^{\prime}$, and for $\boldsymbol{d}^{*}=\boldsymbol{C}\bar{\boldsymbol{Y}}^{*}$, where $\boldsymbol{C}=\begin{bmatrix}\boldsymbol{B} & 0\\ 0 & \boldsymbol{B}\end{bmatrix}_{8\times12}$, $E\left[\boldsymbol{d}^{*}\right]=\boldsymbol{C}E\left[\bar{\boldsymbol{Y}}^{*}\right]=\left(\Delta^{\prime},\Delta^{\prime}\right)^{\prime}$,

where $\Delta=\left(\left(\mu_{11}-\mu_{10}\right),\left(\mu_{12}-\mu_{10}\right),\left(\mu_{21}-\mu_{20}\right),\left(\mu_{22}-\mu_{20}\right)\right)^{\prime}=\left(\Delta_{11},\Delta_{12},\Delta_{21},\Delta_{22}\right)^{\prime}$. Accordingly, Δ_{11} is the true treatment effect of the lower dose for the first endpoint, Δ_{12} is the true treatment effect of the higher dose for the first endpoint, Δ_{21} is the true treatment effect of the lower dose for the second endpoint, and Δ_{22} is the true treatment effect of the higher dose for the second endpoint. The covariance matrix that applies to $\boldsymbol{d}^{*}$ is complicated because the sample sizes n_{2ij+} depend on u_{0}, u_{1}, and u_{2}. With $\boldsymbol{D}_{a}$ as a diagonal matrix with $\boldsymbol{a}=\left(\sigma_{1},\sigma_{1},\sigma_{2},\sigma_{2}\right)^{\prime}$ on the diagonal; unconditionally $Var(\boldsymbol{d}_{1})$ is given in (4).

$$Var\left(\boldsymbol{d}_{1}\right)=\boldsymbol{D}_{a}\begin{bmatrix}v_{111} & v_{11} & c_{11} & c_{10}\\ v_{11} & v_{112} & c_{10} & c_{12}\\ c_{11} & c_{10} & v_{121} & v_{12}\\ c_{10} & c_{12} & v_{12} & v_{122}\end{bmatrix}\boldsymbol{D}_{a}$$

$$=\boldsymbol{D}_{a}\begin{bmatrix}\frac{1}{rn_{10}}+\frac{1}{rn_{11}} & \frac{1}{rn_{10}} & \left[\frac{1}{rn_{10}}+\frac{1}{rn_{11}}\right]\rho & \frac{1}{rn_{10}}\rho\\ \frac{1}{rn_{10}} & \frac{1}{rn_{10}}+\frac{1}{rn_{12}} & \frac{1}{rn_{10}}\rho & \left[\frac{1}{rn_{10}}+\frac{1}{rn_{12}}\right]\rho\\ \left[\frac{1}{rn_{10}}+\frac{1}{rn_{11}}\right]\rho & \frac{1}{rn_{10}}\rho & \frac{1}{rs_{2}n_{10}}+\frac{1}{rs_{2}n_{11}} & \frac{1}{rs_{2}n_{10}}\\ \frac{1}{rn_{10}}\rho & \left[\frac{1}{rn_{10}}+\frac{1}{rn_{12}}\right]\rho & \frac{1}{rs_{2}n_{10}} & \frac{1}{rs_{2}n_{10}}+\frac{1}{rs_{2}n_{12}}\end{bmatrix}\boldsymbol{D}_{a}$$

$$= \begin{bmatrix} \dfrac{\sigma_1^2}{n_{110}}+\dfrac{\sigma_1^2}{n_{111}} & \dfrac{\sigma_1^2}{n_{110}} & \left[\dfrac{1}{n_{110}}+\dfrac{1}{n_{111}}\right]\rho\sigma_1\sigma_2 & \dfrac{1}{n_{110}}\rho\sigma_1\sigma_2 \\[2ex] \dfrac{\sigma_1^2}{n_{110}} & \dfrac{\sigma_1^2}{n_{110}}+\dfrac{\sigma_1^2}{n_{112}} & \dfrac{1}{n_{110}}\rho\sigma_1\sigma_2 & \left[\dfrac{1}{n_{110}}+\dfrac{1}{n_{112}}\right]\rho\sigma_1\sigma_2 \\[2ex] \left[\dfrac{1}{n_{110}}+\dfrac{1}{n_{111}}\right]\rho\sigma_1\sigma_2 & \dfrac{1}{n_{110}}\rho\sigma_1\sigma_2 & \dfrac{\sigma_2^2}{n_{120}}+\dfrac{\sigma_2^2}{n_{121}} & \dfrac{\sigma_2^2}{n_{120}} \\[2ex] \dfrac{1}{n_{110}}\rho\sigma_1\sigma_2 & \left[\dfrac{1}{n_{110}}+\dfrac{1}{n_{112}}\right]\rho\sigma_1\sigma_2 & \dfrac{\sigma_2^2}{n_{120}} & \dfrac{\sigma_2^2}{n_{120}}+\dfrac{\sigma_2^2}{n_{122}} \end{bmatrix}$$

(4)

For (4), ρ represents the correlation between the two endpoints within the treatment groups for the two doses and placebo. The covariance matrix for d_2^* can be consistently estimated by the expression given in (5).

$$\widetilde{Var}(d_2^*)=D_a \begin{bmatrix} v_{211} & v_{21} & c_{21} & c_{20} \\ v_{21} & v_{212} & c_{20} & c_{22} \\ c_{21} & c_{20} & v_{221} & v_{22} \\ c_{20} & c_{22} & v_{22} & v_{222} \end{bmatrix} D_a$$

$$= \begin{bmatrix} \dfrac{\sigma_1^2}{n_{210+}}+\dfrac{\sigma_1^2}{n_{211+}} & \dfrac{\sigma_1^2}{n_{210+}} & \left[\dfrac{1}{n_{210+}}+\dfrac{1}{n_{211+}}\right]\rho\sigma_1\sigma_2 & \dfrac{1}{n_{210+}}\rho\sigma_1\sigma_2 \\[2ex] \dfrac{\sigma_1^2}{n_{210+}} & \dfrac{\sigma_1^2}{n_{210+}}+\dfrac{\sigma_1^2}{n_{212+}} & \dfrac{1}{n_{210+}}\rho\sigma_1\sigma_2 & \left[\dfrac{1}{n_{210+}}+\dfrac{1}{n_{212+}}\right]\rho\sigma_1\sigma_2 \\[2ex] \left[\dfrac{1}{n_{210+}}+\dfrac{1}{n_{211+}}\right]\rho\sigma_1\sigma_2 & \dfrac{1}{n_{210+}}\rho\sigma_1\sigma_2 & \dfrac{\sigma_2^2}{n_{220+}}+\dfrac{\sigma_2^2}{n_{221+}} & \dfrac{\sigma_2^2}{n_{220+}} \\[2ex] \dfrac{1}{n_{210+}}\rho\sigma_1\sigma_2 & \left[\dfrac{1}{n_{210+}}+\dfrac{1}{n_{212+}}\right]\rho\sigma_1\sigma_2 & \dfrac{\sigma_2^2}{n_{220+}} & \dfrac{\sigma_2^2}{n_{220+}}+\dfrac{\sigma_2^2}{n_{222+}} \end{bmatrix}$$

(5)

The estimators d_1 and d_2^* can be evaluated by simulations. Also, unconditionally, $Cov(d_1,d_2^*)=0_{4\times4}$, since the patients in the two periods of the trial are independent. Altogether, we have the consistent estimator for $Var(d^*)$ as $\widetilde{Var}(d^*)$ in (6).

$$\widetilde{Var}(d^*)=\begin{bmatrix} Var(d_1) & \\ & \widetilde{Var}(d_2^*) \end{bmatrix}$$

(6)

In order to weight the results of each period in the trial to produce $g_{ij}=\left(w_j d_{1ij}+(1-w_j)d_{2ij}^*\right)$ for the test statistic of interest for the j-th treatment difference of interest for the i-th endpoint, two different methods of weighting are considered in Section 6.2. In this regard, we note that $\dfrac{n_{1ij}}{n_{1ij}+n_{2ij+}}$ has the simplification given in (7), which will be used in the weighting methods.

$$\frac{n_{1ij}}{n_{1ij}+n_{2ij+}}=\frac{rs_it_jN}{rs_it_jN+(1-r)s_it_jN+u_js_it_jN_+}=\frac{rN}{N+u_jN_+}$$

(7)

We can then define $g_i = (g_{i1}, g_{i2})'$ for the i-th endpoint as given in (8).

$$g_i = \begin{bmatrix} w_1 d_{1i1} + (1-w_1) d^*_{2i1} \\ w_2 d_{1i2} + (1-w_2) d^*_{2i2} \end{bmatrix} \tag{8}$$

Under the alternative hypothesis, $E[g_i \mid H_A] = (\Delta_{i1}, \Delta_{i2})'$. Under the null hypothesis, $E[g_i \mid H_0] = (0,0)'$. Let $\widetilde{Var}(g_{i1}), \widetilde{Var}(g_{i2})$ be consistent estimators of $Var(g_{i1}), Var(g_{i2})$, respectively, where $\widetilde{Var}(g_{i1}) = v_{g_{i1}} = w_1^2 v_{1i1} + (1-w_1)^2 v_{2i1}$ and $\widetilde{Var}(g_{i2}) = v_{g_{i2}} = w_2^2 v_{1i2} + (1-w_2)^2 v_{2i2}$. The test statistics, $b_i = (b_{i1}, b_{i2})'$, are then formed as given in (9).

$$b_i = \begin{bmatrix} \dfrac{g_{i1}}{\sqrt{v_{g_{i1}}}} \\ \dfrac{g_{i2}}{\sqrt{v_{g_{i2}}}} \end{bmatrix} = \begin{bmatrix} b_{i1} \\ b_{i2} \end{bmatrix} \tag{9}$$

Although the unconditional distributions of b_{i1}, b_{i2} are possibly unclear, determinations of p-values can be based on assuming that b_{i1}, b_{i2} follow approximately normal distributions with mean 0 and variance 1 under $H_0 : \Delta_{ij} = 0$, and they can be subsequently evaluated by simulation. Thus, the (upper) one-sided p-value for each test statistic is $p_{ij} = 1 - \Phi(b_{ij})$ where $\Phi(\cdot)$ is the cumulative distribution function of the standard normal distribution.

6.5.2 Technical Details for Simulations

For each combination of the specifications, we randomly sample 10,000 trials.

For each trial, we first randomly determine $\tilde{d}_1 = D_a^{-1} d_1 = (\tilde{d}_{111}, \tilde{d}_{112}, \tilde{d}_{121}, \tilde{d}_{122})'$ with $a = (\sqrt{v_{111}}, \sqrt{v_{112}}, \sqrt{v_{121}}, \sqrt{v_{122}})'$, and it represents the vector of observed standardized treatment differences from placebo for the interim analysis for period 1 in correspondence to sTST low dose, sTST high dose, WASO low dose, and WASO high dose. The applicable four-variate normal distribution for $\tilde{d}_1$ has standardized expected values $\tilde{\Delta} = D_a^{-1} \Delta = (\tilde{\Delta}_{11}, \tilde{\Delta}_{12}, \tilde{\Delta}_{21}, \tilde{\Delta}_{22})'$ and covariance matrix $\Sigma_1 = D_a^{-1} [Var(d_1)] D_a^{-1}$ in (10) where $Var(d_1)$ given in (4). For reasons given in Appendix Sections 6.5.3 and 6.5.4, the covariances that pertain to the two endpoints in (10) are specified as 0 for the comparisons of the two doses to placebo.

$$\Sigma_1 = \begin{bmatrix} v_{111} & v_{11} & 0 & 0 \\ v_{11} & v_{112} & 0 & 0 \\ 0 & 0 & v_{121} & v_{12} \\ 0 & 0 & v_{12} & v_{122} \end{bmatrix} = \begin{bmatrix} \dfrac{1}{n_{110}} + \dfrac{1}{n_{111}} & \dfrac{1}{n_{110}} & 0 & 0 \\ \dfrac{1}{n_{110}} & \dfrac{1}{n_{110}} + \dfrac{1}{n_{112}} & 0 & 0 \\ 0 & 0 & \dfrac{1}{n_{120}} + \dfrac{1}{n_{121}} & \dfrac{1}{n_{120}} \\ 0 & 0 & \dfrac{1}{n_{120}} & \dfrac{1}{n_{120}} + \dfrac{1}{n_{122}} \end{bmatrix} \quad (10)$$

Then, we let $f_{1ij} = \tilde{d}_{1ij}/\sqrt{v_{1ij}}$ for $i = 1, 2$ and $j = 1, 2$ for the two endpoints and two doses, and expression (3) is used to compute the conditional power for each endpoint for each dose at interim for the most stringent one-sided Type I error α for the multiplicity method that corresponds to the four different types of trials that are addressed in Sections 6.3.2, 6.3.3, 6.3.4, and 6.3.5. In this regard, $\alpha = 0.0125$ for the simulations for Sections 6.3.2, 6.3.3, and 6.3.5 in accordance with Figures 6.1, 6.2, and 6.4, respectively, and $\alpha = 0.00625$ for Section 6.3.4 in accordance with Figure 6.3. The simulations used a promising zone specification of 0.30 to 0.80. Let $\tilde{d}_2^* = (\tilde{d}_{211}^*, \tilde{d}_{212}^*, \tilde{d}_{221}^*, \tilde{d}_{222}^*)$ be the vector of observed standardized treatment differences for period 2 of a trial. Simulated samples of $\tilde{d}_2^*$ are from a four-variate normal distribution with mean $\tilde{\Delta} = D_a^{-1}\Delta$, as defined previously, and covariance matrix $\Sigma_2 = D_a^{-1}\left[\widetilde{Var}(d_2^*)\right]D_a^{-1}$ in (11) where $\widetilde{Var}(d_2^*)$ given in (5).

$$\Sigma_2 = \begin{bmatrix} v_{211} & v_{21} & 0 & 0 \\ v_{21} & v_{212} & 0 & 0 \\ 0 & 0 & v_{221} & v_{22} \\ 0 & 0 & v_{22} & v_{222} \end{bmatrix} = \begin{bmatrix} \dfrac{1}{n_{210+}} + \dfrac{1}{n_{211+}} & \dfrac{1}{n_{210+}} & 0 & 0 \\ \dfrac{1}{n_{210+}} & \dfrac{1}{n_{210+}} + \dfrac{1}{n_{212+}} & 0 & 0 \\ 0 & 0 & \dfrac{1}{n_{220+}} + \dfrac{1}{n_{221+}} & \dfrac{1}{n_{220+}} \\ 0 & 0 & \dfrac{1}{n_{220+}} & \dfrac{1}{n_{220+}} + \dfrac{1}{n_{222+}} \end{bmatrix}$$

$$(11)$$

For the weighting of the results of each period in the trial to produce $g_{ij} = \left(w_j \tilde{d}_{1ij} + (1-w_j)\tilde{d}_{2ij}^*\right)$ (for the ith endpoint and j-th treatment difference) for the test statistics of interest, the two different methods described in Section 6.2 are used. We can then define $g_i = (g_{i1}, g_{i2})$ for the ith endpoint as given in (8), and the test statistics $b_i = (b_{i1}, b_{i2})'$ as given in (9); and the (upper) one-sided p-value for each test statistic is $p_{ij} = 1 - \Phi\left(b_{ij}\right)$.

6.5.3 Derivation of Treatment Effect Estimates

For the changes from baseline for the two endpoints at Month 1, Tables 2 and 3 of Herring et al. (2016) provide the least squares means and 95% confidence intervals for the differences between the high dose and placebo (Table 2 of Herring et al.) and the low dose and placebo (Table 3 of Herring et al.). Furthermore, Sun et al. (2018) provide observed estimates for the differences from placebo for each of the endpoints at Month 1 by dose

TABLE 6.11

Effect size estimates based on Tables 2 and 3 in Herring et al. (2016).

Trial	Dose	Measure	Estimate	Average Estimate	Observed Estimate (Sun et al., 2018)
1	LD	sTST	19.6	18.60	18.54
2	LD	sTST	26.3		
1	HD	sTST	16.3	22.95	23.74
2	HD	sTST	20.9		
1	LD	WASO	-26.3	-25.25	-26.59
2	LD	WASO	-29.4		
1	HD	WASO	-26.4	-27.85	-28.54
2	HD	WASO	-24.1		

TABLE 6.12

Standard deviation estimates based on 95% CIs in Supplement of Herring et al. (2016).

Trial	Dose	Measure	Lower	Upper	Length	SE	n	SD
1	Placebo	sTST	17.7	28.4	10.7	2.730	365	52.149
2	Placebo	sTST	16.7	28.1	11.4	2.908	350	54.407
1	LD	sTST	32.8	45.9	13.1	3.342	244	52.201
2	LD	sTST	36.1	50.6	14.5	3.699	219	54.740
1	HD	sTST	37.3	48.0	10.7	2.730	363	52.006
2	HD	sTST	43.1	54.3	11.2	2.857	365	54.586
1	Placebo	WASO	-23.7	-13.6	10.1	2.577	272	42.493
2	Placebo	WASO	-27.5	-17.4	10.1	2.577	271	42.415
1	LD	WASO	-51.2	-38.9	12.3	3.138	185	42.678
2	LD	WASO	-53.8	-39.3	14.5	3.699	133	42.659
1	HD	WASO	-50.1	-39.9	10.2	2.602	275	43.150
2	HD	WASO	-56.9	-46.9	10.0	2.551	280	42.687

level and visit for the pooled trials in their Table A1. Table 6.11 provides a summary of these estimates.

These reported estimates are helpful guides for the possible treatment effects for a future study, and they are used in the simulations for this chapter. In this regard, a reasonable estimate of the effect size of the high dose on the difference from placebo in change from baseline for WASO based on the results from the two trials is −27, and it is 22 for sTST. Also, we note that the effect sizes for the low dose on the two endpoints could be about 85% of those for the high dose; that is, $(0.85 \times -27) = -22.95$ for WASO and $(0.85 \times 22) = 18.7$ for sTST.

The Supplement of Herring et al. (2016) provides the least squares means and 95% confidence intervals (CIs) for changes from baseline for sTST and WASO by treatment group in Table S1. Using the 95% CIs, we compute the standard error estimates by dividing the length of the CI by (2×1.96). Then, based on the applicable sample sizes for each dose group and endpoint at Month 1, we compute the standard deviations of the outcome measures as $\sqrt{n} \times SE$. Table 6.12 includes the standard deviation (SD) estimates for each trial, dose group, and endpoint.

Based on the estimated standard deviations for each trial, dose group, and endpoint in Table 6.12, we will subsequently use 45 and 55 as reasonable estimates of the standard deviations for the WASO endpoint and the sTST endpoint, respectively, for all dose groups. Moreover, for the remainder of the discussion of the suvorexant trials here, as well as for all of the simulations in Section 6.3, we will reverse the sign of WASO so that it has a positive expression, rather than negative.

Ultimately, for sample sizes n_0, n_1, n_2 for placebo, low dose, and high dose, and s_2 as the specified proportion of the sample size for the WASO endpoint, expression (12) presents an approximately multivariate normal distribution for the means of the two endpoints for the differences from placebo for changes from baseline for high dose and low dose, and in (12), ρ denotes the correlation between sTST and WASO for all dose groups for those patients who had measurements for both endpoints.

$$
\begin{pmatrix} \text{sTST LD} \\ \text{sTST HD} \\ \text{WASO LD} \\ \text{WASO HD} \end{pmatrix} \sim N
$$

$$
\left(\begin{pmatrix} 18.7 \\ 22.0 \\ 23.0 \\ 27.0 \end{pmatrix} \begin{bmatrix} \dfrac{3025}{n_1} + \dfrac{3025}{n_0} & \dfrac{3025}{n_0} & \dfrac{2475\rho}{n_1} + \dfrac{2475\rho}{n_0} & \dfrac{2475\rho}{n_0} \\[2ex] \dfrac{3025}{n_0} & \dfrac{3025}{n_2} + \dfrac{3025}{n_0} & \dfrac{2475\rho}{n_0} & \dfrac{2475\rho}{n_2} + \dfrac{2475\rho}{n_0} \\[2ex] \dfrac{2475\rho}{n_1} + \dfrac{2475\rho}{n_0} & \dfrac{2475\rho}{n_0} & \dfrac{2025}{s_2 n_1} + \dfrac{2025}{s_2 n_0} & \dfrac{2025}{s_2 n_0} \\[2ex] \dfrac{2475\rho}{n_0} & \dfrac{2475\rho}{n_2} + \dfrac{2475\rho}{n_0} & \dfrac{2025}{s_2 n_0} & \dfrac{2025}{s_2 n_2} + \dfrac{2025}{s_2 n_0} \end{bmatrix} \right)
$$
(12)

Multiplication of the estimates in (12) by $\boldsymbol{D}_{\tilde{a}}^{-1}$ as the inverse of a diagonal matrix with $\tilde{a} = (55, 55, 45, 45)'$ on the diagonal (together with premultiplication and postmultiplication of their covariance matrix by $\boldsymbol{D}_{\tilde{a}}^{-1}$) provides the approximately multivariate normal distribution in (13) for the standardized effect sizes of the endpoints for the two doses.

$$
\boldsymbol{D}_{\tilde{a}}^{-1} \begin{pmatrix} \text{sTST LD} \\ \text{sTST HD} \\ \text{WASO LD} \\ \text{WASO HD} \end{pmatrix} \sim N \left(\begin{pmatrix} 0.34 \\ 0.40 \\ 0.51 \\ 0.60 \end{pmatrix} \begin{bmatrix} \dfrac{1}{n_1} + \dfrac{1}{n_0} & \dfrac{1}{n_0} & \dfrac{\rho}{n_1} + \dfrac{\rho}{n_0} & \dfrac{\rho}{n_0} \\[2ex] \dfrac{1}{n_0} & \dfrac{1}{n_2} + \dfrac{1}{n_0} & \dfrac{\rho}{n_0} & \dfrac{\rho}{n_2} + \dfrac{\rho}{n_0} \\[2ex] \dfrac{\rho}{n_1} + \dfrac{\rho}{n_0} & \dfrac{\rho}{n_0} & \dfrac{1}{s_2 n_1} + \dfrac{1}{s_2 n_0} & \dfrac{1}{s_2 n_0} \\[2ex] \dfrac{\rho}{n_0} & \dfrac{\rho}{n_2} + \dfrac{\rho}{n_0} & \dfrac{1}{s_2 n_0} & \dfrac{1}{s_2 n_2} + \dfrac{1}{s_2 n_0} \end{bmatrix} \right)
$$
(13)

More simply with $\boldsymbol{S} = \begin{bmatrix} \dfrac{1}{n_1} + \dfrac{1}{n_0} & \dfrac{1}{n_0} \\[2ex] \dfrac{1}{n_0} & \dfrac{1}{n_2} + \dfrac{1}{n_0} \end{bmatrix}$, then the covariance matrix in (13) becomes $\begin{bmatrix} \boldsymbol{S} & \rho \boldsymbol{S} \\ \rho \boldsymbol{S} & \dfrac{1}{s_2} \boldsymbol{S} \end{bmatrix}$.

Sun et al. (2018) provide the covariance structure for the observed estimates for changes from baseline for the differences between the dose groups and placebo in their Table A2. Based on this covariance matrix, we can estimate the correlation between the two endpoints for each dose group (see Appendix Section 6.5.4). Since these estimates are well below 0.10 (when we reverse the sign of WASO to be positive), we henceforth specify $\rho = 0$, and (14) provides the simplified distribution for the two endpoints for the standardized effect sizes relative to placebo for changes from baseline for high dose and low dose.

$$
\boldsymbol{D}_{\bar{a}}^{-1}\begin{pmatrix} \text{sTST LD} \\ \text{sTST HD} \\ \text{WASO LD} \\ \text{WASO HD} \end{pmatrix} \sim N\left(\begin{pmatrix} 0.34 \\ 0.40 \\ 0.51 \\ 0.60 \end{pmatrix}, \begin{bmatrix} \boldsymbol{S} & \boldsymbol{0}_{2\times2} \\ \boldsymbol{0}_{2\times2} & \dfrac{1}{s_2}\boldsymbol{S} \end{bmatrix}\right) \tag{14}
$$

6.5.4 Correlation Derivation

Sun et al. (2018) provide the distribution for sTST LD, sTST HD, WASO LD, and WASO HD given in (15).

$$
\begin{pmatrix} \text{sTST LD} \\ \text{sTST HD} \\ \text{WASO LD} \\ \text{WASO HD} \end{pmatrix} \sim N(\boldsymbol{\eta},\boldsymbol{\Sigma}) \equiv N\left(\begin{pmatrix} 18.54 \\ 23.74 \\ -26.59 \\ -28.54 \end{pmatrix}, \begin{bmatrix} 10.44 & 4.09 & -0.97 & -0.38 \\ 4.09 & 8.12 & -0.38 & -0.75 \\ -0.97 & -0.38 & 10.37 & 3.83 \\ -0.38 & -0.75 & 3.83 & 7.59 \end{bmatrix}\right) \tag{15}
$$

Let $\boldsymbol{a}^* = \left(\sqrt{10.44},\sqrt{8.12},\sqrt{10.37},\sqrt{7.59}\right)'$ be the vector denoting the square root of the variances (i.e., standard deviations) for sTST LD, sTST HD, WASO LD, and WASO HD. Let $\boldsymbol{D}_{a^*}$ be a diagonal matrix with $\boldsymbol{a}^*$ on the diagonal. Therefore, expression (16) provides the correlation matrix derived from the covariance matrix.

$$
\boldsymbol{D}_{a^*}^{-1}\boldsymbol{\Sigma}\boldsymbol{D}_{a^*}^{-1} = \begin{bmatrix} 1.00 & 0.44 & -0.09 & -0.04 \\ 0.44 & 1.00 & -0.04 & -0.10 \\ -0.09 & -0.04 & 1.00 & 0.43 \\ -0.04 & -0.10 & 0.43 & 1.00 \end{bmatrix} \tag{16}
$$

The upper right 2×2 matrix (and also the lower left 2×2 matrix) provides correlations between sTST and WASO that pertain to the differences between low dose and placebo and the differences between high dose and placebo. These correlations are all below 0.10 in absolute value, thereby indicating very weak or no correlation between treatment differences for sTST and WASO. On the other hand, as would usually be expected, the correlations between the treatment difference for low dose and the treatment difference for high dose are about 0.44 for each endpoint separately, and so are moderately strong.

7

Hierarchical Composite Endpoints in COVID-19: The DARE-19 Trial

Samvel B. Gasparyan, Elaine K. Kowalewski, Joan Buenconsejo, and Gary G. Koch

Introduction

The idea of prioritized outcomes for combining different clinical outcomes of patients into a composite endpoint so as to preserve their different natures is applied in clinical trials in multiple therapeutic areas with various names. Examples include the win ratio endpoint in Ferreira et al. (2020) or the desirability of outcome ranking in Evans et al. (2020). *Prioritized outcome composite endpoints* have an ordinal nature meaning that better and worse are defined between the outcomes, but how much better or worse is not defined since the distance between the outcomes is unspecified. In a randomized trial setting, such outcomes are usually analyzed with methods for pairwise comparisons of patients in the active group with patients in the placebo (or control) group for all outcomes included in the definition of prioritization during their *shared follow-up time*. Shared follow-up time means that two patients with differing follow-up times are compared for their common follow-up period, which is the shortest of their two follow-up times.

Hierarchical composite endpoints (HCEs) (Packer 2016) are a special example of prioritized outcome composite endpoints. They have a distinguishing feature of requiring the same fixed follow-up, i.e., the same follow-up for all patients, and they use only the clinically most important event for each patient in the analysis. This seemingly limiting constraint enables comparing patients on a global clinical scale through patients contributing one and only one event to the analysis, with it being their clinically most important event (Gasparyan et al. 2022). Another important characteristic is that HCEs can include outcomes that are indicative of a positive shift in a patient's clinical status, and thus can capture a treatment effect in terms of improving outcomes for patients. This contrasts with many clinical endpoints that include only clinically severe outcomes that the treatment intends to prevent. Hierarchical composite endpoints originated from heart failure (HF) trials (Packer 2001), where the basic idea was to combine outcomes corresponding to the multiple therapeutic goals in treating HF patients. They include reducing the risk of cardiovascular death as well as reducing the burden of recurrent HF hospitalizations and improving symptoms associated with heart failure. Therefore, the combination of these three outcomes into a composite with recognition of their clinical priority can capture the overall treatment effect on clinical outcomes and symptoms.

In this chapter we will discuss the design and analysis of hierarchical composite endpoints as well as trials based on these endpoints. We will motivate the use of the win odds as the analysis method and describe the novel *maraca* plots (Karpefors, Lindholm,

DOI: 10.1201/9781003288640-7

and Gasparyan 2023) as the method of visualization. We will also discuss the principles of constructing such endpoints and how these principles were used to create a novel endpoint in a COVID-19 trial.

The DARE-19 trial (Kosiborod et al. 2021a, b), with its HCE as one of the dual primary endpoints, will be described in detail. This trial used an HCE that adapted a WHO-suggested ordinal endpoint (WHO 2020) so as to capture disease-specific outcomes, combined with outcomes associated with the known profile of the active drug dapagliflozin. We discuss the practical aspects of designing new studies based on an HCE. These practical aspects include sample size, power, minimal detectable effect, standardized effect size, and number needed to treat calculations for an HCE based on the win odds analysis (Gasparyan et al. 2021b; Gasparyan, Kowalewski, and Koch 2022). We also consider the management of missing data and the clinical interpretability of the treatment effect in relation to the notion of the estimand (Gasparyan et al. 2022). Based on these methods, we will discuss the results of DARE-19 for its HCE primary endpoint, the estimand of DARE-19 associated with this HCE, and the visualization of results using the maraca plots.

7.1 Hierarchical Composite Endpoints

7.1.1 Definition and Analysis Method

One of the challenges in designing clinical trials that can inform clinical practice is the selection of a meaningful primary efficacy endpoint. The ideal endpoint should be modifiable by the intervention, clinically important, and relevant in the management of the disease in the target population. Clinical endpoints are generally focused on assessment of the individual components of a patient's status at a specific timepoint. In practice, the totality of such components over the entire treatment period represents a patient's true disease burden. This consideration is especially important for studies of acutely ill and hospitalized patients. Therefore, in assessing the total disease burden, a comprehensive approach is to combine both favorable and unfavorable events which are observed during the treatment period. For example, the scope can include improvements in clinical status such as a shorter hospital stay as well as deterioration in clinical status such as the occurrence of major clinical events. The capture of both improvement and deterioration expands the scope of information for the analysis and thereby provides a more sensitive endpoint to detect the benefit and possibly the overall benefit-risk of an intervention. This approach has the potential to improve the power for treatment comparisons and correspondingly to improve trial design efficiency with smaller sample sizes.

Unlike traditional dichotomous composite endpoints, *hierarchical composite endpoints* (HCEs) (Packer 2001, 2016; Gasparyan et al. 2022) need to have an ordinal nature to distinguish multiple possible favorable and unfavorable outcomes. HCEs consider all defined clinical events within their scope for a given patient and assign higher priority to the clinically most important, usually the most severe, event. Therefore, patients experiencing deterioration regardless of any preceding or subsequent improvements will be assigned to an "unfavorable" outcome in the analysis reflective of the deterioration. For example, a patient who experienced improvement in clinical status but later died will be assigned to the death category because death is the most severe outcome and has the highest priority.

Although this discussion emphasizes the analysis of an HCE with the win odds, and win statistics in general, it is important to note that the analysis method for an HCE is separate from its definition. An HCE is an endpoint that can be analyzed by the win odds, or by another method such as ordinal logistic regression (Harrell 2015). More generally, the win odds is applicable to an endpoint without hierarchical structure, such as skewed numeric data, as a version of the Mann–Whitney–Wilcoxon test (Mann and Whitney 1947; Wilcoxon 1992). Therefore, the definition of an HCE in the protocol of a clinical trial should be a separate consideration from the analysis method, and the statistical analysis plan for such an endpoint can specify either the win odds or other analysis methods for it.

7.1.2 Overview of Win Statistics

Two treatment groups are compared for an ordinal endpoint through a win, loss, or a tie for each patient in the active group compared to each patient in the control group. All possible (overall) combinations are denoted by O, with W denoting the total wins for the active group, L the total losses, and T the total ties, so that $O = W + L + T$. Then the following quantities are called **win statistics.**

- **Win probability** defined as $WP = \dfrac{W + 0.5T}{O}$, that is, the total number of wins, added to half of the total number of ties, divided by the overall number of comparisons.

- **Number needed to treat** defined as $NNT = \dfrac{1}{2WP - 1} = \dfrac{O}{W - L}$ (rounded up to the nearest natural number for interpretation).

- **Win ratio** defined as $WR = \dfrac{W}{L}$.

- **Win odds** defined as $WO = \dfrac{W + 0.5T}{L + 0.5T} = \dfrac{WP}{1 - WP}$.

- **Net Benefit** defined as $NB = \dfrac{W - L}{O} = 2WP - 1 = \dfrac{1}{NNT}$.

Given the overall number of comparisons O, the win proportion WP, and the win ratio WR, it is possible to find the total number of wins and losses.

$$
\begin{aligned}
L &= O * \frac{2WP - 1}{WR - 1}, \\
W &= WR * L = WR * O * \frac{2WP - 1}{WR - 1}, \\
T &= O - W - L = O * \left[1 - (WR + 1)\frac{2WP - 1}{WR - 1} \right].
\end{aligned} \tag{1}
$$

The concept of win probability for binary and continuous outcomes has been described in the paper by Buyse (2010) as "proportion in favor of treatment" (see also Rauch et al. (2014)), while in Verbeeck et al. (2020) it is called the "probabilistic index".

The concept of "win ratio" was introduced in Pocock et al. (2012) but does not account for ties. The win odds is the odds of winning, with ties counted as half wins, following Dong et al. (2020a) (see also Peng (2020); Brunner, Vandemeulebroecke, and Mütze (2021); Gasparyan et al. (2021b)). The same statistic was named Mann-Whitney odds in O'Brien and Castelloe (2006). In Gasparyan et al. (2021a) the "win ratio" was used as a general term for the win odds and included ties in the definition. Dong et al. (2022) suggested consideration of the win ratio, win odds, and net benefit together as win statistics.

   The concept of winning for the active group is the same as concordance for the active group. For two variables, X and Y, this pair is concordant if the observation with the larger value of X also has the better value of Y (Agresti 2013). If X indicates the treatment group with the value 1 for the active group and the value 0 for the control group, and the variable Y is the ordinal value for the analysis, then concordance means that a patient with the active treatment has a better value than a patient with the control, while the discordance means the patient in the active group has a worse value than the control patient. Therefore, the win ratio is the total number of concordances divided by the total number of discordances. The win ratio can be obtained from the Goodman-Kruskal gamma (Kruskal and Goodman 1954), G, as follows: $WR = (1 + G)/(1 - G)$. The net benefit is Somers' D C/R (Somers 1962), while the win odds is the Mann-Whitney odds (Mann and Whitney 1947). Estimation of win statistics in the absence of censoring can be done using the theory of U-statistics (Hoeffding 1948).

7.1.3 Definition and Interpretation of WO

Suppose patients are randomized to one of the two treatment groups, active or control. A variable of interest is measured in both groups and each patient has only one measurement. The values of this variable are assumed to be ordinal. An ordinal variable can either be continuous or ordered categorical. We usually use the convention that a higher value signifies a more favorable outcome, but it can also be the other way around. In order to compare the treatment effect between the groups and to test the treatment effect difference, we define the win probability. We assume that the values of the variable of interest in the active treatment group are independently sampled from a random variable η, while the values of the control group are independently sampled from the random variable ξ, where η and ξ are independent ordinal random variables. We need to estimate the win probability and the corresponding win odds for active treatment against control, using the observed measurements in each treatment group.

The win probability is defined as

$$\theta = \mathbf{P}(\eta > \xi) + 0.5\mathbf{P}(\eta = \xi), \tag{2}$$

where as the win odds is the odds of winning,

$$\kappa = \frac{\theta}{1-\theta} = \frac{\mathbf{P}(\eta > \xi) + 0.5\mathbf{P}(\eta = \xi)}{\mathbf{P}(\eta < \xi) + 0.5\mathbf{P}(\eta = \xi)}, \quad \theta = \frac{\kappa}{\kappa+1}. \tag{3}$$

The win probability is defined as the probability of the random variable η being greater than the random variable ξ plus half of the probability that these random variables are equal. If $\theta > 0.5$ then we say that the active treatment "wins" against the control, meaning that a randomly selected patient from the active group will have a better outcome than a randomly selected patient from the control group with more than 0.5 probability, while $\theta < 0.5$ means that the active treatment "loses" against the control, with a "tie" in case of $\theta = 0.5$. In terms of win odds, a "win", a "loss," or a "tie" are, correspondingly, $\kappa > 1$,

$\kappa < 1$, and $\kappa = 1$. If ξ and η have the same distribution, then the win odds $\kappa = 1$, while κ being different from 1 provides information about locations of the distributions of ξ and η with respect to each other (see subsequent Examples).

Example 2.1 (Normal distribution). Suppose that $\xi \sim \mathcal{N}(m_1, \sigma_1^2)$ and $\eta \sim \mathcal{N}(m_2, \sigma_2^2)$ are independent, normally distributed random variables. Then $\eta - \xi \sim \mathcal{N}(m_2 - m_1, \sigma_1^2 + \sigma_2^2)$. The win probability θ can be calculated using the formula

$$\theta = \Phi\left(\frac{m_2 - m_1}{\sqrt{\sigma_1^2 + \sigma_2^2}}\right), \tag{4}$$

where $\Phi(\cdot)$ is the distribution function of the standard normal random variable.

Consider the case of $\xi \sim N(0, 1)$ and $\eta \sim N(1, 1)$. Then $\theta = 0.76$, and when $\xi \sim N(0, 1)$ but $\eta \sim N(1, 4)$, then $\theta = 0.67$. Therefore, an increase in variance in one of the random variables reduces the win probability.

Example 2.2 (Log-normal distribution). Suppose that ξ, η are independent and log-normally distributed, that is, $\log(\xi) \sim \mathcal{N}(m_1, \sigma_1^2)$ and $\log(\eta) \sim \mathcal{N}(m_2, \sigma_2^2)$ are independent, normally distributed random variables. Then,

$$\theta = \mathbf{P}(\eta > \xi) = \mathbf{P}(\log \eta > \log \xi) = \Phi\left(\frac{m_2 - m_1}{\sqrt{\sigma_1^2 + \sigma_2^2}}\right).$$

So in this case as well the win probability depends on the difference $m_2 - m_1$; since *median* $(\xi) = e^{m_1}$ and *median*$(\eta) = e^{m_2}$, the win probability will be different from 0.5 if there is a difference in medians for two log-normally distributed random variables:

$$\theta = \Phi\left(\frac{\log \dfrac{median(\eta)}{median(\xi)}}{\sqrt{\sigma_1^2 + \sigma_2^2}}\right). \tag{5}$$

Therefore, from (4) (difference in means) and (5) (difference in medians) we see that win odds is a measure of the difference between locations of distributions of two independent random variables.

Example 2.3 (Bernoulli). Suppose that ξ, η are independent and Bernoulli distributed random variables; that is, they take the value 1 ("success"), with probabilities correspondingly q and p, and the value 0 ("failure") with probabilities $1 - q$ and $1 - p$. Then,

$$\theta = \frac{p - q + 1}{2} = \frac{1 - q - (1 - p) + 1}{2}. \tag{6}$$

Therefore, the win probability is different from 0.5 if there is a difference in success probabilities, or the risk difference (difference in failure probabilities) is not 0.

Example 2.4 (Identical distributions). Suppose that ξ, η are independent and identically distributed random variables. Then $\theta = 0.5$ and so $\kappa = 1$. Indeed, in this case, since the random variables are identically distributed and independent, then $\mathbf{P}(\eta > \xi) = \mathbf{P}(\eta < \xi)$; hence $2\mathbf{P}(\eta > \xi) + \mathbf{P}(\eta = \xi) = 1$ and therefore $\theta = 0.5$.

The opposite is not true; the win odds may be 1, but there may still be a difference in distributions between the two random variables. Indeed, in Example 2.1, if we have two independent, normally distributed random variables with the same mean but different variances, then from formula (4) we have that $\theta = 0.5$, but the distributions are clearly different since the variances are different.

Therefore, from (4), (5), (6), and Example 2.4 we see that the win odds is a general method of comparing locations of distributions of two independent, ordinal random variables.

Example 2.5 (Beta-binomial). Suppose that the independent random variables ξ and η are ordinal and have five values that can be denoted by the numbers $1, 2, \ldots, 5$, where a higher value indicates a worse outcome, meaning η wins against ξ if $\eta < \xi$. We will consider the auxiliary continuous variables $\tilde{\xi} \sim Beta(\alpha_0, \beta_0)$ and $\tilde{\eta} \sim Beta(\alpha_1, \beta_1)$, that are independent and have a Beta distribution. We can define the random variables ξ and η as follows:

$$P(\eta = k) = P(0.2(k-1) \le \tilde{\eta} < 0.2k), k = 1, \cdots, 5,$$
$$P(\xi = k) = P(0.2(k-1) \le \tilde{\xi} < 0.2k), k = 1, \cdots, 5. \tag{7}$$

Using this definition, it is straightforward to see that the win probability of the random variable η (denoting the active treatment) against the random variable ξ (denoting control) can be calculated as follows:

$$\theta = P(\eta < \xi) + 0.5P(\eta = \xi)$$
$$= \sum_{k=1}^{5} \left[F_{\tilde{\eta}}(0.2k) - F_{\tilde{\eta}}(0.2(k-1)) \right] \left[1 - \frac{F_{\tilde{\xi}}(0.2k) + F_{\tilde{\xi}}(0.2(k-1))}{2} \right]. \tag{8}$$

Here $F_{\tilde{\eta}}(\cdot)$ and $F_{\tilde{\xi}}(\cdot)$ denote the distribution functions of random variables $\tilde{\eta}$ and $\tilde{\xi}$, respectively. Therefore, simulating values from two Beta distributions and categorizing them using the formula (7) will produce simulated values from the ordinal random variables ξ and η.

The formula (8) can be used to calculate the theoretical win odds for the ordinal random variable η against ξ depending on the parameters of the Beta distribution. One way is to fix values $\alpha_0 = 5$, $\beta_0 = 4$, $\beta_1 = 4$ so that α_1 can be chosen in a way to obtain the prespecified win probability or win odds. For example, in case of $\kappa = 1.10$ we have $\alpha_1 = 4.69$, and similarly for $\kappa = 1.15$, $\alpha_1 = 4.56$; for $\kappa = 1.2$, $\alpha_1 = 4.44$; for $\kappa = 1.25$, $\alpha_1 = 4.33$; and for $\kappa = 1.30$, $\alpha_1 = 4.21$.

Example 2.6 (Proportional hazards). Suppose that ξ, η are independent and denote the survival times in the active and control groups correspondingly. Consider the survival functions of these random variables.

$$S\xi(t) = \mathbf{P}(\xi \ge t), \ S\eta(t) = \mathbf{P}(\eta \ge t).$$

Under the proportional hazards assumption, the hazard ratio HR of the active treatment against the control is constant, and

$$S_\eta(t) = S_\xi(t)^{HR}.$$

TABLE 7.1

Distribution of ordinal values in the ACTT-1 trial.

Scale	Remdesivir, n (%)	Placebo, n (%)
1	99 (23)	76 (19)
2	158 (36)	127 (31)
3	11 (3)	6 (1)
4	23 (5)	20 (5)
5	34 (8)	40 (10)
6	16 (4)	14 (3)
7	60 (14)	72 (18)
8	33 (8)	55 (13)

TABLE 7.2

Remdesivir trial results.

Estimate	LCL	UCL	P	Statistic
0.56	0.53	0.6	0.001	Win proportion
1.29	1.11	1.5	0.001	Win odds
0.13	0.05	0.2	0.001	Net Benefit
8.00	4.00	15.0		NNT

In the case of no censoring and absence of ties, the win odds equals the reciprocal of the hazard ratio.

$$\kappa = \frac{1}{HR}, \quad \theta = \frac{1}{HR+1} \tag{7}$$

Thus, $\theta > 0.5$ and $\kappa > 1.0$ when $HR < 1.0$, whereas $\theta < 0.5$ and $\kappa < 1.0$ when $HR > 1.0$.

7.1.4 REMDESIVIR: Example and Motivation for Analysis by Win Odds

ACTT-1 was a double-blind, randomized, placebo-controlled trial of intravenous remdesivir in adults who were hospitalized with COVID-19 and had evidence of lower respiratory tract infection (Beigel and al. 2020).

Based on a proportional odds model with an eight-category ordinal scale (see Table 7.4), the patients who received remdesivir were found to have higher odds (i.e., more likely than those who received placebo) for better clinical improvement at day 15 (odds ratio (95% CI) was 1.5 (1.2, 1.9), with p = 0.001, for nonadjusted analysis). At day 15 the number of patients with nonmissing clinical status in the remdesivir group was 434, and the same was 410 in the placebo group (see Figure 7.1 and Table 7.1).

Given the reported numbers, calculation is possible for the win odds of the remdesivir group against the placebo group. Every patient in the remdesivir group can be compared with every patient in the placebo group, and the result will be a "win" for the patient in the remdesivir group if the patient's ordinal value is *better* than that of the patient in the placebo group. For the ACTT-1 outcome, the higher the ordinal value, the worse the outcome clinically. Therefore, the WO (95% CI) of remdesivir on day 15 is (see the formula (A12)) $\hat{k}_N = 1.29, (1.11, 1.5), P = 0.001$.

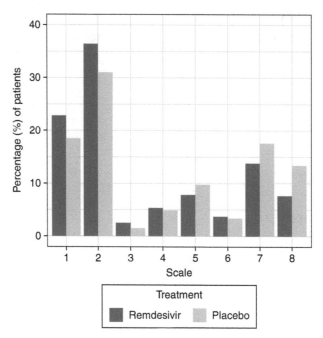

FIGURE 7.1
Comparison of ordinal values in ACTT-1 trial.

TABLE 7.3

Sample size of a COVID-19 trial.

Estimate	Size	Method	Notes
1.20	1272	Win odds	Responder analysis, WP data dependent SD = 0.50
1.29	816	Win odds	SD = 0.5578, data dependent SD for WP
1.29	874	Win odds	SD = 0.5774, data independent SD for WP
1.29	826	Win odds	Formula with ties
1.37	850	Win ratio	Prob. of ties 0.201

This result corresponds (see formula (A14) and Table A.1) to Number Needed to Treat (NNT) of 8, with a 95% CI of (4, 15) and standardized effect size of $SES = 0.227$, where $SD = 0.5578$ (see (A16)). This means that eight patients need to be treated with remdesivir compared to placebo so as to have one patient with a better clinical status at day 15 (see Table 7.2).

If we consider a responder analysis by categorizing the endpoint presented in Table 7.4 to *improvement* (Categories 1 and 2) versus *nonimprovement/deterioration* for the remaining outcomes, then we see that 59% of patients in the remdesivir group have improvement, compared to 50% in the placebo group (see Table 7.1). This result corresponds to a 9% risk reduction or a win odds of 1.2. If we use the reciprocal of the absolute risk reduction to calculate the NNT for the responder analysis, the result is $NNT = 11$. Of note, for the binary random variable, the NNT based on the formula (A14) is equivalent to the reciprocal of the absolute risk reduction (Gasparyan et al. 2021a). Therefore, as expected, the ordinal scale is more sensitive to detect a treatment effect, and so it provides a lower NNT of 8 for the win odds estimate of 1.29. This interpretation can be confirmed by the standardized effect size as well. The responder analysis produces an effect size of 0.2, while the effect size of the win odds analysis is 0.227, and so is 13.5% higher.

The estimated win proportion $\hat{\theta}_N$ has the following standard error $SE = 0.0192$, and it can be used to calculate the sample size of a study designed to detect a win odds of 1.29 (using the formula (A23)). For 90% power, approximately 816 patients will be required to detect the same win odds as in the *ACTT-1* trial with two-sided type I error of 0.05. Using the observed standard error (SE), we can calculate the standard deviation (SD) of the win proportion for the sample size of the study via

$$SD = SE * \sqrt{N} = 0.0192 * \sqrt{844} = 0.5578.$$

This SD estimate is similar to the theoretical standard deviation of the win probability. Thus, for large sample sizes, the SD is stable and depends only on the studied population (for example, the severity of the disease of COVID-19 patients included in the study) and the definition of the endpoint. If a different scale is chosen or the population differs from the one studied in this trial, then the standard deviation will be different as well. As discussed in Section A.4, the data-independent standard deviation estimate of $\frac{1}{\sqrt{3}} = 0.5774$ can be used if no prior information is available to derive the estimated standard deviation. We see that the data-independent standard deviation estimate is larger than the observed standard deviation, and so its use produces a larger sample size estimate, approximately 874 (see Table 7.3).

On the other hand, if we use the sample size calculation formulas accounting for ties (Section A.5), then for the reported numbers by outcomes and treatment groups, we can obtain that 46.2% of comparisons produce a win for the active group, 20.1% are ties and 33.7% are losses. Hence the win ratio is $WR = 1.37$ and the formula (A26) for the win ratio sample size calculation provides the sample size of 850, while the formula (A29) for the win odds sample size calculation provides the sample size of 826 via $Coe f = 0.945$ (Gasparyan, Kowalewski, and Koch 2022).

7.1.5 Analysis Considerations

7.1.5.1 Length of Follow-up

Although an HCE requires fixed follow-up for evaluation, clinical trials using an HCE as the primary endpoint do not necessarily need to have a fixed follow-up design. An HCE can be applicable for one or more fixed follow-up periods within a clinical trial that does not have a fixed follow-up design if that trial has a minimum follow-up period for all patients. For example, an event-driven trial might enroll patients for 1 year and then follow all patients until both a specified number of events have occurred and all patients have at least 1 year of follow-up. For this clinical trial, an HCE could be produced for 1 year of follow-up as a fixed period. Such flexible designs will give the possibility to collect more events for the analysis of secondary, time-to-event-based endpoints in the trial or to assess the robustness of the HCE results with respect to the contribution of components.

An HCE based on an entire fixed follow-up period of a clinical trial can be supplemented with longitudinal assessments of an HCE for fixed intervals within that fixed follow-up period. Such analyses can be conducted to assess the impact of the length of follow-up on the results, and the contribution of the components on the overall results. For example, this analysis can answer the question of whether the win odds in favor of test treatment are

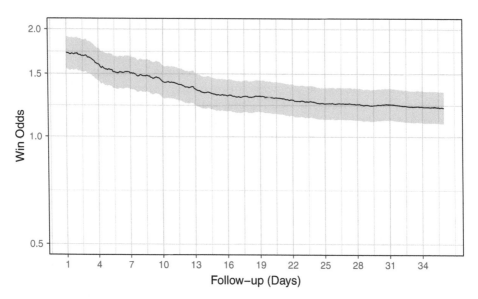

FIGURE 7.2
Win odds depending on the length of follow-up.

homogeneous for these time intervals or whether they have a trend so as to become larger for the later time intervals. Figure 7.2 displays how the win odds depends on the length of follow-up. A similar plot for the win ratio was suggested in Finkelstein and Schoenfeld (2019). The HCE in Figure 7.2 is constructed for one time-to-event outcome (death) and a continuous outcome, which can be considered as change from baseline in a symptoms score measured for patients who are alive at the end of follow-up. In this example, there is a bigger treatment effect on symptoms than on death, but for a longer follow-up, the contribution of death increases, and so the overall treatment effect decreases.

Several papers have explored the impact of the length of follow-up on the analysis of prioritized outcome composite endpoints. As noted in Dong et al. (2020b), prioritized outcome endpoints have advantages relative to traditional endpoints if the clinically more important endpoints tend to occur later and are reasonably frequent. An important consideration is also the impact of the treatment on the clinically most important outcomes (Ferreira et al. 2020). Therefore, for an HCE, as well as for other prioritized outcome composite endpoints, the length of follow-up should be specified with recognition of the time-course of occurrence of each component as well as the potential effect of the treatment on each of those components.

7.1.5.2 Note on Transitivity

Transitivity is a property of a comparison such that patient A having an outcome less than the outcome of patient B so that $A < B$, and patient B having an outcome less than the outcome of patient C so that $B < C$, should imply that $A < C$. Prioritized outcome composite endpoints do not require fixed follow-up time, but rather are based on pairwise comparisons between patients for their *shared follow-up*. This means that the rankings pertain to different times of assessment for different pairs of patients as "shared follow-up time" varies among the pairs. Therefore, comparisons are on the event level only for the shared follow-up time rather than on the patient level. This leads to cases where *transitivity* does not necessarily

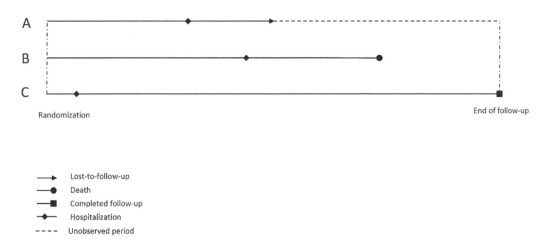

FIGURE 7.3
An example of a nontransitive comparison.

apply and that, as explained above, $A > C$ can occur. Consider the example in Figure 7.3 which illustrates an endpoint consisting of death and hospitalizations. The prioritization is the following: the early death is the worst outcome, followed by repeated hospitalizations, then a late single hospitalization and the most favorable outcome is being event free by the end of fixed follow-up. If we compare patients using the shared follow-up approach then $A < B$ since in their shared follow-up both patients are alive and have only one hospitalization, but A is hospitalized earlier. Similarly, $B < C$ since B experiences death. However, $A > C$ due to the differences in shared follow-up time and C being hospitalized early. If we were to assume that A does not have any other events during their unobserved period, then the comparison would have been $B < C < A$, since B experiences death, while C has an early hospitalization. An HCE avoids this transitivity issue by requiring fixed follow-up. Of course, even for a fixed follow-up period, some patients may have shorter follow-up due to premature study discontinuation. In the HCE analysis, this issue produces missing data, and it can be addressed with the methods of multiple imputation (see Section 2.5.3).

The presence of nontransitive comparisons can affect the estimation of the standard error of the win statistics, and the usual theory of win odds estimation presented in the Appendix may not apply in that case. Another issue with the nontransitive comparisons is how to interpret the results given that these types of comparisons can lead to paradoxical conclusions (Gardner 1970; Savage Jr 1994; Brunner, Vandemeulebroecke, and Mütze 2021).

7.1.5.3 Missingness Associated with HCE

There are two types of missingness associated with HCEs. One type is incomplete assessments of outcomes due to premature study discontinuation such as when patients are lost to follow-up or withdraw consent. Another type is missingness of measurements associated with each outcome that are relevant for further ordering of patients inside each category, such as missing the date an event occurred. For patients who discontinue from the study prematurely, multiple imputation methods can be used to impute events in the interval from study discontinuation to the end of the fixed follow-up period. For example, in Figure 7.4, events can be simulated for the unobserved period for patient A using the estimated distributions of death and hospitalization events from the observed outcomes.

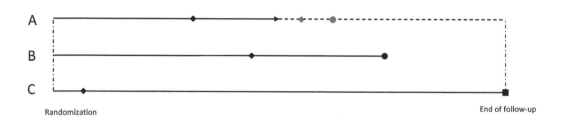

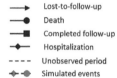

FIGURE 7.4
Imputations for HCE.

Methods are similar to those for time to event outcomes (Zhao et al. 2014). Then, the most severe outcome of all observed and imputed events for a patient can be used in the analysis. If, for example, a hospitalization is imputed for patient *A* (as shown on Figure 7.4 without the occurrence of the death), then the global ordering of patients would be *B* < *A* < *C* since *A* has two hospitalizations and hence loses against *C*. Meanwhile, if both hospitalization and death are imputed for *A* then the global order of patients would be *A* < *B* < *C* since *A* has an earlier death than *B*. This imputation method can be performed several times, and the resulting treatment effect estimates can be combined using Rubin's rule (Rubin 2004).

The second type of missingness can be managed using the median rank within each outcome category to which the patient is assigned (see the example of DARE-19 in Section 3.4.2). Or, in the case of a continuous component of an HCE, methods pertaining to the imputation of continuous outcomes can be used (see Section 5.4 in Gasparyan et al. (2021a) for an example in the heart failure setting with a heart failure symptoms score being a continuous component of an HCE).

7.1.6 Visualization of HCE – Maraca Plots

One of the challenges for the interpretation of an HCE is the lack of proper tools for visualizing the treatment effect captured by the complex nature of the HCE for its combination of events of different types. Graphical representation of the win ratio was considered in Finkelstein and Schoenfeld (2019), but visualization of the HCE itself was still unavailable. Karpefors, Lindholm, and Gasparyan (2023) introduced the novel *maraca* plots for the visualization of an HCE. These plots accommodate multiple time-to-event outcomes and a single continuous outcome. The maraca plots combine violin plots (Hintze and Nelson 1998) with nested box plots (Tukey 1977) to enable visualization of the density of the distribution for the continuous outcome, together with *Kaplan-Meier plots* (Kaplan and Meier 1958) for the time-to-event outcomes. This creates a comprehensive display that clearly shows the treatment effects on each of the HCE components. Outcomes are first ordered according to their clinical importance. In Figure 7.5, outcomes I–IV are time-to-event

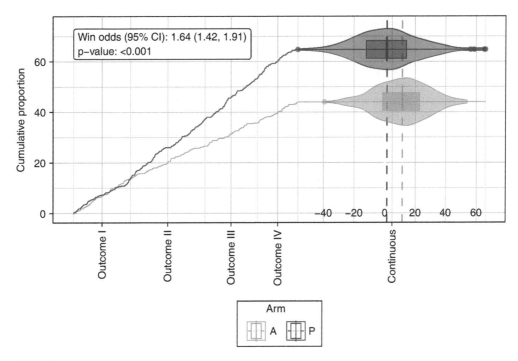

FIGURE 7.5
An example of a maraca plot.

outcomes and the last outcome is continuous. The x-axis shows the clinical importance scale from the most severe outcome on the very left (denoted by outcome I on the plot, and it is usually death) to the most favorable outcome on the right (highest value of the continuous outcome). For outcome I, a simple Kaplan-Meier plot can be constructed for showing the cumulative percentage of patients over the fixed follow-up time with outcome I in the overall population by treatment group. The y-axis shows that the cumulative percentage of patients with outcome I in both treatment groups at the end of the fixed follow-up is about 15% (Figure 7.5). Because of the ordering, patients with outcomes II–IV and patients contributing to the analysis with the continuous outcome are considered as censored at the end of the fixed follow-up period for the analysis of outcome I. Next, for outcome II events, a Kaplan-Meier plot is constructed over the same fixed follow-up time, with outcome I from the first period considered as an event at day 0 for the second period, and patients with outcomes III–IV and the continuous outcome have censoring at the last day of the second period. These new cumulative curves are added to the Kaplan-Meier plots for outcome I, by treatment group. In other words, the Kaplan-Meier plot for outcome II starts where the Kaplan-Meier plot of outcome I ends. This provides the cumulative percentage of patients with outcomes I or II. Similarly, we can construct the plot showing the cumulative percentage of patients with outcomes I–IV. Therefore, the left part of the plot shows clinically severe outcomes that the treatment intends to prevent, and hence the separation of curves is indicative of a treatment effect if the active treatment has a lower cumulative percentage of patients with outcomes I-IV.

In Figure 7.5, the cumulative percentage of outcomes I–IV in the active group is around 45% while it is around 65% in the control group.

The x-axis for the continuous outcomes corresponds to its unit (for example, change from baseline in a symptoms score) and a beneficial treatment effect is characterized by a shift to the right. In the maraca plot, the distribution of the continuous outcome is visualized with a horizontal violin plot and a nested box plot. The associated vertical line shows the median values for the continuous outcome for patients who do not have outcomes I–IV. A higher median value in the active group indicates that the treatment improves the continuous outcome. Indeed, in the active group the median change from baseline is around 11, while in the control group it is around 1, and so the median difference between the two groups is about 10 (Figure 7.5).

Additionally, since each patient contributes to the HCE only once, the widths of each category (time-to-event outcomes and continuous outcome) on the maraca plot correspond to the percentages of that category in the overall population and show the contribution of each component to the composite.

Figure 7.5 shows that the left part (outcomes I–IV) is a little wider than the right part (continuous outcome), and this feature means that the majority of patients contributed to the analysis with outcomes I–IV. The win odds and its 95% confidence interval are calculated with the formula (A12).

The maraca plots are implemented in the maraca package (Martin Karpefors and Samvel B. Gasparyan 2022) in R (R Core Team 2022).

7.2 The DARE-19 Trial

The DARE-19 trial methods and main results were published previously (Kosiborod et al. 2021a,b; Heerspink et al. 2022). Briefly, DARE-19 (NCT04350593) was an international, multicenter, randomized, double-blind, placebo-controlled trial to evaluate the effects of treatment with dapagliflozin for 30 days in hospitalized patients with COVID-19 with respiratory failure, and at least one cardiometabolic risk factor: hypertension, type 2 diabetes, atherosclerotic cardiovascular disease, heart failure, or chronic kidney disease. The trial randomized 1250 patients at 95 centers in 7 countries. The objective of DARE-19 was to investigate if treatment with dapagliflozin could prevent clinical worsening by reducing complications and/or increase the number of patients that recover/leave the hospital without complications.

7.2.1 COVID-19 and its Endpoints

The global pandemic caused by coronavirus disease 2019 (COVID-19) has created worldwide challenges for researchers and incentives to accelerate development of new therapies. With such acceleration, there needs to be accurate and rapid communication of key efficacy and safety findings from clinical trials so that people in need can access life-saving medicines sooner. Important considerations for the communication of scientific findings are clear and precise definitions of clinical outcome endpoints and transparency of underlying statistical assumptions for the estimation of the treatment effect. If possible, clinical outcome endpoints should be consistent across different studies and should be analyzed under the same statistical assumptions in order to have the same quantitative measure for the treatment effect.

TABLE 7.4

WHO Ordinal Scale for COVID-19.

Scale	Category
1	not hospitalized no limitations of activities
2	not hospitalized, limitation of activities home oxygen requirement, or both
3	hospitalized, not requiring supplemental oxygen and no longer requiring ongoing medical care
4	hospitalized, not requiring supplemental oxygen but requiring ongoing medical care
5	hospitalized, requiring any supplemental oxygen
6	hospitalized, requiring noninvasive ventilation or use of high-flow oxygen devices
7	hospitalized, receiving invasive mechanical ventilation or extracorporeal membrane oxygenation (ECMO)
8	death

Most COVID-19-infected patients are asymptomatic or develop mild disease, but some develop respiratory failure requiring hospitalization with significant risk of dying afterward. Treatments for COVID-19 are intended to be curative. An important therapeutic goal of a successful COVID-19 treatment in hospitalized patients is recovery. This is typically defined within a fixed period of time such as 30 days. Recovery in the simplest form is the outcome of discharge from the hospital, and its analysis can be with time-to-event methods or a responder criterion with a specific threshold for defining recovery in terms of the improvement in clinical status compared to baseline (Beigel and al. 2020). However, a binary definition of recovery can have a loss of efficiency and reduction in power for the statistical comparison of treatments. Furthermore, another limitation of using a "response criterion" is the potential arbitrariness in defining an "improvement" threshold unless appropriate methodology is applied, and this justification can require additional data (Natanegera et al. 2021).

A more comprehensive endpoint for COVID-19, which includes patient recovery, is the ordinal scale endpoint presented in Table 7.4. This endpoint was suggested by WHO (WHO 2020). The ordinal scale endpoint represents meaningful patient states ranked by clinical importance (Dodd et al. 2020). It includes clinical status across a wide spectrum of outcomes from death to cure and accounts for significant changes in clinical status such as changes in supplementary oxygen requirements.

7.2.2 Dapagliflozin and the Novel HCE

Although there are several versions of the WHO suggested ordinal scale (see Table 7.4), they are usually for ordinal outcomes that have a seven- or eight-point scale for the vital status, the amount of oxygen support needed, hospital discharge, or limitation of physical activities if discharged. However, all of them share the following important characteristics:

1. They always include death and hospital discharge as unfavorable and favorable outcomes, respectively.
2. They are assessed at a fixed timepoint and therefore do not include events that occur between the baseline and the prespecified timepoint. For example, a 30-day

TABLE 7.5

The DARE-19 HCE.

Order	Category
I	Death
II	More than one new or worsened organ dysfunction events
III	One new or worsened organ dysfunction event
IV	Hospitalized at the end of follow-up (day 30)
V	Discharged from hospital before day 30

    endpoint would assess status only at 30 days and not consider clinical events that happened earlier such as at day 15.

3. Following the previously noted characteristics, they do not prioritize the most severe outcome, but rather use the latest observed outcome in the analysis. The exceptions are death events that may occur at any time within the fixed follow-up.

The WHO ordinal endpoints are an example of the simplest types of HCEs. A limitation is that they do not account for the most severe event for the patient during the entire follow-up period if it is not death. Accordingly, these endpoints are designed to capture the treatment effect of drugs that have antiviral effects and are thus expected to reduce the oxygen support of patients, and the time to hospital discharge.

In contrast, DARE-19 was studying dapagliflozin, an SGLT2i, that has proven benefits on cardiorenal organ protection in the chronic setting, but it does not have known antiviral effects (Wiviott et al. 2019; McMurray et al. 2019; Heerspink et al. 2020; Solomon et al. 2022; Jhund et al. 2022). Therefore, an HCE was tailored to include outcomes that are relevant in the COVID-19 setting and are expected to be affected by the intervention. It included cardiorenal outcomes of COVID-19-related complications and death in order to investigate if dapagliflozin has an organ protective effect in the acute illness setting. Hence, in DARE-19, the HCE shown in Table 7.5 was developed. This endpoint ranks the patients from lowest to highest, where a higher rank represents a better outcome (Gasparyan et al. 2022). This HCE includes both clinical deterioration and clinical improvement in a single metric. Clinical deterioration includes cardio-renal-metabolic organ dysfunction events during the index hospitalization and prolonged hospitalization or death. Clinical improvement includes better clinical status and hospital discharge.

The key difference between the HCE used in DARE-19 and the ordinal scale endpoint suggested by WHO is that the DARE-19 HCE accounts for in-hospital worsening via organ dysfunction events and includes deaths occurring after discharge. For example, patients having in-hospital worsening before hospital discharge will be categorized as recovered by the WHO ordinal scale, but the DARE-19 HCE will rank this patient according to the worst experienced event during the hospitalization.

Therefore, the DARE-19 HCE is an endpoint with a more stringent definition of recovery by capturing the whole disease burden of patients throughout their hospitalization for COVID-19. Almost all patients enrolled in the DARE-19 study had the same baseline severity – hospitalized with COVID-19 with low-flow oxygen support. Therefore, recovery is represented as a measurable and meaningful improvement in clinical status compared to baseline:

1. Discharge from hospital before or at day 30 without in-hospital worsening and alive at day 30; or

2. Still in the hospital at day 30, but without in-hospital worsening during the 30 days of hospitalization and without oxygen support.

Additionally, the suggested ranking (Table 7.5) provides a patient-level ranking through the ordering of all patients into one and only one category. In addition, within each category, the timing of events was used to further rank patients. This can increase statistical power (Dodd et al. 2020) by reducing ties in the rankings and making the resulting HCE more sensitive to the treatment effect. Moreover, patients experiencing more than one event in the same category are further ranked according to the number of events, where more events represent a worse rank. Patients in category IV, hospitalized at the end of follow-up without previous worsening events, are further ranked according to oxygen support requirements at the hospital (IV.1 on high-flow oxygen devices, IV.2 requiring supplemental oxygen, IV.3 not requiring supplemental oxygen).

7.2.3 Estimand Based on COVID-19 HCE

In addition to defining the endpoint, clinical trials' guidelines highlight the importance of defining the estimand. The estimand was introduced by ICH (ICH 2020) as a conceptual framework for the precise definition of the treatment effect as it applies to the clinical question posed by a given clinical trial objective.

For constructing the estimand, assessment should be made for intercurrent events. Intercurrent events are defined as events occurring after treatment initiation with effects on either the measurement of the endpoint or interpretation of the effect of treatment on the endpoint. Examples of intercurrent events include discontinuation of assigned treatment, use of additional or alternative treatment, or death. Any plans on how to address the intercurrent events should be specified. For example, in many settings, the occurrence of a major event during the conduct of the trial may represent a meaningful degree of clinical deterioration that cannot be ignored in any analysis of efficacy. Such intercurrent events, for example, can be included in the definition of a hierarchical composite endpoint by assigning them to an appropriate rank. This is known as the composite strategy of handling intercurrent events.

The primary estimand in DARE-19 for its HCE was the extent to which dapagliflozin (10 mg once daily plus standard of care) improves recovery in adults with cardiometabolic-renal risk factors who were hospitalized with severe respiratory failure due to COVID-19, irrespective of exposure, treatment discontinuation, or concomitant treatment.

Hence, the attributes of the estimand of the DARE-19 trial were the following: the population included the patients who had cardiometabolic or renal risk factors, were hospitalized with severe but not critical COVID-19, and were treated with the standard of care or dapagliflozin 10 mg administered once daily for 30 days in addition to standard of care. Hospital discharge is an intercurrent event for this outcome because the ranking only accounts for organ dysfunction events during the index hospitalization. This is managed with the composite strategy through its inclusion in the definition of the endpoint. The handling of the intercurrent events of initiation of concomitant treatment and study drug discontinuation is reflected in the estimand with the treatment policy strategy, and hence these intercurrent events were disregarded. The corresponding endpoint was the hierarchical composite endpoint of recovery in Table 7.5 and described above. The population level summary was the win odds.

7.2.4 Design of DARE-19

7.2.4.1 Statistical Hypothesis Testing

The HCE described above was one of two dual endpoints in DARE-19. The trial had sufficient sample size to detect a WO of 1.23 at a two-sided significance level of 2.5%, where the overall two-sided significance level of 5% was split between dual primary endpoints (see formula (A23)). A sample size of 1200 patients provided 80% power, and the minimum detectable treatment effect was WO = 1.15 (see formula (A24)), corresponding to number needed to treat of 15. The trial actually randomized 1250 patients at 95 centers in 7 countries.

It was hypothesized that dapagliflozin, which had a cardiorenal organ protective effect, would prevent in-hospital COVID-19-related organ dysfunction events and thus contribute to early recovery, reducing the time to hospital discharge. Therefore, the COVID-19 HCE, as capturing both an effect on prevention of in-hospital organ dysfunction events and improvement in time-to-recovery, would be able to detect a treatment effect on clinically important COVID-19-related outcomes.

7.2.4.2 Management of Missing Data

The two possible types of missingness have been described previously. For all analyses in DARE-19 (primary and supplementary), events with a missing date of occurrence were managed by imputing the ranks of these patients with the median rank of the category for the event. For example, if it is known that the patient died, then this patient is in category I (Table 7.5). Hence, the median rank of the patients who died with known date of death is the imputed rank for the patients who are known to have died with unknown date of death.

Missing occurrences of events were managed in the primary analysis for DARE-19 by censoring, as discussed in the next section, mainly because there were relatively few patients with such missing data. However, as indicated in Section 2.5.3, a multiple imputation method would be preferable if many patients had missing data for occurrences of events.

7.2.4.3 Primary Analysis Method

For the patient-level outcomes of the HCE, Cox proportional hazards regression stratified by country was applied to estimate the WO for the primary analysis. Ties were managed with the Efron method (Cox 1972). The statistical test for this treatment comparison was the stratified log-rank test (Mantel 1966). The rationale for this was the following. In the case of no censoring and no ties, and under the proportionality assumption, the win odds is equal to $1/HR$ for time-to-event outcomes (see Example 2.6). Therefore, for the COVID-19 HCE consisting of multiple time-to-event outcomes and with the presence of negligible censoring, Cox regression could be applied to the outcomes of the HCE to derive the win odds. In this regard, the ordering of outcomes was used as "time" in the Cox regression model and the log-rank test, with higher ranks being less favorable than lower ranks. The advantage of calculating the win odds estimate from Cox regression and using the log-rank test for the primary hypothesis is the capability to address missing events due to incomplete follow-up with censoring. For this purpose, patients who were lost to follow-up were ranked according to their most severe event during their follow-up time in the study with the same derivation method of the HCE as for patients completing the

30 days of follow-up. However, unlike patients completing the 30-day follow-up period of the DARE-19 trial who were included in the analysis as having an "event," patients with this type of missingness were managed as censored in the log-rank test and Cox regression analysis in order to account for their unknown status between the time of discontinuation of follow-up and day 30. The Cox regression model has the advantage of including all patients in the analysis and so was in accordance with the intention-to-treat principle. As noted in Section 2.5, the presence of censoring introduces nontransitive comparisons and hence may make the interpretation of results difficult. While Cox regression can be used in the presence of negligible censoring to include patients in the analysis who are lost to follow-up, a multiple imputation approach would have been better suited to handle the transitivity issue.

As a sensitivity analysis, a direct win odds based on the comparison of ranks of the intervention group versus the placebo group was also produced for only patients with complete follow-up. The confidence interval for the direct WO was constructed using the methods of U-statistics (see (A12)). The resulting win odds was not very different from the win odds obtained from the primary analysis.

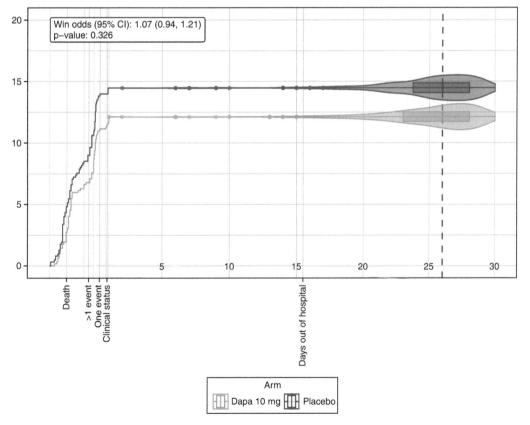

FIGURE 7.6

The maraca plot of DARE-19 HCE.

7.2.4.4 Results

The DARE-19 trial did not achieve statistical significance for either of its dual primary endpoints. The primary endpoint of recovery had a WO of 1.09 (95% CI, 0.97–1.22; p = 0.14) (Kosiborod et al. 2021b). Among the 1250 patients in the DARE-19 trial, 9 patients discontinued the study prematurely and hence could not be explicitly ranked. These patients were ranked based on their observed events before their study discontinuation, and they were included in the primary analysis as censored as described previously. For the direct win odds with exclusion of the 9 patients with premature discontinuation, the WO was 1.07 (95% CI, 0.94–1.21; p = 0.33). In the maraca plot (Figure 7.6) for only the patients who completed the follow-up, the majority of patients are shown to have been discharged from the hospital without experiencing in-hospital organ dysfunction events and are alive on day 30. Although some separation of curves is present for outcomes I–IV, outcome V of not being in the hospital (30 days minus time to discharge from hospital) is not affected by the treatment.

The timing of the events was used to reduce the ties for the pairwise comparisons of patients to determine the win odds. Overall, 7.5% of these comparisons were ties (47.8% were wins for the dapagliflozin group, 44.6% were wins for the placebo group). Although the direct win odds calculation can include patients with premature study discontinuation in the analysis, by classifying their pairwise comparisons to other patients as "tied" when they cannot be classified as better or worse, such management of missing data can have departures from transitivity. However, as for the primary analysis, this consideration would not have a noteworthy impact on the results or interpretation of the treatment effect because of the low number of discontinuations. A win odds of 1.09 means that the odds of a randomly selected patient in the intervention group having a better outcome than a randomly selected patient in the placebo group is 1.09. Therefore, in this case, the number needed to treat is 24 as defined in (A14) (see Table A.1). This means that 24 patients would need to be treated with the intervention treatment rather than with placebo to have one patient with a clinically better outcome. The DARE-19 HCE had patient-level ranks, and so the treatment effect estimate is interpretable on a common clinical scale. More generally, as in the absence of transitivity in the comparison, an NNT = 24 still means that 24 patients need to be treated to have one patient with a better outcome than in the placebo group, but "better" in that case may not have a straightforward clinical scale for interpretation.

7.2.4 Discussion

Hierarchical composite endpoints (HCEs) are a special case for *prioritized outcome composite endpoints* with the distinguishing feature of requiring a fixed follow-up period. HCEs are flexible endpoints, and their construction is feasible in different disease areas and for medicines with different modes of action. They provide clinically meaningful measures of a patient's condition throughout a follow-up period rather than giving priority to the first event or only measurements that pertain to a specific timepoint. Importantly, they can be designed to capture the entire disease burden of the patients by accounting for both improvement and deterioration in clinical status with higher priority for the most severe outcomes.

The concept of HCEs in clinical trials became more commonly incorporated in the heart failure (HF) setting to combine clinical outcome events such as both heart failure hospitalizations and cardiovascular death, with important patient-centered assessments, such as change in symptoms (Packer 2001, 2016). Some of the recent large HF trials used such an HCE in the statistical testing hierarchy. For the DAPA-HF trial (McMurray et al. 2019) and the DELIVER trial (Solomon et al. 2022), an HCE that accounted for change in HF symptoms score at month 8 and death was a secondary endpoint. The EMPULSE trial (Voors et al. 2022) was a study to test the effect of empagliflozin in patients who are in the hospital for acute heart failure. This study used a fixed 90 days of follow-up and had an HCE as a primary endpoint that accounted for change in HF symptoms score at day 90, death, and heart failure events including hospitalizations for heart failure, urgent heart failure visits, and unplanned outpatient visits. We presented the example of the DARE-19 trial (Gasparyan et al. 2022), which constructed an HCE in the COVID-19 setting.

Since all patients fully contribute to an HCE, it can be a more sensitive endpoint to detect treatment effects. The design of a trial with an HCE as the primary endpoint and with the win odds as the primary analysis method, based on HCE's enhanced capability to demonstrate therapeutic efficacy, can potentially lead to more efficient trials with smaller sample size and possibly shorter (fixed) duration relative to studies based only on preventing adverse clinical events. Such trials can be especially important when clinical answers are needed expeditiously, such as during a pandemic. Also, an HCE accounting for both improvement and deterioration could be more important for studies evaluating interventions in acutely ill patients. However, HCEs pertain to scientific questions that are different from those for just adverse clinical events and for which longer-term outcome studies are necessary to investigate effects on chronic diseases in the ambulatory setting. Ultimately, the choice of endpoints depends on multiple factors, including the estimand that accounts for the therapeutic goal, the patient population, and the mechanism of action for the intervention.

A potential limitation of designing trials based on an HCE is its requirement for designs with at least a minimum fixed follow-up period. A fixed follow-up design allows patient-level rankings for which the patients can be ordered according to the ordinal outcomes from a prespecified scale of priority. This property makes the treatment effect interpretable at a common, patient-level clinical scale. With patient-level ranks, the win odds exceeding 1.0 for the intervention treatment compared to control means that the distribution function of the intervention treatment is shifted to the right of the distribution function of the control group (see the maraca plot in Figure 7.5, for separation of curves in the beginning of the x-axis and then shift to the right). Therefore, a shift to the right side of the scale in correspondence to a better clinical outcome means that patients in the intervention group are more likely to have a better clinical outcome. For a ranking without the transitivity property, the univariate distributions of the rankings for each treatment group cannot be compared on a common underlying scale. Hence, the win odds from a transitive comparison not only provides information about relative improvement of the intervention group against the control group but also contains information about a meaningful change on a common clinical scale.

In trials of patients hospitalized with severe COVID-19, an HCE can be defined to include improvement in clinical status as well as deterioration or death. This definition of the HCE provides a strict definition of recovery, and it accounts for in-hospital worsening events and deaths after discharge. Additionally, the timing of all events can be useful to distinguish between patients who recover or experience worsening. This consideration makes the HCE more sensitive to capture the treatment effect. An HCE can be analyzed with the win/Mann-Whitney odds (win ratio with ties) or other win statistics and its use does not require distributional assumptions for estimation such as the proportionality assumption for the proportional odds model. The win odds for an HCE can be useful for designing new trials, and it can provide a clinically meaningful treatment effect estimate with respect to the estimand framework. The use of NNT and standardized effect size for the win odds can lead to consistency of reporting trial results across different therapeutic areas. Maraca plots are useful in visualizing HCE, by exploring the treatment effect on components and over time.

For the definition of an HCE, it is important to include outcomes that are both clinically meaningful in the given disease therapeutic area and are also outcomes that are expected to be affected by the treatment. The example of DARE-19 showed that the inclusion in the HCE of an outcome (hospital discharge) that was the primary contributor to the endpoint and was not correlated with other outcomes that were affected by the treatment effect (see the maraca plot in Figure 7.6) had a negative impact on the study power, and so the overall treatment effect was not statistically significant.

Appendix A. Win Odds

Here we cover the theory of win statistics as based on the theory of *U*-statistics (Hoeffding 1948). This theory is formulated for an HCE without censoring, and so all patients contribute to the analysis. Calculation methods and construction of confidence intervals are discussed for all win statistics, and their connection to well-known statistical tests is summarized (*Fligner-Policello statistic* (Fligner and Policello 1981), *Somers' D C/R* (Somers 1962), *Goodman Kruskal's gamma* (Kruskal and Goodman 1954)). Additionally, for the win odds, methods are provided for adjustment for stratification and/or a numeric covariate (Quade 1967; Koch et al. 1998b; Kawaguchi, Koch, and Wang 2011a; Koch, Sen, and Amara 2004; Gasparyan et al. 2021a; Stokes, Davis, and Koch 2012). Sample size, power, minimum detectable treatment effect, number needed to treat, and standardized effect size calculation formulas are provided for the win odds (Gasparyan et al. 2021a,b; Gasparyan, Kowalewski, and Koch 2022). The chapter ends with software implementation for the calculation of the win odds confidence interval using the SAS software (SAS Institute Inc. 2018) and the package hce (Gasparyan 2022) of the R software (R Core Team 2022). The *maraca* plots are constructed using the R software package maraca (Martin Karpefors and Samvel B. Gasparyan 2022).

A.1 Estimation

To estimate the win odds κ (see equation (3)) of the random variable η against the random variable ξ, under the assumption of independence of these random variables, we observe i.i.d. (independent, identically distributed) samples Y for η and X for ξ in (A1).

$$Y = \left(Y_1, \cdots, Y_{n_2}\right), \quad X = \left(X_1, \cdots, X_{n_1}\right). \tag{A1}$$

We will describe a method of construction of a confidence interval for win odds based on the theory of *U*-statistics (Hoeffding 1948). For the estimation of the win probability and win odds, the samples (A1) of independent, in general, ordinal random variables, can be replaced by numeric samples (Koch et al. 1998b; Gasparyan et al. 2021a,b).

$$Y_2^0 = \left(p_1, p_2, \cdots, p_{n_2} \right), \quad Y_1^0 = \left(q_1, q_2, \cdots, q_{n_1} \right) \tag{A2}$$

Here p_j is the *individual win proportion* of patient j of the active group against the control group, defined as

$$p_j = \frac{1}{n_1} \sum_{i=1}^{n_1} \left(\mathbb{I}\{Y_j > X_i\} + 0.5 \, \mathbb{I}\{X_i = Y_j\} \right). \tag{A3}$$

Here $\mathbb{I}(\cdot)$ is the indicator function which equals 1 if $(\cdot)$ is true, and it equals 0 if $(\cdot)$ is not true. Correspondingly q_i is the *individual win proportion* of patient i of the control group against the active group. The win probability θ (see equation (2)) can be estimated using the Mann-Whitney estimate, which we also call the *win proportion* (WP), since it shows the proportion of all comparisons that resulted in a "win" for the active group (evenly splitting the ties between "wins" and "losses"):

$$\hat{\theta}_N = \frac{1}{n_1 n_2} \sum_{i=1}^{n_1} \sum_{j=1}^{n_2} \left(\mathbb{I}\{Y_j > X_i\} + 0.5 \, \mathbb{I}\{X_i = Y_j\} \right) \tag{A4}$$

where $N = n_1 + n_2$ is the total sample size and the indicator function $\mathbb{I}(\cdot)$ takes the value 1 if the underlying condition is true, 0 otherwise. This estimator is consistent and asymptotically normal.

The estimator for the win odds will be

$$\hat{\kappa}_N = \frac{\hat{\theta}_N}{1 - \hat{\theta}_N}. \tag{A5}$$

Equation (A4) can also be written as

$$\hat{\theta}_N = \frac{1}{n_2} \sum_{j=1}^{n_2} p_j = 1 - \frac{1}{n_1} \sum_{i=1}^{n_1} q_i. \tag{A6}$$

Testing of the null hypothesis of no treatment effect, expressed as $\kappa_0 = 1$, or equivalently, $\theta_0 = 0.5$, can be done using the following Z statistic, which has a standard normal asymptotic distribution.

$$Z_N = \frac{\hat{\theta}_N - \theta_0}{SE}, \quad SE = \sqrt{\frac{var\left(Y_2^0\right)}{n_2} + \frac{var\left(Y_1^0\right)}{n_1}}, \tag{A7}$$

where $var\left(Y_2^0\right)$ and $var\left(Y_1^0\right)$ denote the estimates of the variances

$$var(Y_2^0) = \frac{1}{n_2} \sum_{j=1}^{n_2} (p_j - \hat{\theta}_N)^2, \quad var\left(Y_1^0\right) = \frac{1}{n_1} \sum_{i=1}^{n_1} (q_i - (1 - \hat{\theta}_N))^2 \tag{A8}$$

The $(1 - \alpha)$, $\alpha \in (0, 1)$ level confidence interval (CI) for the win proportion $\hat{\theta}_N$ can be constructed using the formula

$$\left[\hat{\theta}_N - Z_{1-\frac{\alpha}{2}} \cdot SE, \hat{\theta}_N + Z_{1-\frac{\alpha}{2}} \cdot SE \right], \tag{A9}$$

where $Z_{1-\frac{\alpha}{2}}$ is the $\left(1 - \dfrac{\alpha}{2}\right)$-quantile of the standard normal distribution, that is,

$$\mathbf{P}(\zeta < Z_{1-\frac{\alpha}{2}}) = 1 - \frac{\alpha}{2}, \ \zeta \sim N(0.1).$$

Since the function $f(x) = \dfrac{x}{1-x}$, $x \in (0, 1)$ is increasing, the CI for the win odds $\hat{\kappa}_N$ (see (A5)) can be constructed using the formula

$$\left[f\left(\hat{\theta}_N - Z_{1-\frac{\alpha}{2}} \cdot SE \right), f\left(\hat{\theta}_N + Z_{1-\frac{\alpha}{2}} \cdot SE \right) \right]. \tag{A10}$$

It should be noted that the function $f(x)$ is not range-preserving and hence may result in the lower bound of the CI (A10) being less than 0. A better approach (Carr, Hafner, and Koch 1989; Brunner, Vandemeulebroecke, and Mütze 2021; Gasparyan et al. 2021b) is to exponentiate the limits of the CI for $\log\left(\dfrac{\theta}{1-\theta} \right) = \log(\kappa)$:

$$\frac{SE}{\hat{\theta}_N \left(1 - \hat{\theta}_N\right)}. \tag{A11}$$

(A11) provides the approximate standard error for $\log\left(\dfrac{\hat{\theta}_N}{1-\hat{\theta}_N} \right) = \log\left(\hat{\kappa}_N \right)$ from its linear Taylor series (or the δ-method, see Van der Vaart (2000)), where SE is the standard error for $\hat{\theta}_N$ (see (A7)). Using the standard error in (A11) leads to an asymptotic CI in (A12) for the win odds $\hat{\kappa}_N$.

$$\left[\hat{\kappa}_N \cdot e^{-Z_{1-\frac{\alpha}{2}} \cdot \frac{SE}{\hat{\theta}_N \left(1-\hat{\theta}_N\right)}}, \ \hat{\kappa}_N \cdot e^{-Z_{1-\frac{\alpha}{2}} \cdot \frac{SE}{\hat{\theta}_N \left(1-\hat{\theta}_N\right)}} \right]. \tag{A12}$$

Additionally, Kawaguchi, Koch, and Wang (2011a) indicate that consideration of $\log\left(\hat{\kappa}_N \right)$ and its approximate standard error (A11) enable better control of type I error and coverage of confidence intervals for inferences about θ than direct consideration of $\hat{\theta}_N$, particularly when θ was not near 0.5 (see also Carr, Hafner, and Koch (1989) for other related properties of this transformation and for a simulation study).

Therefore, if the standard error of the win proportion is obtained, then the standard error of the logarithm of the win odds can be calculated using the formula (A11) and its asymptotic CI constructed using (A12). The computational challenge of obtaining the standard error (and hence the confidence interval) for the win proportion is to calculate the individual win probabilities Y_1^0, Y_2^0 (see (A2)) given the values X, Y. This can be simplified by the following fact:

Consider the combined sample of two treatment groups $\left(X_1, \cdots, X_{n_1}, Y_1, \cdots, Y_{n_2}\right)$.

$$(R_{11}, \cdots, R_{1n1}, R_{21}, \cdots, R_{2n2})$$

Let denote the respective ranks of the components of this sample. To get the ranks, we need to order these values increasingly. If all the values are different, then the smallest value will have the rank 1 and the largest value will have the highest rank equal to N. If several values are equal, then each one of them will be assigned the mean value of their ranks. The mean method of handling ties has the same meaning as splitting "ties" evenly between "wins" and "losses" in equation (A3). If we introduce ranks in the active group separately, $\left(\tilde{R}_{21}, \cdots, \tilde{R}_{2n_2}\right)$, then the individual win proportion p_j of patient j in the active group will be the rank of that patient in the combined sample minus the rank of that patient in its own (active) group, divided by the number of patients in the other (control) group, that is,

$$p_j = \frac{R_{2j} - \tilde{R}_{2j}}{n_1}. \tag{A13}$$

Therefore, instead of doing all possible comparisons between the patients in two groups, we can just rank patients in the combined sample and then in their respective groups to get their individual win proportions using equation (A13). The win proportion can then be calculated by taking the average of these values (see equation (A6)):

$$\hat{\theta}_N = \frac{1}{n_2} \sum_{j=1}^{n_2} p_j = \frac{1}{n_1 n_2} \sum_{j=1}^{n_2} \left(R_{2j} - \tilde{R}_{2j}\right).$$

Another convenient formula to calculate the win proportion is

$$\hat{\theta}_N = \frac{1}{2} + \frac{\bar{R}_2 - \bar{R}_1}{N}, \quad N = n_1 + n_2,$$

where $\bar{R}_k = \frac{1}{n_k} \sum_{j=1}^{n_k} R_{kj}, k = 1, 2.$

To illustrate the coverage properties of the WO CI, Gasparyan et al. (2021b) conducted a simulation study using categorization of variables from Beta distributions (see Example 2.5). The simulation study indicated that the coverage probability of the CI for WO has consistently good performance for different values of WO and different sizes of the sample.

A.2 Number Needed to Treat

As suggested by Gasparyan et al. (2021a), a transformation of the win probability can define number needed to treat (NNT) and its estimate can be based on the win proportion. Additionally, we can construct a CI for the NNT, and we will introduce standardized effect size (SES) for the win proportion. These measures provide alternative ways to describe the observed treatment effect.

For the win probability θ, the NNT v (which takes the values 1, 2, 3, …) can be defined as

$$v = \frac{1}{2\theta - 1}, \theta \in \left(\frac{1}{2}, 1\right].$$

In terms of the win odds κ the NNT can be written as $v = \frac{k+1}{k-1}$.

TABLE A.1

Number Needed to Treat (NNT) based on the win odds.

Win Odds	NNT
1.05	41
1.1	21
1.15	15
1.2	11
1.25	9
1.3	8
1.35	7
1.4	6
1.45	6
1.5	5
2	3
3	2
-	1

For the case of $\theta > 0.5$, or equivalently, $\kappa > 1$, v corresponds to NNT to benefit, while in case of $\theta < 0.5$, replacing θ by $(1 - \theta)$ for v corresponds to NNT to harm, and the following observations are applicable to that case as well. NNT to benefit and NNT to harm are useful metrics as supportive tools in benefit-risk assessments in regulatory deliberations (Mendes, Alves, and Batel-Marques 2017).

An estimator for the NNT and SES for the win proportion (win odds) can be calculated with formula (A14).

$$NNT = \frac{1}{2\hat{\theta}_N - 1}, \quad SES = \frac{2\hat{\theta}_N - 1}{SD}. \tag{A14}$$

NNT is the number of patients needed to be treated by the active treatment compared to control to have one patient with a better outcome. Therefore, it is always an integer, and so if the calculated value is not an integer, it should be rounded up. For example, suppose that $\hat{\theta}_N = 0.6$, which corresponds to win odds of $\hat{\kappa}_N = 1.5$. In this case, $NNT = 5$ (see Table A.1). With 5 patients per treatment group, there are 25 pairings of a test treatment patient with a control patient; among them, 15 are wins for the test treatment and 10 are wins for the control. Thus, the average number of wins per test treatment patient is 3 and the average number of wins per control treatment patient is 2; so $NNT = 5$ means that the average number of wins per test treatment patient will exceed the average number of wins per control patient by 1 when there are 5 patients per treatment group.

To construct a CI for the NNT we can use the range-preserving CI $[\hat{\kappa}^L, \hat{\kappa}^U]$ for the win odds (see (A12)) and directly apply the transformation $\pi(x) = \frac{x+1}{x-1}$, and it provides the following CI in (A15).

$$[LL1_{NNT}, UL1_{NNT}] = \left[\frac{\hat{\kappa}^U + 1}{\hat{\kappa}^U - 1}, \frac{\hat{\kappa}^L + 1}{\hat{\kappa}^L - 1}\right]. \tag{A15}$$

On the other hand, from the standard error SE of the win proportion $\hat{\theta}_N$ (see (A7)) and application of the δ-method (Van der Vaart 2000), a CI for the NNT can be constructed.

Indeed, consider the transformation $g(v) = \log(v - 1)$. Applying the δ-method, we will find the standard error of the estimator $\log(NNT - 1)$ to equal $SE = \dfrac{NNT}{1 - \hat{\theta}_N}$, and the CI for the NNT in (A16) is based on this result.

$$[LL2_{NNT}, UL2_{NNT}] =$$
$$= \left[(NNT - 1) \cdot e^{-Z_{1-\frac{\alpha}{2}} \cdot SE \cdot \frac{NNT}{1-\theta_N}} + 1, (NNT - 1) \cdot e^{Z_{1-\frac{\alpha}{2}} \cdot SE \cdot \frac{NNT}{1-\theta_N}} + 1 \right]. \tag{A16}$$

To illustrate the coverage properties of the CI for the NNT Gasparyan et al. (2021b) conducted a simulation study using categorization of variables from Beta distributions (see Example 2.5). The CI (A16) for the NNT based on the δ-method had better coverage than the direct CI (A15) of the NNT and therefore should be preferred. The CI for NNT based on the δ-method, while very useful and informative, should be used with caution, since its coverage probability can be lower than 95%, especially for small sample sizes or large treatment effects (higher values of WO).

A.3 Hypothesis Testing

The null hypothesis of no treatment effect for the win odds κ (see (3)) can be written as

$$\mathcal{H}_0: \quad \kappa = 1, \tag{A17}$$

while the two-sided alternative hypothesis of $\kappa \neq 1$ means that the distributions of the two random variables are shifted. In this regard, $\kappa > 1$ means that the distribution of the random variable η is shifted to the right compared to the distribution of the random variable ξ, and so it has "wins" with greater values with a higher probability, under the assumption that higher values mean better outcomes. The null hypothesis (A17) is equivalent to the null hypothesis in (A18) for the win probability θ (see (2)).

$$\mathcal{H}_0': \quad \theta = 0.5. \tag{A18}$$

With the formula from (A7) for the Z-statistic, an asymptotic test of level $\alpha \in (0, 1)$ for the hypothesis (A17) (equivalently, the hypothesis (A18)) is shown in (A19).

$$\psi_\alpha = \mathbb{I}\left\{ \left| \frac{\hat{\theta}_N - \theta_0}{SE} \right| \geq Z_{1-\frac{\alpha}{2}} \right\} \tag{A19}$$

Here $\mathbb{I}(\cdot)$ is the indicator function which equals 1 if $(\cdot)$ is true and equals 0 if $(\cdot)$ is not true; also $Z_{1-\frac{\alpha}{2}}$ is the $\left(1 - \dfrac{\alpha}{2}\right)$-quantile of the standard normal distribution and $\theta_0 = 0.5$. The standard error can be estimated with the formula (A7), (A8).

A.4 Power and Sample Size Calculation

Since the statistical test (A19) uses the standard error (SE) of the win proportion $\hat{\theta}_N$, it is applicable also under the alternative hypothesis $\theta \neq \theta_0 = 0.5$ for calculating the power of that test. For a given alternative θ, the power of the win proportion test will be

$$\pi_\theta\left(\psi_\alpha\right) = P_\theta\left(\left|\frac{\hat{\theta}_N - \theta_0}{SE}\right| \geq Z_{1-\frac{\alpha}{2}}\right) \approx \Phi\left(-Z_{1-\frac{\alpha}{2}} - \frac{\theta - \theta_0}{SE}\right) + \Phi\left(-Z_{1-\frac{\alpha}{2}} + \frac{\theta - \theta_0}{SE}\right), \qquad \text{(A20)}$$

where $\Phi(\cdot)$ is the cumulative distribution function of the standard normal distribution, and $Z_{1-\frac{\alpha}{2}}$ is the $\left(1 - \frac{\alpha}{2}\right)$-quantile of that distribution so that the test asymptotically has significance level α under $\mathcal{H}_0$ in (A17).

In the parametric case, the distribution functions of random variables η and ξ are assumed to belong to a family of distributions, and the following convergence can be used to derive tests:

If $\frac{n_1}{N} \to \gamma$, as $n_1 \to +\infty$, $n_2 \to +\infty$, then the win proportion is also asymptotically normal (Bebu and Lachin 2016, Van der Vaart (2000)):

$$\sqrt{N}\left(\hat{\theta}_N - \theta\right) \Rightarrow \mathcal{N}\left(0, \frac{1}{1-\gamma}\sigma_{10}^2 + \frac{1}{\gamma}\sigma_{01}^2\right).$$

Here,

$$\sigma_{10}^2 = \mathbb{C}ov\left(\mathbb{1}(\xi < \eta),\, \mathbb{1}(\xi' < \eta)\right) = \mathbf{P}(\xi < \eta, \xi' < \eta) - \mathbf{P}(\xi < \eta)^2,$$

$$\sigma_{01}^2 = \mathbb{C}ov\left(\mathbb{1}(\xi < \eta),\, \mathbb{1}(\xi < \eta')\right) = \mathbf{P}(\xi < \eta, \xi < \eta') - \mathbf{P}(\xi < \eta)^2,$$

where ξ' has the same distribution as ξ, η' has the same distribution as η. All ξ, ξ', η, η' are independent.

Therefore, if the distributions of random variables ξ and η are known, the formulas above can be used to calculate the asymptotic variance of the win proportion and hence the power of the win proportion test. We will next provide sample size and power calculation formulas when the distribution functions are unknown.

For the design of a new study for an HCE with analysis by a win odds, the formula (A20) can be used to calculate the sample size for a given power and a given alternative, without any distributional assumptions, and it is also applicable if the standard error SE of the win proportion is known from previous studies. Here we describe how the value for the standard error SE can be determined. Consider the case of no ties (the distributions of ξ and η are continuous). Under the rank sum null hypothesis and balanced allocation of treatment ($n_1 = n_2 = N/2$), the Wilcoxon statistic (see (A48), which is further described in Section A.7.4) can be written as (see also Kawaguchi, Koch, and Wang (2011a))

$$Z^W = \sqrt{N}\sqrt{\frac{N}{\sqrt{N}+1}}\frac{\left(\hat{\theta}_N - 0.5\right)}{1/\sqrt{3}}.$$

Therefore,

$$\sqrt{N}\left(\hat{\theta}_N - 0.5\right) \Rightarrow \mathcal{N}\left(0, \frac{1}{3}\right). \qquad \text{(A21)}$$

The result in (A21) means that the asymptotic variance of the win proportion is $1/3$, under the null hypothesis, when there are no ties and for balanced allocation of treatments.

Under the alternative hypothesis, the asymptotic variance will be smaller. The same is true in the presence of ties since a large amount of ties will decrease the asymptotic variance. Therefore, the value of $1/\sqrt{3}$ is an upper bound for the standard deviation, and it can be used in the majority of cases since it is data independent. Particularly, it can be used for sample size calculations. Formula (A20), using $SE = SD/\sqrt{N} = 1/\sqrt{3N}$, provides

$$
\begin{aligned}
\pi_\theta(\psi_\alpha) &\approx \Phi\left(-Z_{1-\frac{\alpha}{2}} - \frac{\sqrt{N}}{SD}(\theta-\theta_0)\right) + \Phi\left(-Z_{1-\frac{\alpha}{2}} + \frac{\sqrt{N}}{SD}(\theta-\theta_0)\right) \\
&= \Phi\left(-Z_{1-\frac{\alpha}{2}} - \sqrt{3N}(\theta-\theta_0)\right) + \Phi\left(-Z_{1-\frac{\alpha}{2}} + \sqrt{3N}(\theta-\theta_0)\right).
\end{aligned}
\tag{A22}
$$

Formula (A22) can be used to calculate the sample size N for given power π_0.

$$
N = SD^2 \frac{\left(Z_{1-\frac{\alpha}{2}} - Z_{1-\pi_0}\right)^2}{(\theta-\theta_0)^2} = \frac{1}{3}\frac{\left(Z_{1-\frac{\alpha}{2}} - Z_{1-\pi_0}\right)^2}{(\theta-\theta_0)^2},
\tag{A23}
$$

where $Z_{1-\frac{\alpha}{2}}$ and $Z_{1-\pi_0}$ are the $\left(1-\frac{\alpha}{2}\right)$ and $(1-\pi_0)$-quantile of the standard normal distribution, respectively. For example, if a new study is designed to detect a win odds of $\kappa = 1.25$, which corresponds to a win probability of

$$
\theta = \frac{\kappa}{\kappa+1} = \frac{1}{1/\kappa+1} = 0.5556
$$

with 90% power ($\pi_0 = 0.9$) and two-sided $\alpha = 0.05$, then the required sample size is $N = 1135$ (see Table A.2), which corresponds to about 570 per treatment group with balanced allocation. Figure A.1 shows the dependence of the win odds test power on the sample size for the win odds values $\kappa = 1.15, 1.2, 1.25, 1.3$.

Moreover, for a given sample size, it is possible to calculate the minimum detectable win odds value using the formula (A23). Indeed, the minimum detectable treatment effect corresponds to 50% power ($\pi_0 = 0.5$), and thereby $Z_{1-\pi_0} = 0$ and

$$
\theta = \theta_0 + \frac{Z_{1-\frac{\alpha}{2}}}{\sqrt{3N}} = 0.5 + \frac{Z_{1-\frac{\alpha}{2}}}{\sqrt{3N}}.
\tag{A24}
$$

TABLE A.2

Sample size based on the win odds test, alpha = 0.05.

Win Odds	Win Probability	Power = 80%	Power = 90%
1.10	0.5238	4616	6179
1.15	0.5349	2151	2879
1.20	0.5455	1267	1696
1.25	0.5556	848	1135
1.30	0.5652	616	824
1.35	0.5745	472	632
1.40	0.5833	377	505
1.45	0.5918	311	416
1.50	0.6000	262	351

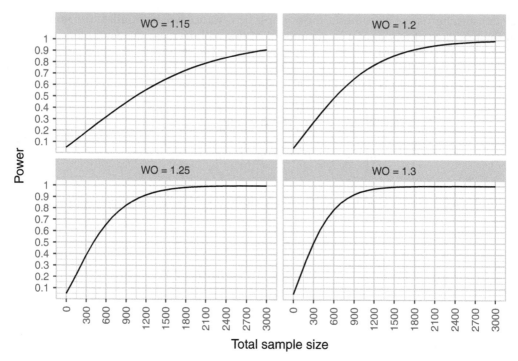

FIGURE A.1

Win odds test power as a function of sample size, for the win odds values 1.15, 1.2, 1.25, 1.3.

TABLE A.3

Minimum detectable win odds for a given sample size.

Sample Size	Win Odds	Win Probability
100	1.59	0.6132
500	1.23	0.5506
1000	1.15	0.5358
1250	1.14	0.5320
1500	1.12	0.5292
2000	1.11	0.5253
3000	1.09	0.5207
4000	1.07	0.5179
7200	1.05	0.5133

From (A24), the minimum detectable win odds values are summarized in Table A.3 for a two-sided alpha of 0.05 and the data-independent standard deviation estimate.

The previous formulas (A21), (A22), (A23), (A24) use the data-independent standard deviation estimate. The standard deviation depends on the definition of the endpoint (ordinal scale) and the studied population. If prior study data are available (for example, Phase 2 trial data for the same endpoint in the same disease area), the standard deviation can be estimated based on actual data, instead of a data-independent estimate, and then used to inform the design of a Phase 3 trial.

A.5 Sample Size in the Presence of Ties

Yu and Ganju (Yu and Ganju 2022) have presented a straightforward sample size formula for a *win ratio* endpoint. This formula relies on an asymptotic variance estimate of the win ratio estimate

$$Var(\ln(WR)) \approx \frac{\sigma^2}{N} = \frac{1}{N} \frac{4(1 + p_{ties})}{3k(1-k)(1-p_{ties})}, \tag{A25}$$

where k denotes the proportion of patients allocated to one group. It has the following form:

$$N \approx \frac{\sigma^2 (Z_{1-\alpha} + Z_{1-\beta})^2}{[\ln(WR)]^2}, \tag{A26}$$

where α refers to the one-sided significance level (type I error rate), β refers to the type II error rate, and Z refers to the quantile value from the standard normal distribution. First note that this formula implicitly assumes that the null hypothesis is $WR = 1$. Second, from formula (1) we see that the proportion of ties p_{ties} in (A25) can be calculated if both WR and WO are given, and so

$$Pties = 1 - (WR + 1) \frac{2WP - 1}{WR - 1}$$

where $WP = \dfrac{WO}{WO + 1}$ is the win proportion $\left(WO = \dfrac{WP}{1 - WP} \right)$.

In Gasparyan, Kowalewski, and Koch (2022) a generalization of the formula (A23) has been provided for nonbalanced randomization and the presence of ties. Additionally, the generalized sample size calculation formula for win odds has been compared to the sample size formula (A26) for the win ratio. Both are general formulas that can incorporate unbalanced randomization and ties. In the case of no ties, $WO = WR$ and both formulas produce similar results. The main difference between these formulas is how the alternative hypothesis is formulated (such as in terms of a win odds or a win ratio). The following examples are from Gasparyan, Kowalewski, and Koch (2022).

Both methods rely on the theory of U-statistics for deriving their results. For comparison of these formulas, the same notation as in (Yu and Ganju 2022) is used. For the case of 1:1 randomization with $k = 0.5$, the formula (A23) can be rewritten as

$$N \approx Var(WP) \frac{(Z_{1-\alpha} + Z_{1-\beta})^2}{[WO/(WO+1) - 0.5]^2} = \frac{4}{3} \frac{(Z_{1-\alpha} + Z_{1-\beta})^2}{[(WO-1)/(WO+1)]^2}. \tag{A27}$$

Here, $Var(WP)$ is the asymptotic variance of $WP = WO/(WO + 1)$ or the win proportion (total number of comparisons resulting in a win for active group, plus half of the total number of ties divided by the product of sample sizes).

With $k = 0.5$ and (for now) taking also $p_{ties} = 0$ in (A25) we can transform the formula (A26) as follows:

$$N \approx \frac{16}{3} \frac{\left(Z_{1-\alpha}+Z_{1-\beta}\right)^2}{[\ln(WR)]^2}. \tag{A28}$$

Example A.1 (Continuous distributions). In the case of continuous distributions (when there are no ties), the win odds and the win ratio are the same, and so the formulas (A27) and (A28) differ only by denominators $(WO-1)/(WO+1)$ and $\ln(WO)/2$. The former is always less than the latter, and so the formula (A28) will provide a smaller sample size, which could be an advantage. The difference between these two quantities increases as WO moves away from 1, but for $WO = 2$, it is 1/3 versus 0.347, or a 4% increase in sample size (if the formula (A27) is used instead of formula (A28)). Therefore, the increase in sample size with (A28) relative to (A27) will be even less than this for WO values lower than 2 (for the case of absence of ties).

It should be noted that (A27) can be generalized to include unbalanced randomization and ties. The asymptotic variance of the win proportion $Var(WP) = 1/3$ used in the formula (A27) is derived from the *Wilcoxon-Mann-Whitney U-test* for the case with no ties (see Section 5.3 in Gasparyan et al. (2021b)). Suppose that ordinal values of two treatment groups are ranked (with ties managed with the average method which corresponds to considering ties as half wins) and W denotes the sum of all ranks in the active group (the *Wilcoxon rank sum statistic*). Then, the following formula can be used to construct the asymptotic test for the win proportion (Gasparyan et al. 2021b):

$$Z^W = \frac{k(1-k)N^2(WP-0.5)}{\sqrt{Var(W)}}$$

In this regard, Woolson and Clarke (2011) provide a formula for the variance of the *Wilcoxon rank sum statistic* in the presence of ties.

$$Var(W) = \frac{k(1-k)}{12}N^2(N+1)\left[1-\frac{1}{N(N^2-1)}\sum_{i=1}^{s}t_i(t_i^2-1)\right].$$

Here $1, \ldots, s$ denote unique values with ties from the sample size of N, while t_i is the total number of tied values (both groups combined) to the value i. Therefore, the squared standard error of the win proportion will be

$$SE(WP)^2 \approx \frac{1}{N}\frac{1}{12k(1-k)}\left[1-\sum_{i=1}^{s}\left(\frac{t_i}{N}\right)^3\right].$$

We see again that in the case of no ties ($s = N$), $N * SE(WP)^2$ has the limit

$$\frac{1}{12k(1-k)},$$

which, in the case of 1:1 randomization, produces the value for the asymptotic variance 1/3 described in (A23) (Gasparyan et al. 2021b). For example, for 2:1 randomization, the asymptotic variance would be 3/8 (see Table A4 for sample size calculation for a 2:1 randomization via (A29) with $k = 2/3$ and $Coef = 1.0$).

TABLE A.4

Sample size based on the win odds test, 2:1 randomization.

Win Odds	Win Probability	Power = 80%	Power = 90%
1.10	0.5238	5193	6951
1.15	0.5349	2419	3239
1.20	0.5455	1425	1908
1.25	0.5556	954	1277
1.30	0.5652	693	927
1.35	0.5745	531	711
1.40	0.5833	424	568
1.45	0.5918	349	468
1.50	0.6000	295	395

Using this formula for $SE(WP)$, the sample size formula (A23) (or (A27)) can be updated as follows:

$$N \approx \frac{1}{3k(1-k)}\left[1 - \sum_{i=1}^{s}\left(\frac{t_i}{N}\right)^3\right]\frac{\left(Z_{1-\alpha} + Z_{1-\beta}\right)^2}{[(WO-1)/(WO+1)]^2}. \tag{A29}$$

Here t_i/N is the proportion of values i in the total sample size N, which more easily can be used than the proportion p_{tie} of ties in the pairwise comparisons. The coefficient $Coef = 1 - \sum_{i=1}^{s}\left(\frac{t_i}{N}\right)^3$ is close to 1 in cases where s is large and $Coef = 1$ can still be used as a conservative value to avoid the risk of underpowered trials.

Example A.2 (Case with 50% ties). If it is expected that one of the categories will have approximately 50% of the distribution (i.e., $(t_i/N) = 0.5$), then

$$Coef \approx 1 - 0.5^3 = 0.875,$$

the sample size (A27) can be decreased by at least 12.5%. In the case of 50% ties the formula (A28) will be multiplied by 3 via (A26), while if the ties increase to 80% the multiplicative factor will become 9. The formula (A27) is affected by ties through the definition of WO since it includes ties as half wins (the WO will be closer to 1 in the presence of more ties and hence a larger sample size would be required).

Consider the following example of a clinical trial comparing two treatments for an ordinal outcome. Suppose that 30% of pairwise comparisons resulted in a win for the active treatment, 20% resulted in a loss, and 50% in ties. In this case, the win ratio is $WR = 1.5$, while the win odds is $WO = 1.222$. Suppose a new trial with 1:1 randomization allocation is to be conducted to detect, with 90% power, the same treatment effect. The sample size formula (A28) (multiplied by 3 because of 50% ties) provides a sample size of approximately 1020 (two groups combined). The formula (A27) provides a sample size of approximately 1400 (since the formula (A27) is conservative, particularly with respect to the extent of ties). Note that the formula (A29) mitigates this problem by allowing the reduction of sample size in the case where the extent of ties for each value can be estimated in advance. Multiplying the sample size estimate of 1400 from (A27) by 0.875 will produce a sample size of 1225.

The formula (A29) seems to have the disadvantage of being more conservative since it produces a larger sample size, but that's because *WR* in the case of a substantial amount of ties can exaggerate the degree of dissimilarity of two distributions that are being compared (see Brunner, Vandemeulebroecke, and Mütze 2021). However, the formula (A29) uses *WO* in the calculations and its use can be a more reasonable way of comparing two distributions. Therefore, the main difference between the two formulas (A26) and (A29) is how the alternative hypothesis is formulated (in terms of *WR* or *WO*).

Example A.3 (Trichotomous). Consider two trichotomous distributions which take values 1, 2, 3 (a higher value signifying a favorable outcome). Suppose that the observed proportions in the control group are $p_1 = 0.07$, $p_2 = 0.9$, $p_3 = 0.03$, while in the active group the proportions are $p_1 = 0.03$, $p_2 = 0.9$, $p_3 = 0.07$. These specifications imply 13.09% wins for the active treatment, 81.42% ties, and 5.49% losses. The win ratio is $WR = 2.3843$, while the win odds is $WO = 1.1645$. In this case $t_1 = 0.05N$, $t_2 = 0.9N$, $t_3 = 0.05N$; therefore for 90% power at one-sided $\alpha = 0.025$, the formula (A26) provides a sample size of 725, while the formula (A29) provides the sample size of 657.

A.6 Adjusted and Stratified Win Odds

The theory of analysis of covariance of ordered categorical data for randomized studies is extensively formulated in Koch et al. (1982); Koch et al. (1990); Koch et al. (1998a); and Kawaguchi, Koch, and Wang (2011b) (see also Kawaguchi and Koch (2015b)). Below we present the stratification and adjustment of win odds according to Gasparyan et al. (2021a).

A.6.1 Stratified Win Odds

In the stratified analysis, we suppose that each treatment group is divided into two separate subgroups, called strata (we are considering only the case of two strata). The measurements of subjects in different strata have different distributions, even inside the same treatment group. Therefore the model assumes that the measurements of each treatment group are characterized by two random variables each (here as before, η denotes the active group, whereas ξ denotes the control group).

$$(\xi, \xi'), (\eta, \eta').$$

The numbers of observations in each treatment group by strata are given in Table A.5. For each stratum, the win probability is defined as

$$\theta = \mathbf{P}(\eta > \xi) + 0.5\mathbf{P}(\eta = \xi) \text{ and } \theta' = \mathbf{P}(\eta' > \xi') + 0.5\mathbf{P}(\eta' = \xi')$$

The stratified win probability is defined as

$$\theta^{str} = \omega\theta + (1 - \omega)\theta', \omega \in (0,1).$$

TABLE A.5

Numbers of observations in each treatment group by strata.

	Strata I	Strata II
Active	n_{A1}	n_{A2}
control	n_{P1}	n_{P2}

Instead of the weights, we will sometimes specify only the coefficients ω_1, ω_2 per stratum, and the weights can be calculated using the formula

$$\omega = \frac{\omega_1}{\omega_1 + \omega_2}, 1 - \omega = \frac{\omega_2}{\omega_1 + \omega_2}.$$

For each stratum separately, we can construct the win proportions (A4), denoted correspondingly by $\hat{\theta}_N$ and $\hat{\theta}'_N$. A general method of combining these estimates is to use the weighted sum of the estimates in each stratum as

$$\hat{\theta}_N^{str} = \omega \hat{\theta}_N + (1 - \omega)\hat{\theta}'_N. \tag{A30}$$

The variance of the stratified estimator can be calculated using the formula (since observations in different strata are independent)

$$var\left(\hat{\theta}_N^{str}\right) = \omega^2 var\left(\hat{\theta}_N\right) + (1 - \omega)^2 var\left(\hat{\theta}'_N\right). \tag{A31}$$

The variances of the win proportions inside each stratum can be estimated with (A7).

$$var\left(\hat{\theta}_N\right) = SE^2 \text{ and } var\left(\hat{\theta}'_N\right) = SE'^2$$

The weights can be estimated with the *Mantel-Haenszel* weights (Mantel and Haenszel (1959), see also Appendix II in Koch et al. (1998b); Agresti (2013)), where the coefficients are defined as

$$w_1 = \frac{n_{A1}n_{P1}}{n_1}, w_2 = \frac{n_{A2}n_{P2}}{n_2}. \tag{A32}$$

Here we have denoted the total number of observations in each stratum by

$$n_1 = n_{A1} + n_{P1}, \quad n_2 = n_{A2} + n_{P2}.$$

This will give the following estimates of the weights:

$$w = \frac{\dfrac{1}{n_{A2}} + \dfrac{1}{n_{P2}}}{\dfrac{1}{n_{A1}} + \dfrac{1}{n_{A2}} + \dfrac{1}{n_{P1}} + \dfrac{1}{n_{P2}}}, \quad 1 - w = \frac{\dfrac{1}{n_{A1}} + \dfrac{1}{n_{P1}}}{\dfrac{1}{n_{A1}} + \dfrac{1}{n_{A2}} + \dfrac{1}{n_{P1}} + \dfrac{1}{n_{P2}}}.$$

Note that the weight estimate w for the first stratum uses the reciprocals of numbers of observations in the second stratum.

If a balanced design between the treatment groups and the strata is applicable, that is, $n_{A1} = n_{A2} = n_{P1} = n_{P2}$, then both weights would be 0.5, and so the stratified win proportion would be just the average win proportion of the two strata. While in the case of the treatment groups having the same proportion in both strata,

$$n_{A1} = np_1 = \frac{n_1}{2}, \ n_{A2} = np_2 - \frac{n_2}{2},$$

that is, only balanced allocation of treatments within a stratum is present (for a stratified randomization), but one stratum may have larger sample size than the other, then $w = \dfrac{n_1}{n_1 + n_2}$, the larger stratum will get larger weight.

Another possible choice of coefficients is

$$w_1^0 = \frac{n_{A1} n_{P1}}{n_1 + 1}, \quad w_2^0 = \frac{n_{A2} n_{P2}}{n_2 + 1}, \tag{A33}$$

which corresponds to the *van Elteren* weights (Van Elteren 1960).

The standard error (A31) can be used to construct an asymptotic confidence interval for a given significance level for the stratified win odds (A30), either with (A32) or (A33) for the weights. The formulas (A30), (A31) can be easily extended for the case of $m > 2$ strata. Indeed, the stratified win proportion in this case can be estimated using the formula (A34)

$$\hat{\theta}_N^{str} = \sum_{j=1}^{m} \frac{w_j}{w} \hat{\theta}_N^{(j)}, \quad w_j = \frac{n_{Aj} n_{Pj}}{n_{Aj} + n_{Pj}}, w = \sum_{j=1}^{m} w_j. \tag{A34}$$

While the standard error of the stratified win proportion can be calculated with the formula (A35)

$$\left(SE^{str} \right)^2 = \sum_{j=1}^{m} \frac{w_j^2}{w^2} \left(SE^{(j)} \right)^2. \tag{A35}$$

Here $\hat{\theta}_N^{(j)}$ is the win proportion in the stratum j, while $SE^{(j)}$ is its standard error.

A.6.2 Adjusted Win Odds

In the case that a numeric covariate is available at randomization, the win odds may be adjusted by this covariate. Suppose we observe ordinal analysis values from two treatment groups with associated numeric baseline covariates

$$(Y, Y^*), \ (X, X^*), \tag{A36}$$

where Y, X are the ordinal values for the active and control groups correspondingly (see (A1)) with their numeric baseline covariates defined as

$$Y^* = \left(Y_1^*, \cdots, Y_{n_2}^* \right), X^* = \left(X_1^*, \cdots, X_{n_1}^* \right).$$

Here again using the formulas (A3), we can replace the ordinal samples (A36) with the samples of individual win proportions

$$\left(Y^0, Y^* \right), \left(X^0, X^* \right),$$

where the individual proportions p_j and q_i are calculated with the formulas (A2), without taking into consideration the values of the covariates. Consider the mean values, the variances of the response variables and covariates, as well as the covariances between the response variables and covariates

$$\bar{X}^* = \frac{1}{n_1}\sum_{i=1}^{n_1} X_i^*, \quad \bar{Y}^* = \frac{1}{n_2}\sum_{j=1}^{n_2} Y_j^*,$$

$$var\left(X^*\right) = \frac{1}{n_1}\sum_{i=1}^{n_1}\left(X_i^* - \bar{X}^*\right)^2, \quad var\left(Y^*\right) = \frac{1}{n_2}\sum_{j=1}^{n_2}\left(Y_j^* - \bar{Y}^*\right)^2,$$

$$\mathbb{C}ov\left(X^0, X^*\right) = \frac{1}{n_1}\sum_{i=1}^{n_1}\left(q_i - \left(1 - \hat{\theta}_N\right)\right)\left(X_i^* - \bar{X}^*\right),$$

$$\mathbb{C}ov\left(Y^0, Y^*\right) = \frac{1}{n_2}\sum_{j=1}^{n_2}\left(p_j - \hat{\theta}_N\right)\left(Y_j^* - \bar{Y}^*\right), \tag{A37}$$

Then, the *adjusted win proportion* can be defined as

$$\hat{\beta}_N = \hat{\theta}_N - \frac{\bar{Y}^* - \bar{X}^*}{\dfrac{var\left(Y^*\right)}{n_2} + \dfrac{var\left(X^*\right)}{n_1}}\left[\frac{\mathbb{C}ov\left(Y^0, Y^*\right)}{n_2} + \frac{\mathbb{C}ov\left(X^0, X^*\right)}{n_1}\right]. \tag{A38}$$

This estimator provides the win proportion of the active group against the control group adjusted for the mean difference in covariates (Koch et al. 1998b; Gasparyan et al. 2021a). The adjustment for covariates provides more powerful tests for the treatment comparison through the variance reduction. It also accounts for possible random group differences in covariate values so that the observed treatment effect is not driven by the random difference in covariates.

The asymptotic variance of this estimator can be calculated as follows:

$$SE_{\beta}^2 = \frac{var\left(Y^0\right)}{n_2} + \frac{var\left(X^0\right)}{n_1} - \frac{\left[\dfrac{\mathbb{C}ov\left(Y^0, Y^*\right)}{n_2} + \dfrac{\mathbb{C}ov\left(X^0, X^*\right)}{n_1}\right]^2}{\dfrac{var\left(Y^*\right)}{n_2} + \dfrac{var\left(X^*\right)}{n_1}}. \tag{A39}$$

Here the variances $var(Y^0)$ and $var(X^0)$ are estimated using the formulas (A8). The adjusted win odds and its confidence interval can be calculated using the formulas (A11), (A12)

$$\hat{k}_N^{\beta} = \frac{\hat{\beta}_N}{1 - \hat{\beta}_N} \in \left[\hat{k}_N^{\beta} \cdot e^{-Z_{1-\frac{\alpha}{2}} \cdot \frac{SE_{\beta}}{\hat{\beta}_N\left(1-\hat{\beta}_N\right)}}, \hat{k}_N^{\beta} \cdot e^{Z_{1-\frac{\alpha}{2}} \cdot \frac{SE_{\beta}}{\hat{\beta}_N\left(1-\hat{\beta}_N\right)}}\right].$$

This result is applicable to any numeric covariate including dummy covariates with the values 0 and 1. The method can be extended to the case of ordinal covariates by replacing the mean difference $\left(\bar{Y}^* - \bar{X}^*\right)$ by a win proportion minus 0.5, where the win proportion is defined by pairwise comparisons of the values of covariates.

A.6.3 Stratified Win Odds with Adjustment

Here we will describe how to estimate the win odds in the presence of stratified analysis and with adjustment by a numeric covariate (Koch et al. 1998b). *Stratified win odds with (stratified) adjustment* first calculates the stratified win odds and then adjusts for a covariate that is stratified as well. For the rank ANCOVA (analysis of covariance) (Quade 1967), there is first adjustment for the ranks using the continuous covariate followed by the stratified analysis on residuals. This consideration is essentially the main difference in hypothesis testing between rank ANCOVA and stratified win odds with adjustment as explained in Gasparyan et al. (2021a).

Similar to (A34) if there are $j = 1, \ldots, m$ strata, then we can calculate the stratified win odds with adjustment using the given weights $\dfrac{w_j}{w}$

$$\hat{\beta}_N^{str} = \sum_{j=1}^{m} \frac{w_j}{w} \hat{\theta}_N^j -$$
$$- \frac{\sum_{j=1}^{m} \frac{w_j}{w} \left(\bar{Y}^* - \bar{X}^* \right)_j}{\sum_{j=1}^{m} \frac{w_j^2}{w^2} \left(\frac{var\left(Y^*\right)}{n_2} + \frac{var\left(X^*\right)}{n_1} \right)_j} \left[\sum_{j=1}^{m} \frac{w_j^2}{w^2} \left(\frac{\mathbb{C}ov\left(Y^0, Y^*\right)}{n_2} + \frac{\mathbb{C}ov\left(X^0, X^*\right)}{n_1} \right) \right]_j. \quad (A40)$$

The standard error of this win odds can be calculated as follows:

$$\left(SE_\beta^{str}\right)^2 = \sum_{j=1}^{m} \frac{w_j^2}{w^2} \left(SE^{(j)}\right)^2 - \frac{\left[\sum_{j=1}^{m} \frac{w_j^2}{w^2} \left(\frac{\mathbb{C}ov\left(Y^0, Y^*\right)}{n_2} + \frac{\mathbb{C}ov\left(X^0, X^*\right)}{n_1} \right) \right]_j^2}{\sum_{j=1}^{m} \frac{w_j^2}{w^2} \left(\frac{var\left(Y^*\right)}{n_2} + \frac{var\left(X^*\right)}{n_1} \right)_j}. \quad (A41)$$

Here all calculations are done in each stratum separately. $SE^{(j)}$ is the standard error of the nonadjusted win proportion in the stratum j. The *stratified win odds with adjustment* and its confidence interval can be calculated as follows:

$$\hat{k}_\beta^{str} = \frac{\hat{\beta}_N^{str}}{1 - \hat{\beta}_N^{str}} \in \left[\hat{k}_\beta^{str} \cdot e^{-Z_{1-\frac{\alpha}{2}} \cdot \frac{SE_\beta^{str}}{\hat{\beta}_N^{str}\left(1-\hat{\beta}_N^{str}\right)}}, \hat{k}_\beta^{str} \cdot e^{Z_{1-\frac{\alpha}{2}} \cdot \frac{SE_\beta^{str}}{\hat{\beta}_\beta^{str}\left(1-\hat{\beta}_\beta^{str}\right)}} \right].$$

A.7 Statistics Related to Win Odds

A.7.1 Placements and the Fligner-Policello Test

In Gasparyan et al. (2021a), the statistic from the *Fligner-Policello (FP)* (Fligner and Policello 1981) test was used to construct the *FP* confidence interval for the win proportion. This confidence interval will correspond to the hypothesis test based on the *FP* test. Moreover, the *FP* confidence interval is related to the confidence interval based on the theory of *U*-statistics, from equations (A7) and (A8). This means that software where the *FP* test is implemented, e.g., proc npar1way in SAS, can provide the win odds confidence interval by utilizing this relationship. We will provide the SAS software implementation in Section A.8.2.2 for the FP confidence interval for WP.

The statistics $n_1 p_j$ and $n_2 q_i$, which are the number of wins for patients in active and control groups, respectively (see (A3)), are called *placements*. If we denote the vectors of placements by

$$y = \left(n_1 p_1, \cdots, n_1 p_{n_2}\right) \text{ and } x = \left(n_2 q_1, \cdots, n_2 q_{n_1}\right), \tag{A42}$$

then the Fligner-Policello *(FP)* statistic is

$$Z_N^0 = \frac{SUM_y - SUM_x}{2\sqrt{Std_x^2 \left(n_x - 1\right) + Std_y^2 \left(n_y - 1\right) + MEAN_x MEAN_y}}. \tag{A43}$$

In (A43), *SUM* denotes the sum and *MEAN* denotes the mean for the corresponding placements in the two treatment groups; the *Std* are the consistent estimators of standard errors for placements and $n_x = n_1$ and $n_y = n_2$. As was shown in (Gasparyan et al. 2021a), this statistic can be expressed in terms of the win proportion (equation (A6)) as

$$Z_N^0 = \frac{\hat{\theta}_N - \frac{1}{2}}{SE_0}, \quad SE_0^2 = SE^2 + \frac{1}{n_1 n_2} \hat{\theta}_N \left(1 - \hat{\theta}_N\right). \tag{A44}$$

Therefore, from the *FP* statistic, it is possible to construct a confidence interval for the win proportion, although it will always be wider than the CI based on the *U*-statistic (since *SE* < SE_0, see (A7), (A8)).

A.7.2 Somers' D C/R and Net Benefit

The win proportion and its asymptotic standard error (based on the theory of *U*-statistics) can also be obtained from *Somers' D C/R* statistic (Σ_D) (Somers 1962) as noted in *Section 4.3.3* and *Section 14.6* of Stokes, Davis, and Koch (2012). Indeed, Σ_D is the difference between the number of concordances and the number of discordances, divided by the overall number of comparisons. Thus, *Somers' D C/R* is the *net benefit*. Therefore,

$$WP = \frac{\Sigma_D + 1}{2}, \quad SE = \frac{ASE}{2}, \tag{A45}$$

where *SE* is the standard error of *WP* based on the theory of *U*-statistics (see (A7),(A8)), while *ASE* is the asymptotic standard error of *Somers' D C/R* statistic. This means that in all software where this statistic is implemented (for example, in proc freq of the SAS software), the win odds and its CI can be derived, as is shown in Section A.8.2.4.

A.7.3 Goodman-Kruskal Gamma and Win Ratio

Here we provide win ratio confidence intervals based on the *Goodman-Kruskal gamma, G* (Kruskal and Goodman 1954), and its standard error. Since

$$G = \frac{C - D}{C + D}$$

where *C* denotes twice the number of concordant pairs of observations and *D* denotes twice the number of discordant pairs of observations (see Section 5.4.1, Stokes, Davis, and

Koch 2012); it follows that $\dfrac{C}{D} = \dfrac{1+G}{1-G}$. When G pertains to the comparison of two groups for an ordinal endpoint, C and D represent wins and losses for the active group relative to the control group, and so the win ratio equals

$$WR = \frac{C}{D} = \frac{wins}{losses} = \frac{1+G}{1-G}$$

Accordingly, the CI for gamma can be transformed into a CI for *WR*. As noted in Carr, Hafner, and Koch (1989), using the transformation $\log\!\left(\dfrac{C}{D}\right)$, we can obtain the standard error of $\log(WR)$, denoted by $SE_{\log(WR)}$, from the standard error of G, denoted by SE_G. The corresponding CI would be range preserving. Indeed, applying the δ-method, we obtain the standard error of the $\log(WR)$ by the following formula:

$$SE_{\log(WR)} = \frac{2}{WR(1-G)^2}SE_G = \frac{(WR+1)^2}{2WR}SE_G.$$

And the confidence interval for the win ratio can be calculated as follows:

$$\left[WR\cdot e^{-Z_{1-\frac{\alpha}{2}}SE_{\log(WR)}}, WR\cdot e^{Z_{1-\frac{\alpha}{2}}SE_{\log(WR)}} \right].$$
(A46)

This result means that in all software that provide G and SE_G (for example, using the `measures` option in `proc freq` of the SAS software), the win ratio and its CI can be derived. The standard error of the G can be calculated as follows:

$$SE_G^2 = \frac{16}{(C+D)^4}\sum_i \sum_j n_{ij}\left(C_{ij}D - D_{ij}C\right)^2.$$

Here i denotes the treatment group, while j denotes the unique ordinal values in the overall population. C is twice the number of total concordances for the active group and D is twice the number of discordances for the active group, together with C_{ij} and D_{ij} as the corresponding numbers for the unique j value in the treatment group i.

Note that Yu and Ganju (2022) have provided a simple formula (A25) approximating the standard error of the logarithm of the win ratio, and it uses only the proportion of ties in all pairwise comparisons. This formula also can be used to construct an asymptotic confidence interval for the win ratio.

A.7.4 Relationship to the Wilcoxon Rank Sum Test

Gasparyan et al. (2021a) also explored the relationship of the Wilcoxon rank sum test and the test based on (A7). Both statistics test the null hypothesis of equality of the distributions of ξ and η, and in terms of the win probability (2), it implies $\theta = 0.5$. Hence, the win proportion test can be used instead of the Wilcoxon rank sum test since the former also provides an estimate and confidence interval associated with the test. The Z statistic from the Wilcoxon rank sum test is

$$Z^W = \frac{\sum_{j=1}^{n_2} R_{2j} - n_2 \bar{R}}{\sqrt{\frac{n_1 n_2}{N} var(R)}}, \tag{A47}$$

where $\bar{R}$ is the average and $var(R)$ is the variance of the combined sample of ranks, under the null hypothesis of equality of distributions (all possible assignments of ranks to the two groups are equally likely). With $n_2 \bar{R} = \frac{n_2(N+1)}{2}$ applied, and denoting $W = \sum_{j=1}^{n_2} R_{2j}$, we obtain from (A47) the following expression

$$Z^W = \frac{W - \frac{n_2(N+1)}{2}}{\sqrt{var(W)}} = \frac{n_1 n_2 \left(\hat{\theta}_N - 0.5\right)}{\sqrt{var(W)}}$$

Here $var(W) = \frac{n_1 n_2 (N+1)}{12}$ when there are no ties (Lehmann and D'Abrera 1975); therefore

$$Z^W = \sqrt{\frac{12 n_1 n_2}{N+1}} \left(\hat{\theta}_N - 0.5\right). \tag{A48}$$

Both the Wilcoxon test and the win odds test under the null hypothesis of $\theta = 0.5$ and the absence of ties have the same asymptotic variance (equal to $1/3$ in the case of balanced randomization, see (A21)), but nonasymptotically the standard errors differ (Gasparyan et al. 2021a). Usually, the Wilcoxon rank sum test is used in combination with medians of samples X and Y for a continuous endpoint. The treatment effect is estimated by the Hodges-Lehmann estimator (Lehmann and D'Abrera (1975)), and it is the median of all possible differences of values of X and Y samples. This estimator is only possible to calculate if the observed values are numeric and not ordinal so that the difference of values is defined. For the confidence interval construction methods see Hollander, Wolfe, and Chicken (2013).

A.7.5 Relationship to Ordinal Logistic Regression

In this section, we are considering the proportional odds form of an ordinal logistic regression model (*Chapter 9*, Stokes, Davis, and Koch (2012), Harrell (2015)). Consider the combined sample of two treatment groups

$$Z = (X_1, \cdots, X_{n1}, Y_1, \cdots, Y_{n2}),$$

and denote the sample $J = (J_1, ..., J_N)$, $N = n_1 + n_2$ of values 1 and 0 where 1 corresponds to the values from Y (active treatment) and 0 corresponds to the values from X (control). Since Z takes ordinal values, we can denote levels of these values by $0, 1, 2, ..., k$. Then, the proportionality of odds assumption is stated as follows:

$$P(Z \le j \mid J) = \frac{1}{1 + \exp\left(-\left(\alpha_j + J\beta\right)\right)}, \quad j = 0, \cdots, (k-1). \tag{A49}$$

There are k intercepts (a_j, $j = 1, \ldots, k$), one for each level of the response variable and common coefficients for the treatment effect (β). If we denote the odds of having level less than or equal to j in two groups by

$$Odds(Y, j) = \frac{P(Z \le j \mid J = 1)}{P(Z > j \mid J = 1)}, \quad Odds(X, j) = \frac{P(Z \le j \mid J = 0)}{P(Z > j \mid J = 0)},$$

then, from (A49), we obtain

$$\frac{Odds(Y, j)}{Odds(X, j)} = e^{\beta}, j = 0, \cdots, (k-1). \tag{A50}$$

The "common" odds ratio (A50) corresponds to an odds ratio from a binary logistic regression if we categorize all values less than or equal to j to category 1 and other values to category 2. Therefore, the odds of having values less than or equal to j is assumed to be proportional in the two treatment groups, for all j. This means that the treatment effect is the same regardless of how we categorize ordinal values into binary categories.

The statistical test based on the ordinal logistic regression with one binary covariate is asymptotically equivalent to the Wilcoxon rank sum test and the win odds test (Whitehead 1993). The difference between the methods is that the ordinal logistic regression involves the proportional odds assumption (A49), (A50). Additionally, in the win odds approach, missingness can be managed in a very simple way by considering patients with missing values as tied to every other value in the pairwise comparisons for forming the winner. Accordingly, the win odds method may be better suited for related sensitivity analyses than the proportional odds model, particularly if departures from proportional odds are more evident in sensitivity analyses than analyses with a primary method.

A.8 Software Implementation

Some current limitations for the use of the win odds analysis methods are that the power and sample size calculations for the U-statistic-based win odds test are not straightforward. Furthermore, confidence interval calculation is not implemented in some commonly used statistical software in clinical trials, such as the SAS software (SAS Institute Inc. 2018). We describe the implementation of the win odds analysis in the SAS software through the use of the well-known *Fligner-Policello* test (Fligner and Policello 1981) and *Somers' D C/R* statistic (Section 4.3.3, Stokes, Davis, and Koch 2012). We also describe the package hce (Gasparyan 2022) which provides R software implementation (R Core Team 2022) of the win odds calculations.

A.8.1 Example

To illustrate the software implementation, we use the *resp* dataset available in *Chapter 15 of Categorical data analysis using SAS* (Stokes, Davis, and Koch 2012). The *resp* dataset contains information for 111 patients randomized into two treatment groups – the active group and the control group. As *resp* is a patient-level dataset, each row corresponds to one patient. The patient global ratings of symptom control are measured at visits 1, 2, 3, and 4. The five categories are the following: 4 = excellent, 3 = good, 2 = fair, 1 = poor, 0 = terrible. We will use *visit 4* (which is renamed to *AVAL*, to denote the analysis value) for scores to determine the treatment effect on symptoms.

The null hypothesis is that there is no treatment effect on symptoms at visit 4, that is, $\theta = 0.5$; or equivalently, in terms of the win odds, $\kappa = 1$. The alternative hypothesis can be formulated as $\kappa > 1$; it means that in the active group there is a positive treatment effect on the symptoms at visit 4.

A.8.2 SAS Implementation

Below we define *ID* by enumerating the rows and choose *visit 4* values as analysis values (*AVAL*).

```
data resp;
    set resp;
    ID=_N_;
    AVAL=visit4;
run;
```

A.8.2.1. The Fligner-Policello (FP) test. In this section we will use the relationship (A44) of the win proportion test and the Fligner-Policello test to derive the confidence interval (CI) for the win odds.

The Fligner-Policello test is implemented in proc npar1way. It can be calculated with the following code:

```
proc npar1way data=resp FP;
    class treatment;
    var AVAL;
    ods output FPPlacements=FPPlacements FPTest=FPTest
                             FPBoxPlot=FPBoxPlot;
run;
```

The *FP* option on the procedure statement requests the Fligner-Policello test. The output of this procedure consists of two datasets and a boxplot:

Here we will derive the statistics in the dataset *FPTest*, using the statistics from the dataset *FPPlacements*. As described in the documentation of proc npar1way, the Z statistic of the Fligner-Policello test can be calculated from the formula (A43). The reported difference is the difference of the sums of placements.

$$Diff = SUM_A - SUM_P = 1900.5 - 1177.5 = 723.$$

TABLE A.6

The dataset FPPlacements (Fligner-Policello Placements).

Treatment	N	Sum	Mean	StdDev
A	54	1900.5	35.19444	14.30675
P	57	1177.5	20.65790	15.61511

TABLE A.7

The dataset FPTest (Fligner-Ploicello Test).

Fligner-Policello Test	
Difference (A – P)	723
Statistic (Z)	2.2759
One-Sided p value	0.0114
Two-Sided p value	0.0229

Hence, from (A43) we obtain

$$Z = \frac{1900.5 - 1177.5}{2\sqrt{14.306753^2(54-1) + 15.615113^2(57-1) + 35.194444 * 20.657895}} = 2.275889.$$

And the two-sided p value for the test based on this statistic can be calculated from the following statement:

```
p=2*(1-PROBNORM(2.275889));
```

The two-sided p-value is 0.0229. The dataset *FPPlacements* contains descriptive statistics for the placements (A42), and they can be obtained from the individual win proportions (see (A2)). Given the dataset *FPPlacements* we are able to replicate the results of the dataset *FPTest*. This calculation can be achieved with the following code, which also includes the calculations described in the subsequent discussion.

```
proc iml;
  use FPPlacements;
  varNames = {"N" "Sum" "Mean" "StdDev"};
  read all var varNames into fpA where (Class = "A");
  read all var varNames into fpP where (Class = "P");
  close FPPlacements;
  Z = (fpA[2] - fpP[2]) /
  (2*sqrt((fpP[4]**2)*(fpP[1]-1)
        (fpA[4]**2)*(fpA[1]-1)+(fpP[3]*fpA[3]))));
        p = 2*(1-probnorm(Z)); print Z p;
  WP = (fpA[2] - fpP[2])/(2*fpA[1]*fpP[1])+0.5;
  print WP;
  WP_mean_A = fpA[3]/fpP[1];
  WP_mean_P = 1 - fpP[3]/fpA[1]; print WP mean A WP mean P;
  SE_0 = sqrt(fpA[4]**2*(fpA[1]-1)/(fpA[1]**2*fpP[1]**2)
        + fpP[4]**2*(fpP[1]-1)/(fpA[1]**2*fpP[1]**2)
        +WP*(1-WP)/(fpA[1]*fpP[1])));
  print SE_0;
  Z_N_0 = (WP-0.5)/SE_0;
  print Z_N_0;
  alpha = 0.05;
  C = Probit(1-alpha/2);
  WP_lower = WP - C*SE_0;
```

```
WP upper = WP + C*SE_0;
print WP WP_lower WP_upper;
kappa = WP/(1-WP);
kappa_lower = kappa*exp(-C*SE_0/(WP*(1-WP)));
kappa_upper = kappa*exp(C*SE_0/(WP*(1-WP)));
print kappa kappa lower kappa upper;
SE = sqrt((fpA[4]**2)*(fpA[1]-   1)/((fpA[1]**2)*(fpP[1]**2)) +
           (fpP[4]**2)*(fpP[1]-1)/((fpA[1]**2)*(fpP[1]**2)));
print SE;
WP_lower alt = WP - C*SE;
WP_upper alt = WP + C*SE;
print WP lower_alt;
print WP upper_alt;
Z_N = (WP-0.5)/SE;
print Z_N;
p = 2*(1-probnorm(Z_N));
print p;
kappa_lower_alt = kappa*exp(-C*SE/(WP*(1-WP)));
kappa_upper_alt = kappa*exp(C*SE/(WP*(1-WP)));
print kappa kappa lower alt kappa upper alt;
quit;
```

A.8.2.2. FP confidence interval for WP. Although the *FP* test provides only a *p-value* without an estimate and corresponding confidence interval, (A44) shows that the *FP* test corresponds to a test for the win proportion with the corresponding confidence interval, as constructed from the standard error SE_0. One way of deriving the win proportion is to use the *Diff* in the dataset *FPTest*:

$$WP = \frac{Diff}{2n_A n_p} + 0.5 = \frac{723}{2*57*54} + 0.5 = 0.617446.$$

Another way would be to use the means reported in the dataset *FPPlacements*:

$$WP = \frac{MEAN_A}{n_p} = 1 - \frac{MEAN_P}{n_A} = \frac{35.194444}{57} = 1 - \frac{20.657895}{54} = 0.617446.$$

To construct the *FP* confidence interval for this estimate, we use the formula (A43) for the standard error:

$$SE_0 = \sqrt{\frac{Std_A^2\left(n_A-1\right)}{n_A^2 n_P^2} + \frac{Std_P^2\left(n_P-1\right)}{n_A^2 n_P^2} + \frac{WP\left(1-WP\right)}{n_A n_P}},$$

which yields

$$SE_0 = \sqrt{\frac{14.306753^2\left(54-1\right)}{54^2 * 57^2} + \frac{15.615113^2 *\left(57-1\right)}{54^2 * 57^2} + \frac{0.617446*\left(1-0.617446\right)}{54*57}},$$

that is, $SE_0 = 0.051605$. To verify that this standard error corresponds to the Z statistic given in the dataset *FPTest*, we can use the formula

$$Z_N^0 = \frac{WP - \frac{1}{2}}{SE_0} = \frac{0.617446 - 0.5}{0.051605} = 2.275889,$$

and it is the same Z value reported in the dataset *FPTest*. Using the 0.975 quantile of the standard normal distribution, which is 1.96 via the following code,

```
alpha = 0.05;
C = PROBIT(1-alpha/2);
```

we can derive an asymptotic 95% confidence interval for the win proportion from the formula (A9), and it is

$$0.617446 \ (0.516303, 0.71859).$$

The asymptotic 95% confidence interval does not contain the win probability under the null hypothesis, which is 0.5, and so the null hypothesis is rejected by a test of asymptotic type I error level 5%. This is also confirmed by the two-sided p-value of 0.022853 reported in the dataset *FPTest* being less than 0.05. The corresponding *FP* confidence interval for the win odds (by applying (A12)) is

$$\hat{k}_N = 1.614, [1.052, 2.477], P = 0.0229.$$

As expected this confidence interval is wider than that in (A51).

A.8.2.3. U-Statistic-based confidence interval. In this section, we will replicate the confidence interval (A51) using the output dataset *FPPlacements* of proc npar1way. The standard error SE in (A7) can be calculated as follows:

$$SE = \sqrt{\frac{14.306753^2 (54-1)}{54^2 * 57^2} + \frac{15.615113^2 * (57-1)}{54^2 * 57^2}} = 0.050856,$$

therefore,

$$Z_N = \frac{WP - \frac{1}{2}}{SE} = \frac{0.617446 - 0.5}{0.05085564} = 2.309407,$$

and so $(0.517771, 0.717122)$ is the corresponding 95% CI for the win proportion. The p-value can again be calculated from the Z statistic

```
p=2*(1-PROBNORM(2.309407));
```

Transforming the SE with (A12) we will obtain the *U*-statistic-based 95% CI for the win odds:

$$\hat{\kappa}_N = 1.614, \quad [1.058, 2.461], \quad P = 0.0209. \tag{A51}$$

A.8.2.4. Somers' D C/R. Since *Somers' D C/R* is implemented in proc freq (the measures option) of the SAS software, we obtain the *SE* in (A7) for the win proportion from formula (A45). Note that proc freq by default will order treatments alphabetically and choose the first as the reference group. In our case, it is treatment "A". Hence we obtain the win proportion of the control group against the active group. We can define treatment order (*TRT_ORD*) to obtain the win proportion of the active group.

```
data resp0;
   set resp;
   if treatment = "A" then TRT ORD=2;
   else TRT_ORD = 1;
run;

proc freq data = resp0;
   tables TRT_ORD*AVAL/ measures;
   ods output Measures = Measures0;
run;

data measures;
   set measures0;
   where statistic = "Somers' D C|R";
   value = (value + 1)/2;
   ASE = ASE/2;
   alpha = 0.05;
   C = PROBIT(1 - alpha/2);
   LCL = value - C*ASE;
   UCL = value + C*ASE;
   Z = abs(value - 0.5)/ASE;
   p = 2*(1 - PROBNORM(Z));
run;
```

The obtained output dataset is presented in Table A8.

A.8.3 The Package hce in R

In the R software (R Core Team 2022), the U-statistic-based confidence intervals, as well as power and sample size calculations, are implemented in the package hce (Gasparyan 2022). Consider the following R code:

TABLE A.8
Output from freq procedure.

Value	ASE	LCL	UCL	Z	p
0.617446	0.050856	0.517771	0.717122	2.309407	0.020921

```
calcWINS(visit4 ~ treatment, data = resp, ref = "P")

## $summary
##    WIN LOSS TIE TOTAL          Pties
## 1 1548 825   705 3078   0.2290448343
##
## $WP
##               WP          LCL          UCL          Pvalue
## 1 0.6174463938 0.5177711697 0.7171216178 0.0209209837
##
## $NetBenefit
##     NetBenefit          LCL          UCL          Pvalue
## 1 0.2348927875 0.03554233949 0.4342432356 0.0209209837
##
## $WO
##            WO          LCL          UCL          Pvalue
## 1 1.614012739 1.058380359 2.461343032 0.0209209837
##
## $WR1
##            WR         LCL1         UCL1          Pvalue1
## 1 1.876363636 1.077446672 3.267670306 0.02618122256
##
## $WR2
##            WR         LCL2         UCL2          Pvalue2
## 1 1.876363636 1.09077802 3.227733261 0.02297080054
##
## $gamma
##         gamma          LCL          UCL          Pvalue
## 1 0.3046776233 0.0530547175 0.556300529 0.01763363276
##
## $SE
##           WP_SE NetBenefit_SE  logWR_SE1  logWR_SE2     gamma_SE
## 1 0.05085564062 0.1017112812 0.2830366388 0.2767624561 0.1283813926
##
## $formula
## [1] "visit4 ~ treatment"
##
## $ref
## [1] "A vs P"
##
## $Input
##   alpha WOnull
## 1  0.05  1
```

As is shown previously, it is possible to calculate the win proportion, net benefit, win odds, win ratio, Goodman Kruskal's gamma, and their confidence intervals using only the function calcWINS() from the package hce. For the win ratio, two confidence intervals are provided, with the first based on formula (A46) and the second based on (A25) for *Var*(ln(*WR*)) and transformation of the confidence interval for ln(*WR*) to the confidence interval for *WR*.

The package sanon (Kawaguchi and Koch 2015a) provides the win proportion and its CI calculation as well.

```
library(sanon)
data(resp, package = "sanon")
fit <- sanon(visit4 ~ grp(treatment, ref = "P"), data = resp)
```

The win proportion, its standard error, and the confidence interval can be extracted from the fitted model by the subsequent formulas.

```
alpha <- 0.05 # the significance level
N <- nrow(resp) #111, total number of patients
WP <- fit$xi #0.617446 the win proportion
SE1 <- fit$se # SE calculated in sanon, 0.051086
SE <- SE1* sqrt((N-1)/N) # SE U-statistics, 0.050856
Z <- (WP - 0.5)/SE
CI <- c(WP = WP, LCL = WP - SE*qnorm(1 - alpha/2),
        UCL = WP + SE*qnorm(1-alpha/2), p.value=2*(1-pnorm(Z)))
CI
```

```
##          WP          LCL          UCL       p.value
## 0.6174463938 0.5177711697 0.7171216178 0.0209209837
```

Note that in the package sanon, the standard error SE_1 is calculated using the formula $SE_1 = \sqrt{\dfrac{N}{N-1}} SE$. Here, $N = 111$ is the total sample size of the combined treatment groups. For a large sample size, the coefficient above tends to 1, and so SE_1 (which is based on the theory for one sample U-statistics) from sanon and SE from the theory of two-sample U-statistics will be very similar, but always $SE_1 > SE$. The confidence interval based on SE_1 is

```
output <- as.data.frame(confint(fit)$ci)
output$p <- fit$p
output
```

```
##            Estimate          Lower          Upper              p
## visit4 0.6174463938 0.5173191256 0.7175736619 0.02150600985
```

The package sanon provides calculation of covariate-adjusted and stratified win proportion as well.

The package DescTools (Signorelli et al. 2022) provides implementations for *Somers' D C/R*, *Goodman Kruskal's gamma*, and the total number of concordances and discordances, among other rank-based measures.

```
library(DescTools)
resp$TRTP <- ifelse(resp$treatment == "A", 1, 0)
Tab <- table(resp$visit4, resp$TRTP)
SomersDelta(Tab, conf.level = 0.95)
```

```
## somers              lwr.ci          upr.ci
## 0.23489278752 0.03600178218 0.43378379287
```

```
GoodmanKruskalGamma(Tab, conf.level = 0.95)

##          gamma        lwr.ci        upr.ci
## 0.3046776233 0.0530547175 0.5563005290


ConDisPairs(Tab)

## $pi.c
##      [,1] [,2]
## [1,]   53    0
## [2,]   45   12
## [3,]   33   15
## [4,]   24   32
## [5,]    0   41
##
## $pi.d
##      [,1] [,2]
## [1,]    0   45
## [2,]    1   42
## [3,]    9   25
## [4,]   21   16
## [5,]   30    0
##
## $C
## [1] 1548
##
## $D
## [1] 825
```

Acknowledgment

We thank our collaborators for the presented results, especially Mikhail N. Kosiborod, Jan Oscarsson, Daniel Lindholm, Olof Bengtsson, Folke Folkvaljon, Russell Esterline, Martin Karpefors, and John Adler.

References

Agresti, A. 2013. *Categorical Data Analysis, 3rd Ed*. USA: John Willey and Sons.

Bebu, I, and JM Lachin. 2016. "Large sample inference for a win ratio analysis of a composite outcome based on prioritized components." *Biostatistics* 17 (1): 178–187. https://doi. org/10.1093/ biostatistics/kxv032.

Beigel, JH, KM Tomashek, LE Dodd, AK Mehta, Barry S. Zingman et al. 2020. "Remdesivir for the treatment of Covid-19 — final report." *New England Journal of Medicine* 383 (19): 1813–1826. https://doi.org/10.1056/ NEJMoa2007764.

Brunner, E, M Vandemeulebroecke, and T Mütze. 2021. "Win odds: an adaptation of the win ratio to include ties." *Statistics in Medicine* https://doi.org/10.1002/ sim.8967.

Buyse, M. 2010. "Generalized pairwise comparisons of prioritized outcomes in the two-sample problem." *Statistics in Medicine* 29 (30): 3245–3257.

Carr, GJ, KB Hafner, and GG Koch. 1989. "Analysis of rank measures of association for ordinal data from longitudinal studies." *Journal of the American Statistical Association* 84 (407): 797–804.

Cox, DR. 1972. "Regression models and life-tables." *Journal of the Royal Statistical Society: Series B (Methodological)* 34 (2): 187–202.

Dodd, LE, D Follmann, J Wang, F Koenig, LL Korn, C Schoergenhofer, M Proschan, et al. 2020. "Endpoints for randomized controlled clinical trials for COVID-19 treatments." *Clinical Trials* 17 (5): 472–482.

Dong, G, DC Hoaglin, J Qiu, RA Matsouaka YW Chang, J Wang, and M Vandemeulebroecke. 2020a. "The win ratio: on interpretation and handling of ties." *Statistics in Biopharmaceutical Research* 12 (1): 99–106.

Dong, G, B Huang, Y-W Chang, Y Seifu, J Song, and DC Hoaglin. 2020b. "The win ratio: Impact of censoring and follow-up time and use with nonproportional hazards." *Pharmaceutical Statistics* 19 (3): 168–177.

Dong, G, B Huang, J Verbeeck, Y Cui, J Song, M Gamalo-Siebers, D Wang, et al. 2022. "Win statistics (win ratio, win odds, and net benefit) can complement one another to show the strength of the treatment effect on time-to-event outcomes." *Pharmaceutical Statistics* 22 (1): 20–33.

Evans, SR, M Knutsson, P Amarenco, GW Albers, PM Bath, H Denison, P Ladenvall, et al. 2020. "Methodologies for pragmatic and efficient assessment of benefits and harms: application to the SOCRATES trial." *Clinical Trials* 17 (6): 617–626.

Ferreira, JP, PS Jhund, K Duarte, BL Claggett, SD Solomon, S Pocock, MC Petrie, F Zannad, and JJV McMurray. 2020. "Use of the win ratio in cardiovascular trials." *Heart Failure* 8 (6): 441–450.

Finkelstein, DM, and DA Schoenfeld. 2019. "Graphing the win ratio and its components over time." *Statistics in Medicine* 38 (1): 53–61.

Fligner, MA, and GE Policello. 1981. "Robust rank procedures for the Behrens-Fisher problem." *Journal of the American Statistical Association* 76 (373): 162–168.

Gardner, M. 1970. "Paradox of nontransitive dice and elusive principle of indifference." *Scientific American* 223 (6): 110.

Gasparyan, SB. 2022. *HCE: Design and Analysis of Hierarchical Composite Endpoints*. R package version 0.5.0, https://CRAN.R-project.org/package=hce.

Gasparyan, SB, F Folkvaljon, O Bengtsson, J Buenconsejo, and GG Koch. 2021a. "Adjusted win ratio with stratification: calculation methods and interpretation." *Statistical Methods in Medical Research* 30 (2): 580–611.

Gasparyan, SB, EK Kowalewski, F Folkvaljon, O Bengtsson, J Buenconsejo, J Adler, and GG Koch. 2021b. "Power and sample size calculation for the win odds test: application to an ordinal endpoint in COVID-19 trials." *Journal of Biopharmaceutical Statistics* 31 (6): 765–787.

Gasparyan, SB, EK Kowalewski, and GG Koch. 2022. "Comments on 'Sample size formula for a win ratio endpoint' by RX Yu and J. Ganju." *Statistics in Medicine* 41 (14): 2688–2690.

Gasparyan, SB, J Buenconsejo, EK Kowalewski, J Oscarsson, OF Bengtsson, R Esterline, GG Koch, O Berwanger, and MN Kosiborod. 2022. "Design and analysis of studies based on hierarchical composite endpoints: insights from the DARE-19 Trial." *Therapeutic Innovation & Regulatory Science* 56 (5): 785–794.

Harrell, FE. 2015. *Regression Modeling Strategies: With Applications to Linear Models, Logistic and Ordinal Regression, and Survival Analysis*. London: Springer.

Heerspink, HJL, BV Stefánsson, R Correa-Rotter, GM Chertow, T Greene, F-F Hou, JFE Mann, et al. 2020. "Dapagliflozin in patients with chronic kidney disease." *New England Journal of Medicine* 383 (15): 1436–1446.

Heerspink, HJL, RHM Furtado, O Berwanger, GG Koch, F Martinez, O Mukhtar, S Verma, et al. 2022. "Dapagliflozin and kidney outcomes in hospitalized patients with COVID-19 infection: an analysis of the dare-19 randomized controlled trial." *Clinical Journal of the American Society of Nephrology* 17 (5): 643–654.

Hintze, JL, and RD Nelson. 1998. "Violin plots: a box plot-density trace synergism." *The American Statistician* 52 (2): 181–184.

Hoeffding, W. 1948. "A class of statistics with asymptotically normal distribution." *The Annals of Mathematical Statistics* 19 (3): 293–325. https://doi.org/10.1214/aoms/1177730196.

Hollander, M, DA Wolfe, and E Chicken. 2013. "E9 (R1) addendum on estimands and sensitivity analysis in clinical trials to the guideline on statistical principles for clinical trials." John Wiley & Sons/ICH. https://database.ich.org/sites/default/files/E9-R1_Step4_Guideline_2019_1 203.pdf.

Jhund, PS, T Kondo, JH Butt, KF Docherty, BL Claggett, AS Desai, M Vaduganathan, et al. 2022. "Dapagliflozin across the range of ejection fraction in patients with heart failure: a patient-level, pooled meta-analysis of DAPA-HF and DELIVER." *Nature Medicine* 28 (9): 1956–1964.

Kaplan, EL, and P Meier. 1958. "Nonparametric estimation from incomplete observations." *Journal of the American Statistical Association* 53 (282): 457–481.

Karpefors, M and SB Gasparyan. 2022. *Maraca: The Maraca Plot: Visualization of Hierarchical Composite Endpoints in Clinical Trials*. R package version 0.4.0, https://CRAN.R-project.org/pack age=maraca.

Karpefors, M, D Lindholm, and SB Gasparyan. 2023. "The maraca plot: a novel visualization of hierarchical composite endpoints." *Clinical Trials* 20 (1): 84–88.

Kawaguchi, A, GG Koch, and X Wang. 2011a. "Stratified multivariate Mann–Whitney estimators for the comparison of two treatments with randomization based covariance adjustment." *Statistics in Biopharmaceutical Research* 3 (2): 217–231.

Kawaguchi, A, GG Koch, and X Wang. 2011b. "Stratified multivariate Mann–Whitney estimators for the comparison of two treatments with randomization based covariance adjustment." *Statistics in Biopharmaceutical Research* 3 (2): 217–231.

Kawaguchi, A, and GG Koch. 2015a. "Sanon: an R package for stratified analysis with nonparametric covariable adjustment." *Journal of Statistical Software* 67 (9). https://doi.org/10.18637/jss. v067.i09.

Kawaguchi, A, and GG Koch. 2015b. "Sanon: an R package for stratified analysis with nonparametric covariable adjustment." *Journal of Statistical Software* 67: 1–37.

Koch, GG, IA Amara, GW Davis, and DB Gillings. 1982. "A review of some statistical methods for covariance analysis of categorical data." *Biometrics* 563–595.

Koch, GG, GJ Carr, IA Amara, ME Stokes, and TJ Uryniak. 1990. "Categorical data analysis." *Statistical Methodology in the Pharmaceutical Sciences* 13:389–473.

Koch, GG, CM Tangen, J-W Jung, and IA Amara. 1998a. "Issues for covariance analysis of dichotomous and ordered categorical data from randomized clinical trials and non-parametric strategies for addressing them." *Statistics in Medicine* 17 (15–16):1863–1892.

Koch, GG, CM Tangen, J-W Jung, and IA Amara. 1998b. "Issues for covariance analysis of dichotomous and ordered categorical data from randomized clinical trials and non-parametric strategies for addressing them." *Statistics in Medicine* 17 (15–16): 1863–1892.

Koch, GG, PK Sen, and I Amara. 2004. *Log-Rank Scores, Statistics, and Tests*.

Kosiborod, M, O Berwanger, GG Koch, F Martinez, O Mukhtar, S Verma, V Chopra, et al. 2021a. "Effects of dapagliflozin on prevention of major clinical events and recovery in patients with respiratory failure because of COVID-19: Design and rationale for the DARE-19 study." *Diabetes, Obesity and Metabolism* 23 (4): 886–896.

Kosiborod, MN, R Esterline, RHM Furtado, J Oscarsson, SB Gasparyan, GG Koch, F Martinez, et al. 2021b. "Dapagliflozin in patients with cardiometabolic risk factors hospitalised with COVID-19 (DARE-19): a randomised, double-blind, placebo-controlled, phase 3 trial." *The Lancet Diabetes & Endocrinology* 9 (9): 586–594.

Kruskal, WH, and L Goodman. 1954. "Measures of association for cross classifications." *Journal of the American Statistical Association* 49 (268): 732–764.

Lehmann, EL, and HJM D'Abrera. 1975. *Nonparametrics: Statistical Methods Based on Ranks*. San Francisco, CA: Holden-Day.

Mann, HB, and DR Whitney. 1947. "On a test of whether one of two random variables is stochastically larger than the other." *The Annals of Mathematical Statistics* 50–60.

Mantel, N. 1966. "Evaluation of survival data and two new rank order statistics arising in its consideration." *Cancer Chemother Rep* 50: 163–170.

Mantel, N, and W Haenszel. 1959. "Statistical aspects of the analysis of data from retrospective studies of disease." *Journal of the National Cancer Institute* 22 (4): 719–748.

McMurray, JJV, SD Solomon, SE Inzucchi, L Køber, MN Kosiborod, FA Martinez, P Ponikowski, et al. 2019. "Dapagliflozin in patients with heart failure and reduced ejection fraction." *New England Journal of Medicine* 381 (21): 1995–2008.

Mendes, D, C Alves, and F Batel-Marques. 2017. "Number needed to treat (NNT) in clinical literature: an appraisal." *BMC Medicine* 15 (1): 1–13.

Natanegera, F, N Zariffa, J Buenconsejo, R Liao, F Cooner, D Lakshminarayanan, S Ghosh, JS, and M Gamalo. 2021. "Statistical opportunities to accelerate development for COVID-19 therapeutics." *Statistics in Biopharmaceutical Research* 1–17. https://doi.org/10.1080/19466315.2020.1865195.

O'Brien, RG, and JM Castelloe. 2006. *Exploiting the Link Between the Wilcoxon–Mann–Whitney Test and a Simple Odds Statistic*. Cary, NC: SAS Institute Inc. http://www2.sas.com/proceedings/sugi31/209-31.pdf.

Packer, M. 2016. "Development and evolution of a hierarchical clinical composite end point for the evaluation of drugs and devices for acute and chronic heart failure: a 20-year perspective." *Circulation* 134 (21): 1664–1678.

Packer, M. 2001. "Proposal for a new clinical end point to evaluate the efficacy of drugs and devices in the treatment of chronic heart failure." *Journal of Cardiac Failure* 7 (2): 176–182.

Peng, L. 2020. "The use of the win odds in the design of non-inferiority clinical trials." *Journal of Biopharmaceutical Statistics* 30 (5): 941–946.

Pocock, SJ, CA Ariti, TJ Collie, and D Wang. 2012. "The win ratio: a new approach to the analysis of composite endpoints in clinical trials based on clinical priorities." *European Heart Journal* 33 (2): 176–182.

Quade, D. 1967. "Rank analysis of covariance." *Journal of the American Statistical Association* 62 (320): 1187–1200.

Rauch, G, A Jahn-Eimermacher, W Brannath, and M Kieser. 2014. "Opportunities and challenges of combined effect measures based on prioritized outcomes." *Statistics in Medicine* 33 (7): 1104–1120.

R Core Team. 2022. *R: A Language and Environment for Statistical Computing, version 4.2.2*. Vienna, Austria: R Foundation for Statistical Computing. https://www.R-project.org/.

Rubin, DB. 2004. *Multiple Imputation for Nonresponse in Surveys*. Vol. 81. John Wiley & Sons.

Savage Jr, RP. 1994. "The paradox of nontransitive dice." *The American Mathematical Monthly* 101 (5): 429–436.

Signorell, A, Aho, K, Alfons, A, Anderegg N, Aragon T, Arachchige C et al. 2022. *DescTools: Tools for Descriptive Statistics*. R package version 0.99.47, https://cran.r-project.org/package=DescTools.

Solomon, SD, JJV McMurray, B Claggett, et al. 2022. "Dapagliflozin in heart failure with mildly reduced or preserved ejection fraction." *New England Journal of Medicine* 387 (12): 1089–1098.

Somers, RH. 1962. "A new asymmetric measure of association for ordinal variables." *American Sociological Review* 799–811.

Stokes, ME, CS Davis, and GG Koch. 2012. *Categorical Data Analysis Using SAS®*. 3rd ed. Cary, NC: SAS Institute Inc. http://support.sas.com/rnd/app/stat/cat/edition3/samples/.

SAS Institute Inc. 2018. *SAS/STAT®: 15.1 User's Guide*. Cary, NC: SAS Institute Inc.

Tukey, JW. 1977. *Exploratory Data Analysis*. Vol. 2. Reading, MA: Addison-Wesley.

Van der Vaart, AW. 2000. *Asymptotic Statistics*. Vol. 3. Cambridge: Cambridge University Press.

Van Elteren, PH. 1960. "On the combination of independent two sample tests of Wilcoxon." *Bull Inst Intern Staist* 37: 351–361.

Verbeeck, J, V Deltuvaite-Thomas, B Berckmoes, T Burzykowski, M Aerts, O Thas, M Buyse, and G Molenberghs. 2020. "Unbiasedness and efficiency of non-parametric and UMVUE estimators of the probabilistic index and related statistics." *Statistical Methods in Medical Research* 0962280220966629.

Voors, AA, CE Angermann, JR Teerlink, SP Collins, M Kosiborod, J Biegus, JP Ferreira, et al. 2022. "The SGLT2 inhibitor empagliflozin in patients hospitalized for acute heart failure: a multinational randomized trial." *Nature Medicine* 28 (3): 568–574.

Whitehead, J. 1993. "Sample size calculations for ordered categorical data." *Statistics in Medicine* 12 (24): 2257–2271. https://doi.org/10.1002/sim.4780122404.

WHO, R&D. 2020. *WHO R&D Blueprint Novel Coronavirus (COVID-19) Therapeutic Trial Synopsis.* WHO. https://www.who.int/blueprint/priority-diseases/key-action/COVID-19_Treatment_Trial_Design_Master_Protocol_synopsis_Final_18022020.pdf.

Wilcoxon, F. 1992. "Individual comparisons by ranking methods." In *Breakthroughs in Statistics*, 196–202. London: Springer.

Wiviott, SD, I Raz, MP Bonaca, O Mosenzon, ET Kato, A Cahn, MG Silverman, et al. 2019. "Dapagliflozin and cardiovascular outcomes in type 2 diabetes." *New England Journal of Medicine* 380 (4): 347–357.

Woolson, RF, and WR Clarke. 2011. *Statistical Methods for the Analysis of Biomedical Data.* John Wiley & Sons. Yu, Ron Xiaolong, and Jitendra Ganju. 2022. "Sample size formula for a win ratio endpoint." *Statistics in Medicine* 41 (6): 950–963.

Zhao, Y, AH Herring, H Zhou, MW Ali, and GG Koch. 2014. "A multiple imputation method for sensitivity analyses of time-to-event data with possibly informative censoring." *Journal of Biopharmaceutical Statistics* 24 (2): 229–253.

8

Deep Learning Constructed Statistics with Application to Adaptive Designs for Clinical Trials

Tianyu Zhan

Introduction

Adaptive designs of clinical trials allow for prospectively planned modifications to one or more aspects of the design based on accumulating data from subjects in the trial (Food and Drug Administration, 2019). Properly conducted adaptive designs have several advantages over traditional nonadaptive designs, for example, statistical efficiency, ethical considerations, and early decisions to reduce the overall costs (Bretz et al., 2009; Food and Drug Administration, 2019). Clinical trial optimization is usually conducted in practice to find a feasible, complex, and innovative clinical trial with proper design features for a particular problem. Several works have been proposed to find the optimal design based on specific optimization criteria (Simon, 1989; Dmitrienko et al., 2016; Zhang et al., 2016). Another perspective is to find a better hypothesis testing strategy with higher power given a specific design, in addition to current methods mainly focused on type I error rates control (Bauer and Kohne, 1994; Cui et al., 1999; Mehta and Pocock, 2011).

As a direct optimization, one can evaluate several candidate methods under working assumptions and then propose the best one. However, such a method may not be optimal or even have worse performance when observed data deviate. Another systematic method was proposed in Zhan and Kang (2022) to offer a possible solution to this problem. Test statistics are constructed by deep learning to enhance power under a controlled type I error rate for a specific adaptive clinical trial design. This computational method can automatically leverage machine intelligence to perform hypothesis testing, and its decision function is prespecified before the actual trial conduct.

In this book chapter, we review this deep learning–guided hypothesis testing method of constructing test statistics and estimating critical values in Section 2. This approach is applied to a response adaptive randomization design and a sample size reassessment design in Section 3. Discussions are provided in Section 4.

DOI: 10.1201/9781003288640-8

8.1 Proposed Methods

8.1.1 Setup

We consider a composite hypothesis testing problem in typical clinical trials using two groups of independent data x_j, $j = p, t$, where $j = 1$ denotes placebo and $j = 2$ denotes active treatment group. The parameter of interest θ_j is considered a scaler quantity, while the nuisance parameter η_j is a vector of dimension w in the group j. The null hypothesis H_0 is to be tested against an alternative hypothesis H_1 with a one-sided type I error rate controlled at α:

$$H_0 : \theta_1 = \theta_2, \quad \text{versus} \quad H_1 : \theta_1 < \theta_2. \tag{1}$$

We define a set of sufficient statistics $t^{(s)} = \left\{ \hat{\theta}(x_1), \hat{\theta}(x_2), \hat{\eta}(x_1), \hat{\eta}(x_2) \right\}$ of dimension $w^{(s)}$, where $\hat{\theta}(x_j)$ and $\hat{\eta}(x_j)$ are sufficient statistics of their true parameters θ_j and η_j, respectively, based on data x_j from the distribution function $f(x; \theta_j, \eta_j)$, for group $j = 1, 2$. The superscript "(s)" indicates that $t^{(s)}$ is utilized in the formulation of statistics.

We formulate the hypothesis testing in the context of a binary classification problem to categorize whether data are sampled from H_1 or from H_0. Following the formulation motivated by simple hypothesis testing as discussed in Zhan and Kang (2022), we intend to identify a statistic $d\{t^{(s)}\}$ for composite hypothesis testing such that

$$d\left\{\mathbf{t}^{(s)}\right\} = \text{logit}\left[\Pr\left\{y = 1 \mid \mathbf{t}^{(s)}\right\}\right], \tag{2}$$

where $y \in (0, 1)$ is a latent variable indicating if data are drawn from H_0 or H_1. The critical value c to control type I error rates at α under H_0 satisfies

$$\Pr_{H_0}\left[d\left\{\mathbf{t}^{(s)}\right\} > c\right] = \alpha \tag{3}$$

However, the functional form of $d\{t^{(s)}\}$ in (2) may be intractable. The computation of the critical value c in (3) requires additional investigation, because the distribution of $d\{t^{(s)}\}$ under H_0 in a finite sample can be unknown. In the next section, we review a two-stage method to construct statistics and corresponding critical values by deep neural networks (DNNs) proposed in Zhan and Kang (2022).

8.1.2 Approximating the Test Statistics via DNN

DNN defines a mapping $y = q(t; \psi)$ and learns the value of the parameters ψ that result in the best function approximation of output label y based on input data t (Goodfellow et al., 2016). We train a DNN to approximate the test statistic $d\{t^{(s)}\}$ in (2) by using Monte Carlo samples.

We define $\Theta_1 \subseteq \mathbb{R}$, $\Theta_2 \subseteq \mathbb{R}$, $H_1 \subseteq \mathbb{R}^w$, and $H_2 \subseteq \mathbb{R}^w$ as neighborhoods of the true values of θ_1, θ_2, η_1, and η_2, respectively. We simulate A sets of features $\{\theta_{1,a}, \theta_{2,a}, \eta_{1,a}, \eta_{2,a}\}_{a=1}^{A}$ from uniform distributions in their corresponding parameter spaces. Then within each set a, for $a = 1, \ldots, A$, we simulate B_0 samples under H_0 with distribution $f(x; \theta_{1,a}, \eta_{1,a})$ for group 1 and $f(x; \theta_{1,a}, \eta_{2,a})$ for group 2, and generate B_1 samples under H_1 with distribution $f(x; \theta_{1,a}, \eta_{1,a})$ for group 1 and $f(x; \theta_{2,a}, \eta_{2,a})$ for group 2. In each sample $b \in (1, \ldots, \{A \times [B_0 + B_1]\})$, we computer the vector of sufficient statistics $t_b^{(s)} = \left\{ \hat{\theta}(x_{1,b}), \hat{\theta}(x_{2,b}), \hat{\eta}(x_{1,b}), \hat{\eta}(x_{2,b}) \right\}$ to obtain training data. The classification label $y_b^{(s)}$ takes value of either 0 or 1, where the event $\left\{ y_b^{(s)} = k \right\}$ indicates a sample being drawn from the distribution under H_k, for $k = 0, 1$.

Next, we train the test statistic DNN (TS-DNN) with the *ReLU* function $\text{ReLU}(u) = \max(0, u)$ as the inner-layer activation function and the *sigmoid* function $\text{sigmoid}(u) = 1/[1 + \exp(-u)]$ as the last-layer activation function. In the training process, DNN seeks a solution $\widehat{\psi}^{(s)}$ which maximizes the log-likelihood function:

$$\widehat{\psi}^{(s)} = \arg\max_{\psi^{(s)}} \sum_{b=1}^{A \times (B_0 + B_1)} \left(\left\{ 1 - y_b^{(s)} \right\} \log \left[1 - p \left\{ t_b^{(s)}; \psi^{(s)} \right\} \right] + y_b^{(s)} \log p \left\{ t_b^{(s)}; \psi^{(s)} \right\} \right), \tag{4}$$

where $p\{t^{(s)}; \psi^{(s)}\} = \text{sigmoid}\,[q\{t^{(s)}; \psi^{(s)}\}]$, $q\{t^{(s)}; \psi^{(s)}\}$ is the linear predictor of DNN, and $\psi^{(s)}$ is a stack of the weight and the bias parameters from all layers in DNN. DNN obtains $\widehat{\psi}^{(s)}$ by (4) such that $\text{sigmoid}\left[q\left\{ t^{(s)}; \widehat{\psi}^{(s)} \right\} \right]$ approximates the unknown classification probability $\Pr \{y = 1 | t^{(s)}\} = \text{sigmoid}\,[d\{t^{(s)}\}]$ in (2). Training data are normalized with mean zero and unit standard deviation. Tuning of hyperparameters is based on procedures discussed in Zhan (2022).

8.1.3 Approximating the Critical Values via DNN

In the second stage, we train another DNN to estimate the critical value c in (3) based on simulated samples under H_0.

We construct the training data as $\left\{ t_a^{(c)} \right\}_{a=1}^A$ of dimension $(1 + 2 \times w)$ and size A, where $t_a^{(c)} = \left(\theta_{1,a}, \eta_{1,a}, \eta_{2,a} \right)$ are the simulation design features from the previous section. The superscript "(c)" in $t^{(c)}$ and other notations indicate that they pertain to the estimation of critical values. Given a $t_a^{(c)}$, we simulate B' null data under H_0 with group 1 data from $f(x; \theta_{1,a}, \eta_{1,a})$ and group 2 data from $f(x; \theta_{1,a}, \eta_{2,a})$. Their test statistics based on the TS-DNN in the first stage are computed at $\left\{ q\left[t_{b'}^{(s)}; \widehat{\psi}^{(s)} \right] \right\}_{b'=1}^{B'}$. The output label $y_a^{(c)}$ is set at the empirical upper α quantile in those test statistics to satisfy (3). We train a critical value DNN (CV-DNN) $q\left\{ t^{(c)}; \widehat{\psi}^{(c)} \right\}$ to estimate $y_a^{(c)}$ by *linear* function as the last-layer activation function, and the mean squared error (MSE) as the loss function.

A diagram is provided in Zhan and Kang (2022) to streamline this two-stage method of approximating the test statistics and estimating the critical values training two different DNNs (Figure 8.1).

8.1.4 Hypothesis Testing Based on Observed Data

With observed data $\tilde{x}_1$ from group 1 and $\tilde{x}_2$ from group 2, we first obtain the input data for the TS-DNN at $\tilde{t}^{(s)} = \left\{ \hat{\theta}(\tilde{x}_1), \hat{\theta}(\tilde{x}_2), \tilde{\eta}(\tilde{x}_1), \tilde{\eta}(\tilde{x}_2) \right\}$ and then compute its test statistic

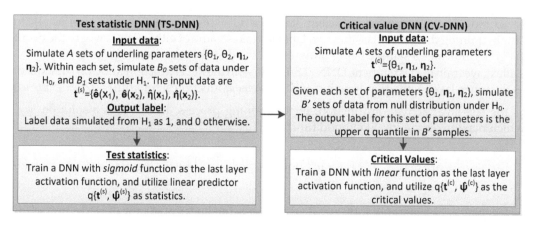

FIGURE 8.1

Diagram in Zhan and Kang (2022) of the two-stage DNN method.

$q\left\{\tilde{t}^{(s)}; \widehat{\psi}^{(s)}\right\}$. Let $\tilde{\theta}(x)$ and $\tilde{\eta}(x)$ be unbiased or consistent estimators for θ and η, respectively. The critical value is computed at $q\left\{\tilde{t}^{(c)}; \widehat{\psi}^{(c)}\right\}$, where $\tilde{t}^{(c)} = \left\{\tilde{\theta}(\tilde{x}_{12}), \tilde{\eta}(\tilde{x}_1), \tilde{\eta}(\tilde{x}_2)\right\}$ and $\tilde{x}_{12} = \left(\tilde{x}_1, \tilde{x}_2\right)$. Finally, H_0 in (1) is rejected if $q\left\{\tilde{t}^{(s)}; \widehat{\psi}^{(s)}\right\} > q\left\{\tilde{t}^{(c)}; \widehat{\psi}^{(c)}\right\}$, but not rejected otherwise.

8.2 Case Studies

8.2.1 Response Adaptive Block Randomization

In the response adaptive block randomization (RABR) design, subjects are more likely to be randomized to better-performing treatment groups based on a prespecified block randomization vector (Zhan et al., 2021). RABR is robust in achieving a desired final sample size per group to meet regulatory requirements and has easy implementation with the interactive response technology (IRT) for randomization. The usual unweighted statistic (UWS) is shown to have a controlled one-sided type I error rate for pairwise comparison in RABR. Compared with the weighed statistic (WS), UWS is easier to compute and more feasible in designs with sequential adaptation. In this section, we apply the proposed method to this RABR to construct another statistic with deep learning to seek a higher power.

For illustration purposes, we consider an RABR with a single active treatment group and a placebo with one interim adaptation. Binary endpoint is considered with $\theta_1 = 0.47$ as assumed as the response rate for placebo and $\theta_2 = 0.6$ for treatment based on a motivating example of the Adaptive COVID-19 Treatment Trial (ACTT; National Institutes of Health, 2020). The burn-in period has a size of $M = 400$ and fixed equal randomization probabilities for two groups. After observing interim data, standardized response rates in Zhan et al.

(2021) are computed at R_2 for the treatment group and R_1 for the placebo group. If $R_2 - R_1$ > 1.9, which means that the standardized treatment effect is larger than a certain clinically meaningful difference, the randomization probability to the treatment group is increased from 1/2 to 2/3 with a second stage sample size of 400. Otherwise, if the treatment effect is not promising, the second-stage sample size is decreased to 40 with equal randomization probabilities. We denote $x_j^{(h)}$ as the vector of observed binary data of size $n^{(h)}$ for group j, $j = 1, 2$ at stage h, $h = 1, 2$.

To implement our proposed method, we consider $\Theta = (0.15, 0.8)$ to cover the true $\theta_1 = 0.47$ and $\theta_2 = 0.6$. We simulate $A = 500$ features with θ_1 from Θ and further set θ_2 under H_1 at a value for our approach to reach approximately 90% power. We choose $B_0 = B_1 = 10^4$. The input vector for the TS-DNN is $t^{(s)} = \left[\hat{\theta}\{x_1^{(1)}\}, \hat{\theta}\{x_2^{(1)}\}, \hat{\theta}\{x_1^{(2)}\}, \hat{\theta}\{x_2^{(2)}\}, n_1^{(2)}, n_2^{(2)} \right]$, where $\hat{\theta}\{x\}$ is the sample mean of x. By cross-validation, the final DNN structure is selected as the one with the smallest validation error from six candidate structures, which are all combinations of the number of layers at 2 and 3, and the number of nodes per layer at 50, 100, and 150. The number of epochs is 10, the batch size is 10^4, and the dropout rate is 0.1. In the CV-DNN, the training data is of size A with $t^c = (\theta_1)$, and the output is computed on $B' = 10^6$ samples under H_0. A number of epochs at 10^3, a batch size of 10, and a dropout rate of 0.1 are utilized in this DNN training. With observed data in the first stage $\tilde{x}_{12}^{(1)} = \left\{ \tilde{x}_1^{(1)}, \tilde{x}_2^{(1)} \right\}$, we use $\hat{\theta}\left\{ \tilde{x}_{12}^{(1)} \right\}$ to estimate the critical value.

In Table 8.1, we evaluate the type I error rate and power of the proposed DNN method versus the weighted statistics (WS) (Bauer and Kohne, 1994; Cui et al., 1999) with equal weights and the unweighted statistics (UWS) with a nominal critical value (Zhan et al., 2021). All three methods have type I error rates controlled at 0.05 under H_0, where the common θ in two groups takes the values 0.37, 0.47, and 0.57. Under H_1 with $\theta_1 = 0.47$, DNN is more powerful than WS and UWS under three scenarios considered. UWS has the smallest power because it has the most conservative error rate among the three methods.

TABLE 8.1

DNN consistently achieves a higher power than WS (weighted statistics) and UWS (unweighted statistics) in RABR.

θ_1	θ_2	Type I Error Rate		
		DNN	WS	UWS
0.37	0.37	5.1%	5.1%	3.6%
0.47	0.47	4.8%	5.1%	3.3%
0.57	0.57	4.8%	5.1%	3.7%
θ_1	θ_2	Power		
		DNN	WS	UWS
0.47	0.58	83.0%	81.9%	80.0%
	0.60	92.4%	91.8%	90.6%
	0.62	97.2%	96.9%	96.3%

TABLE 8.2

DNN consistently achieves a higher power than WS (weighted statistics) and UWS (unweighted statistics) with a fine-tuned critical value of 0.034 in an adaptive design with sample size reassessment.

θ_1	θ_2	Type I Error Rate		
		DNN	WS	UWS
0.17	0.17	4.9%	5.0%	4.5%
0.27	0.27	5.1%	5.0%	4.8%
0.37	0.37	4.9%	5.0%	4.8%
0.47	0.47	4.9%	5.0%	5.2%
θ_1	θ_2	Power		
		DNN	WS	UWS
0.27	0.39	87.4%	82.9%	83.6%
0.27	0.40	91.3%	85.9%	86.4%
0.27	0.41	93.8%	88.2%	88.5%

8.2.2 Sample Size Reassessment

This section showcases the application of our method in adaptive clinical trials with sample size reassessment based on the Multiple Sclerosis and Extract of Cannabis (MUSEC) trial (Zajicek et al., 2012) as investigated in Zhan and Kang (2022).

In Table 8.2, we study the type I error rates under H_0 where the common θ in two groups takes the values 0.17, 0.27, 0.37, and 0.47 around the true $\theta_p = 0.27$. All three methods have type I error rates controlled at the nominal level of 0.05. On power evaluation, we fix θ_1 in the placebo group at 0.27 and consider varying θ_2 of the treatment group at 0.39, 0.4, and 0.41. Under the true $\theta_2 = 0.4$, DNN consistently has higher power than WS and UWS.

8.3 Discussions

The application of the proposed method is not limited to adaptive designs but can be extended to group sequential designs or other two-sample hypothesis testing problems in general (Zhan and Kang, 2022). The generalization to multiple endpoints follows the computational framework in historical data borrowing (Zhan et al., 2022). Some future works include nonparametric testing, Bayesian hypothesis testing, etc.

The current method has some limitations that require additional investigations to seek potential improvement. Firstly, the proposed statistic does not have a straightforward functional form to be communicated externally. One can conduct backward engineering to identify an approximate functional representation with better interpretation. Moreover, extensive computational resources are required to obtain test statistics and critical values by training deep learning models. A more unified neural network may be trained to cover a class of problems, or transfer learning can be utilized to solve a new hypothesis-testing problem based on knowledge gained in solving existing ones.

References

Bauer, P. and Kohne, K. (1994). Evaluation of experiments with adaptive interim analyses. *Biometrics*, 1029–1041.

Bretz, F., Koenig, F., Brannath, W., Glimm, E., and Posch, M. (2009). Adaptive designs for confirmatory clinical trials. *Statistics in Medicine*, 28(8): 1181–1217.

Cui, L., Hung, H. J., and Wang, S.-J. (1999). Modification of sample size in group sequential clinical trials. *Biometrics*, 55(3): 853–857.

Dmitrienko, A., Paux, G., Pulkstenis, E., and Zhang, J. (2016). Tradeoff-based optimization criteria in clinical trials with multiple objectives and adaptive designs. *Journal of Biopharmaceutical Statistics*, 26(1): 120–140.

Food and Drug Administration. (2019). Adaptive Design Clinical Trials for Drugs and Biologics Guidance for Industry. www.fda.gov/regulatory-information/search-fda-guidance-docume nts/adaptive-design-clinical-trials-drugs-and-biologics-guidance-industry.

Goodfellow, I., Bengio, Y., and Courville, A. (2016). *Deep Learning*. MIT Press.

Mehta, C. R. and Pocock, S. J. (2011). Adaptive increase in sample size when interim results are promising: a practical guide with examples. *Statistics in Medicine*, 30(28): 3267–3284.

National Institutes of Health. (2020). Adaptive COVID-19 Treatment Trial (ACTT). https://clinica ltrials.gov/ct2/show/NCT04280705.

Simon, R. (1989). Optimal two-stage designs for phase ii clinical trials. *Controlled Clinical Trials*, 10(1): 1–10.

Zajicek, J. P., Hobart, J. C., Slade, A., Barnes, D., Mattison, P. G., Group, M. R., et al. (2012). Multiple sclerosis and extract of cannabis: results of the MUSEC trial. *Journal of Neurology, Neurosurgery & Psychiatry*, 83(11): 1125–1132.

Zhan, T. (2022). DL 101: Basic introduction to deep learning with its application in biomedical related fields. *Statistics in Medicine*, 41(26): 5365–5378.

Zhan, T., Cui, L., Geng, Z., Zhang, L., Gu, Y., and Chan, I. S. (2021). A practical response adaptive block randomization (RABR) design with analytic type I error protection. *Statistics in Medicine*, 40(23): 4947–4960.

Zhan, T. and Kang, J. (2022). Finite-sample two-group composite hypothesis testing via machine learning. *Journal of Computational and Graphical Statistics: A Joint Publication of American Statistical Association, Institute of Mathematical Statistics, Interface Foundation of North America*, 31(3): 856–865.

Zhan, T., Zhou, Y., Geng, Z., Gu, Y., Kang, J., Wang, L., Huang, X., and Slate, E. H. (2022). Deep historical borrowing framework to prospectively and simultaneously synthesize control information in confirmatory clinical trials with multiple endpoints. *Journal of Biopharmaceutical Statistics*, 32(1): 90–106.

Zhang, L., Cui, L., and Yang, B. (2016). Optimal flexible sample size design with robust power. *Statistics in Medicine*, 35(19): 3385–3396.

9

Predicting Phase III Results by Incorporating Historical Data Using Bayesian Additive Regression Trees (BART) Extensions

Bradley Hupf, Yinpu Li, Rachael Liu, and Jianchang Lin

Introduction

In drug development, phase III clinical trials are crucial to demonstrate the effectiveness of investigational treatment. However, they usually are extremely long in study duration and expensive in cost. To mitigate the potential risk of negative outcomes, sponsors have developed various metrics and approaches to predict the phase III study results through early phase clinical trials data. In addition, as other external data sources including real-world data (e.g., electronic health records, claims data, registries) and historical data have rapidly surged in recent years, there is an increasing interest and need from drug developers to leverage all available information to have more robust decision making in drug development. Incorporating those external data could potentially contribute to a more precise treatment effect size estimation and subsequentially lead to more robust quantitative decision making including phase III study results predictions.

Survival outcomes, e.g., progression-free survival (PFS) or overall survival (OS), are commonly used primary endpoints in many disease areas, especially in oncology. The Cox proportional hazards model is commonly used for survival regression problems when incorporating patient information. However, in practice, the relationships between regressors and the response could be complex. These include nonlinear functions of the covariates, interactions, collinearity, existence of irrelevant features that results in high-dimensional feature space, and violation of proportional hazards assumption. On the other hand, machine learning techniques offer flexible modeling of relationships of covariates to response of interests. In this work, we address and extend the usefulness of machine learning techniques in predicting phase III results. We demonstrate the machine learning techniques' ability and advantages to accommodate data from complex regression models with a sequence of simulation studies that could incorporate historical data.

The remainder of the paper is organized as follows. In Section 9.1, we will review the survival models and describe the CoxBART models. In Section 9.2, we demonstrate how CoxBART performs across multiple simulation scenarios. And in Section 9.3 we illustrate the application of CoxBART on a generated real data example. We conclude in Section 9.4 with a discussion.

DOI: 10.1201/9781003288640-9

9.1 Methods

9.1.1 Survival Model

Let (T_i, C_i) denote the survival and censoring times, respectively, for $i = 1,...,N$. We observe data $D = \{(Y_i, \delta_i, X_i) : i = 1,...,N\}$ where $Y_i = min(T_i, C_i)$ is the observed (right-censored) survival time, $\delta_i = I(T_i \le C_i)$ is the censoring indicator, and $X_i \in \mathbb{R}^P$ is a vector of covariates. Our goal is to model the conditional survival function $S_0(t \mid x)$ of T_i conditional on X_i. Other relevant quantities include the corresponding cumulative hazard function $H_0(t \mid x) = -\log S_0(t \mid x)$ and the hazard function $h_0(t \mid x) = dH_0(t \mid x)$. Throughout this work we assume that the censoring time C_i is independent of T_i given X_i. The response is the indicator of patients in a trial whose tumor is destroyed or significantly reduced by a treatment.

We consider the nonparametric conditional survival analysis problem, where our goal is to assess the impact of P predictors $x = (x_1,...,x_P)$ on the survival function $S(t \mid x) = \mathbb{P}(T > t \mid X = x)$ and the hazard function $h(t \mid x) = -d \log S(t \mid x)$. The time-constant predictors x may include treatments and prognostic markers in a clinical study. A popular semiparametric model in survival analysis is the Cox proportional hazards model [1] $h(t \mid x) = \lambda(t) \exp\{x^\top \beta\}$, where $\lambda(t)$ is a nonparametric baseline hazard model. Instead of this restrictive assumption, methods based on decision trees [2] construct a partition of the predictor space X and estimate $S(t \mid x)$ separately for each equivalence class. Decision trees are also used as building blocks for ensemble methods. For example, the random survival forests algorithm [3] aggregates many decision trees together to obtain a flexible estimate of $S(t \mid x)$. Models based on Bayesian additive regression trees (BART) have also been proposed.

9.1.2 Survival Analysis in General

Incorporating patient's subject-level data offers the potential to make the survival inference more informative and the predicted survival results more accurate. When incorporating the patient subject-level information, the survival time conditions on a vector of predictor variables, X, are expressed as $S(t \mid X)$. Survival analysis has been studied by many; however, most take a proportional hazards approach [1, 4, 5]. We take an approach that is tantamount to discrete-time survival analysis [6, 7, 8]. Relying on the capabilities of machine learning techniques, we do not stipulate a linear relationship with the covariates nor proportional hazards. In the most popular Cox models a linear structure is assumed to relate the predictors to the survival time t. This incarnation of the Cox regression model is computationally straightforward but makes restrictive parametric assumptions regarding linearity.

9.1.2.1 The Cox Model

For a given patient i, the hazard function $h(t|X_i)$ in the Cox model follows the proportional hazards assumption given by

$$h(t|X_i) = h_0(t)\exp\{X_i^\top \beta\},$$

for $i = 1, 2, \cdots, N$, where the baseline hazard function, $h_0(t)$, can be an arbitrary non-negative function of time. The Cox model is a semiparametric model due to the fact that its baseline hazard function is unspecified. And this makes it impossible to fit the model using standard likelihood function. Instead, we proceed with partial likelihood. With reference to the Cox assumption and the presence of censoring, the partial likelihood is defined as

$$\mathcal{L}(\beta) = \prod_{j=1}^{N} \left[\frac{\exp(X_j \beta)}{\sum_{i \in R_j} \exp(X_i \beta)} \right]^{\delta_j}.$$

The maximum partial likelihood estimator can be used along with the numerical Newton-Raphson method to iteratively find an estimator $\hat{\beta}$ which minimizes the partial likelihood.

9.1.2.2 Machine Learning Methods

As more machine learning methods become available, there have been many alternatives to some of these stringent parametric assumptions. Tree-based methods stand out among the competitors. The RSF (random survival forest) approach extends random forests [9] to right-censored survival data. The key idea of the RSF algorithm is to grow a binary survival tree T and construct the ensemble cumulative hazard function (CHF). Each terminal node of the survival tree contains the observed survival times and the binary censoring information for patients who fall in that terminal node. For all of the patients in terminal node b, let $t_{1,b} < t_{2,b} < \cdots < t_{N(b),b}$ be the $N(b)$ distinct event times. The CHF estimate for node b is the Nelson-Aalen estimator $\hat{\Lambda}_b = \sum_{\{l:t_{l,b} \leq t\}} d_{l,b} / R_{l,b}$, where $d_{l,b}$ and $R_{l,b}$ are the number of events and size of the risk set at time point $t_{l,b}$, respectively. All patients within node l then have the same CHF estimate. To compute the CHF for a patient with covariates X_i, one can drop X_i down the tree and obtain the Nelson-Aalen estimator for X_i's terminal node, $\Lambda(t | X_i) = \hat{\Lambda}_h(t)$ if $X_i \in b$. The out-of-bag (OOB) ensemble CHF for each individual, $\lambda^{OOB}(t | X_i)$, can be calculated by dropping OOB data down a survival tree built from in-bag samples, recording i's node and its CHF and taking the average of all of the recorded CHFs. The patient-specific survival curve can be computed as 1 minus the estimated ensemble OOB CHF summed over survival times until t, conditioning on X_i, that is,

$$S(t | X_i) = 1 - \sum_{j:T_j \leq t} \hat{\Lambda}^{OOB}(T_j | X_i)$$

9.1.3 Bayesian Additive Regression Trees

Bayesian additive regression tree (BART) is a Bayesian nonparametric, machine learning, ensemble predictive modeling method for continuous, binary, categorical, and time-to-event outcomes. Furthermore, BART is a tree-based, black-box method that fits the outcome to an arbitrary random function f of the covariates. The BART technique is relatively computationally efficient as compared to its competitors, though large sample sizes can be demanding, see [10]. It provides a flexible approach to fitting a variety of regression models while avoiding strong parametric assumptions. The sum-of-trees model is embedded in a Bayesian inferential framework to support uncertainty quantification and provide a principled approach to regularization through prior specification. BART models an unknown function $f(x)$ as a sum of M decision trees $\sum_{m=1}^{M} \text{Tree}(x; \mathcal{T}_m, \mathcal{M}_m)$ where $\mathcal{T}_m$ denotes the tree topology and splitting rules of the tree and $\mathcal{M}_m$ denotes the predicted response for each leaf node. For detailed reviews of BART, see [11] and [12]. The function $\text{Tree}(x; \mathcal{T}_m, \mathcal{M}_m)$ returns μ_{ml} if x is associated to leaf node l of tree m. Each tree induces a partition of the predictor space $\mathcal{X}$ such that $g(x)$ is constant on each equivalence class of the partition. A schematic showing a particular decision tree with the induced partition over $\mathcal{X} = [0,1]^2$ is given in Figure 9.1. We divide the decision tree nodes into a collection of leaf nodes $l \in \mathcal{L}$ and branch nodes $b \in \mathcal{B}$, where $\mathcal{L}$ consists of the nodes with no children. Associated to each branch b is a decision rule of the form $\left[X_{jb} \leq C_b \right]$, while each leaf l is associated to a prediction μ_{ml}.

Assuming the data to arise from a model with additive Gaussian errors, the response is modeled as

$$Y = f(x) + \epsilon = \sum_{m=1}^{M} \text{Tree}(x; \mathcal{T}_m, \mathcal{M}_m) + \epsilon, \text{ where } \epsilon \sim N(0, \sigma^2).$$

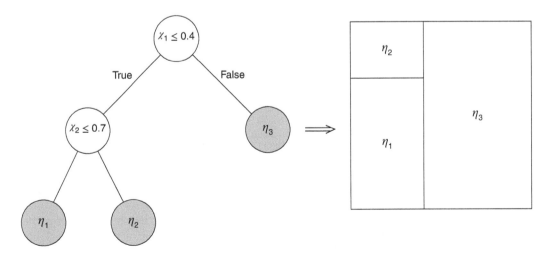

FIGURE 9.1
Left: an example of a decision tree with two variables $X = (X_1, X_2)$. *Right*: the piecewise-constant function induced from the decision tree, taking values η_1, η_2, and η_3 depending on the value of X.

Many machine learning methods avoid overfitting through tuning parameters. For the decision tree–based method, the researcher could prespecify the maximum depth for individual trees or limit the number of observations in each leaf node to constrain each to be a weak learner. In boosting tree algorithms, the fit from each tree is typically multiplied by a small number to shrink the sum of the fit across trees toward zero. This tuning parameter is generally chosen together with the total number of trees via cross-validation. Similar to boosting, BART provides a related but alternative strategy to avoid overfitting that lets the data speak more naturally [13]. The trees are encouraged to be small and the parameters are shrunk toward zero, so each tree-parameter pair constitutes a weak learner. Specifically, we write $f \sim \text{BART}(\pi_T, \pi_M)$ for the BART prior with prior $T_m \overset{\text{i.i.d.}}{\sim} \pi_T$ and $\mu_{ml} \overset{\text{i.i.d.}}{\sim} \pi_M$ given $\{T_m\}$. It is standard to take π_M to be Normal $(0, \sigma^2)$ where $\sigma_\mu \propto M^{-1/2}$; this is conditionally conjugate and ensures that $\text{Var}\{g(x)\} = M\sigma^2$ does not depend on the number of trees M. We take π_T to be the prior described by [14], which can be sampled by initializing T_m with a single root note of depth $d = 0$. This node is then made branch with probability $\gamma/(1+d)^\beta$ and a leaf node otherwise; if the node is a branch node, we add its two children at depth $d+1$. This process then iterates over all the nodes of depth $d = 1, 2, \ldots$ until all of the nodes at some depth are leaf nodes. Bayesian variable selection techniques applicable to BART have been studied by [15], [16], [17], and [18]. We use the following prior to the splitting rules throughout this chapter. First $j_b \sim$ Categorical (s) for some probability vector s. Then, given j_b and the values of (j_b', C_b') for the ancestor nodes of b, we set $C_b \sim$ Uniform (L_j, R_j) where $\prod_{j=1}^{P}(L_j, R_j)$ is the hyperrectangle of x-values which are associated with branch b. Following [19], we set $s \sim$ Dirichlet $(\alpha/P, \ldots, \alpha/P)$ and in our illustrations use $\alpha/(\alpha+P) \sim$ Beta $(0.5, 1)$. This prior for s encourages the model to concentrate on models with a small number of relevant predictors.

$$[s_1, \cdots, s_P] \mid \theta \sim Dirichlet\left(\frac{\theta}{P}, \cdots, \frac{\theta}{P}\right)$$

$$\frac{\theta}{\theta+\rho} \sim Beta(a, b)$$

In summary, BART learns the relationship between the covariates, X, and the response variable arriving at the true formula in the spirit of machine learning while not burdening the user to prespecify the functional form of f nor the interaction terms among the covariates. By specifying an optional sparse Dirichlet prior, BART is capable of variable selection: a form of learning which is especially useful in high-dimensional settings. In the class of ensemble predictive models, BART's out-of-sample predictive performance is competitive with other leading members of this class. Due to its membership in the class of

Bayesian nonparametric models, BART not only provides an estimate of the function but naturally generates the uncertainty as well. And BART was designed to be very flexible via its prior arguments while providing the user robust, low information, default settings that will likely produce a good fit without resorting to computationally demanding cross-validation. BART itself is relatively computationally efficient, but larger data sets will naturally take more time to estimate.

9.1.4 Proposed Survival Analysis with BART Extensions

We propose a model using the BART framework, which we refer to as CoxBART. It is based on a Bayesian interpretation of the Cox partial likelihood.

CoxBART borrows the Cox proportional hazard structure while allowing BART to model the unknown relationship between the covariates and survival rather than assuming a linear relationship as in the standard Cox proportional hazard model.

Consider the proportional hazards model $h(t \mid x) = \lambda(t)\exp\{g(x)\}$ where $\lambda(t)$ is the baseline hazard and $g(x)$ is unknown, with $g(x)$ estimated using the Cox partial likelihood

$$\text{PL}(g) = \prod_{i:\delta_i=1} \frac{exp\{g(X_i)\}}{\sum_{j \in \mathcal{R}_i} exp\{g(X_j)\}} \quad \text{where } \mathcal{R}_i = \{j : Y_j \geq Y_i\} \text{ is the set of subjects at-risk of failure}$$

at time Y_i. Letting Π denote the prior, we define the pseudoposterior

$$\Pi(dg \mid \mathcal{D}_N) = \frac{\text{PL}(g)\,\Pi(dg)}{\int \text{PL}(g)\,\Pi(dg)}$$

This expression arises under an improper prior for $\Lambda(t)$. Consider a discrete time proportional hazards model $S(t \mid x) = exp\left\{e^{g(x)} \sum_{t_i \leq t} \phi_i\right\}$. Ref. [32] shows that PL (g) is the integrated likelihood of $g(x)$ when the parameters ϕ_i are given an improper data-dependent prior where the t_i's are set equal to the observed values of the Y_i's and

$\pi(\phi_1, \cdots, \phi_N) \propto \sum_{i=2}^{N} \delta_i \phi_i^{-1} + (1-\delta_i)\delta_0(\phi_i)$, where $\delta_0(\cdot)$ is a point-mass at 0. The likelihood of (ϕ, g) is

$$\prod_{i=1}^{N} \phi_i^{\delta_i} \exp\left[\delta_i g(X_i) - \exp\{g(X_i)\} \sum_{j:Y_j \leq Y_i} \phi_j\, \delta_j\right]$$

$$= \prod_{i:\delta_i=1}^{N} \phi_i \exp\left[g(X_i) - \phi_i \sum_{j \in \mathcal{R}_j} \exp(g(X_i))\right]$$

The conditional distribution of $(\phi_1, \cdots, \phi_N, \mathcal{D})$ given g under this model is

$$\pi(\phi_1, \cdots, \phi_N, \mathcal{D}|g) = \prod_{i:\delta_i=1} \exp\left[g(X_i) - \phi \sum_j \exp\{g(X_i)\}\right].$$

(1)

From the expression in (1) above, $\phi_i \overset{ind}{\sim} \text{Gamma}\left(1, \sum_{j \in \mathcal{R}_i} exp\{g(X_i)\}\right)$ given $(g, \mathcal{D})$. Integrating

out ϕ, we obtain $\text{PL}(g)$. We refer to this model with $g \sim \text{BART}(\pi_T, \pi_M)$ as CoxBART. CoxBART is a nonparametric model in the sense that $g(x)$ is nonparametric, but we do assume proportional hazards. It is more flexible than the usual Cox linear model, where $g(x) = x^\top \beta$. CoxBART is interesting due to the common use of the proportional hazards assumption in practice while introducing more flexibility through the nonparametric form. A related model is given by [23]; however, this model only satisfies the proportional hazards assumption conditional on latent variables.

Using the default choice of π_T in original BART, the only remaining parameters to choose are (α_μ, β_μ) in the prior $\mu_{ml} \sim \log \text{Gamma}(\alpha_\mu, \beta_\mu)$. To impose that μ_{ml} has mean 0, we set $\log(\beta-\mu) = \psi(\alpha_\mu)$ where $\psi(\alpha)$ is the digamma function $\frac{d}{d\alpha}\log\Gamma(\alpha)$. The variance of μ_{ml} is given by $\sigma_\mu^2 = \psi'(\alpha_\mu)$ where $\psi'(\alpha)$ is the trigamma function. We set $\sigma_\mu \sim \text{Half-Cauchy}\left(0, \frac{1.5}{\sqrt{M}}\right)$ and update σ_μ using slice sampling ([32]). We note that the required special functions ψ, ψ' and $(\psi')^{-1}$ are all straightforward to calculate numerically. The simple approximation $\alpha_\mu = \sigma_\mu^{-2} + 1/2$ and $\beta_\mu = \sigma_\mu^{-2}$ given by [33] also works well when σ_μ is small.

9.2 Simulation Section

In this section, we illustrate the applicability of different models for survival prediction in situations when the regression relationships between the survival times and the covariates are nonlinear and complex, with and without proportional hazards. A series of examples are performed via repeated-data simulation to investigate the performance of the machine learning approach compared to long-standing traditional methods. We will assess the ability of the proposed models to capture nonlinear relationships and to assess what one loses when CoxBART is used when the proportional hazards assumption fails. Techniques being considered include:

Cox-Linear Regression: This semiparametric model fit with the log-linear link tilting the baseline hazard $h(t|x) = h_0(t)\exp(x^\top \beta)$. We set two linear regression models based on Cox's partial likelihood. The first one, *CoxLinear$_0$*, only uses the patients' response as the only covariate, and the second *CoxLinear* uses the full set of patients' information. It's rare to use the first model in reality when other covariates are available; we use *CoxLinear$_0$* only as a benchmark to show that incorporating patients' personal information is beneficial in terms of predicting better survival results. The method is available in the software **R** via `survival::coxph`;

Random Survival Forest: The random survival forest algorithm ([3]) fit with `randomForestSRC::rfsr` in **R**. This fits a fully nonparametric model to the survival function and does not invoke any model assumptions (e.g. Cox' proportional assumption).

CoxBART: BART implementation of Cox partial likelihood, with default priors for BART.

We assess the performance of each model according to how well they estimate the conditional survival function $S(t|x)$. As a measure of accuracy, we consider the average integrated squared distance between the estimated survival function $\hat{S}(t|x)$ and the true survival function $S_0(t|x)$, $MSE = \int \int\limits_{i=1}^{T_{max}} \left(\hat{S}(t|x) - S_0(t|x)\right)^2 dt\, F_X(dx)$, where

the F_X is the true distribution of the predictors and T_{max} is the maximum of all observed survival times in the sample. As MSE in this case has no closed form, we approximate

the integral numerically on the test set as $N^{*-1} \sum\limits_{i=1}^{N^*} \int\limits_0^{T_{max}} \left(\hat{S}(t|X^*) - S_0(t|X^*)\right)^2 dt$, where the

$\int \cdot dt$ integral is computed numerically on the time grid, and the star symbol $\cdot^*$ relates to the test set (internal data set, or another holdout set). We consider the following simulation examples for the true hazard function.

S1: Semiparametric Exponential/Nonlinear exponential
Assuming the semiparametric exponential form of the hazard function $h(t|x) = \exp\{f(x)\}$:

- $f_{ctr}(x) = \sin(\pi x_1 x_2) + 2(x_3 - 0.5)^2 + x_4 + 0.5x_5$
- $f_{trt}(x) = 0.5(\sin(\pi x_1) + \sin(\pi x_2)) - 2.5(x_3 - 0.5)^2 - 1.2x_4 + 0.5x_5 x_2^2$

- Features: $x_1, x_2, x_3 \sim Unif(0,1)$; $x_4 \sim Bin(p_x)$ response indicator, where the probability of response depends on the patient's features: $p_x = expit(g(X)), g(X) = \frac{1}{10}x_1 x_3 + |x_2 - 1| - 0.5$; this setting guarantees that the p_x

approximately ranges between 0.38 and 0.64; $x_5 \sim Bin(0.5)$; $x_j, j > 5 \sim Unif(0,1)$.

S2: Nonparametric/Nonlinear Cox
Assuming $h(t|x) = \exp\{f(x)\}h(t)$, with response indicator being a function of patient-level information:

- $f_{ctr}(x) = \sin(\pi x_1 x_2) + 2(x_3 - 0.5)^2 + x_4 + 0.5x_5$
- $f_{trt}(x) = 0.5(\sin(\pi x_1) + \sin(\pi x_2)) - 2.5(x_3 - 0.5)^2 - 1.2x_4 + 0.5x_5 x_2^2$

- Features: $x_1, x_2, x_3 \sim Unif(0,1)$; $x_4 \sim Bin(p_x)$ response   indicator, where the probability of response depends on the patient's features: $p_x = expit(g(X)), g(X) = \frac{1}{10}x_1 x_3 + |x_2 - 1| - 0.5$; this setting guarantees that the p_x

  approximately ranges between 0.38 and 0.64; $x_5 \sim Bin(0.5)$; $x_j, j > 5 \sim Unif(0,1)$.

S3: Weibull Semiparametric with Cox's assumption violated

This simulation setting was modified based on the example from [10], which strongly violates the proportional hazards assumption.

- The survival time T_i in the control group has a Weibull distribution with rate $\kappa(x) = 0.7 + 1.3x_7$ and scale parameter $1 + 0.25\sum_{j=1}^{6} x_j + 2.5\, x_7$.

- The survival time T_i in the treatment group has a Weibull distribution with $\kappa(x) = 0.7 + 1.3x_7$ and scale parameter $1.25 + 0.25(x_1 + 0.4x_2 + 1.5x_3 + 1.2x_4 + x_5 + x_6) + 4x_7$.

- Features: $x_1, x_2, x_3, x_5, \cdots, x_{10} \sim Unif(0, 1)$; $x_4 \sim Bin(p_x)$ response indicator, where the probability of response depends on the patient's features: $p_x = expit(g(X)), g(X) = \frac{1}{10}x_1 x_3 + |x_2 - 1| - 0.5$; this setting guarantees that the p_x

  approximately ranges between 0.38 and 0.64.

For each simulation setting we took $N = 300$ and $P = 10$. The purpose of S1 and S2 is to assess how much benefit we have if we use a more complicated semiparametric model, CoxBART, instead of the conventional CoxLinear, and how competitive it is comparing to other machine learning methods like the pure data-driven RSF, when the proportional hazards assumption holds. Setting S3 is designed to assess how much is lost using CoxBART when the proportional hazards assumption fails. Figure 9.2 displays randomly sampled true survival curves for the three settings. We could see that survival curves are overlapped between the treatment arm and the control arm. For S3, the treatment effect is not significant compared to the control group at an earlier stage.

  We assess the performance of each model according to how well they estimate the conditional function $S(t|x)$. As a measure of accuracy, we consider the average integrated squared distance between the estimated survival function $\hat{S}(t|x)$ and the true survival function. We use $N' = 100$ new subjects and approximated the empirical integration over time t using a grid of size 500. Results are given in Table 9.1. The CoxBART performs best in either the mean or the median accuracy for S1 and S2, where Cox's proportional hazard assumption holds. When such model assumption is violated in S3, the CoxBART performs reasonably well.

  We conclude that the proposed method is generally effective for situations when the semiparametric Cox's proportional linear regression model $h(t|x) = h_0(t)\exp\{x^\top \beta\}$ fails. For situations where the nonparametric proportional hazard assumption holds, i.e., the hazard function has the specific form of $h(t|x) = \lambda \exp\{f(x)\}$, the CoxBART performs the best due to its capabilities of capturing complicated structures from the data through novel

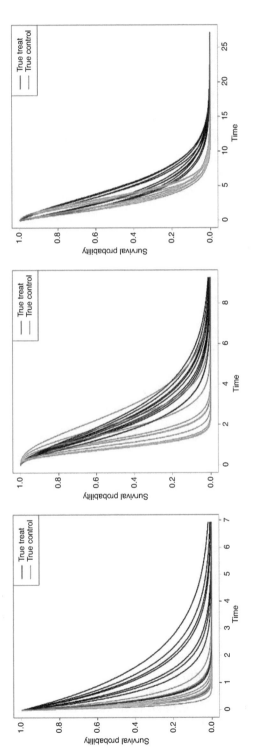

FIGURE 9.2

Randomly selected samples of survival functions $S(t \mid X_i)$ for 10 samples of X_i for each treatment arm. *Left*: S1; *Middle* S2; *Right*: S3.

TABLE 9.1

Results of the simulation experiment for S1, S2, and S3. Each entry is the integrated mean squared error when estimating the survival function. All accuracy results are relative to the best-performing method; that is, the best-performing method has the result 1.00.

Setting	Method	Average Time (mins)	Integrated Mean Squared Error for Treatment Group		Integrated Mean Squared Error for Control Group	
			Mean	Median	Mean	Median
S1	CoxBART	2.45	1.04	**1.00**	**1.00**	**1.00**
	RSF	5.03	1.25	1.54	1.44	1.45
	CoxLinear$_0$	0.06	**1.00**	1.26	2.27	2.33
	CoxLinear	0.06	1.46	1.83	1.15	1.20
S2	CoxBART	3.31	1.05	**1.00**	**1.00**	**1.00**
	RSF	2.66	1.04	1.26	1.45	1.50
	CoxLinear$_0$	0.01	**1.00**	1.25	2.55	2.67
	CoxLinear	0.01	1.58	2.00	1.79	1.81
S3	CoxBART	3.38	**1.00**	**1.00**	1.27	1.19
	RSF	2.75	1.21	1.20	**1.00**	**1.00**
	CoxLinear$_0$	0.01	2.36	2.40	1.88	1.93
	CoxLinear	0.02	1.24	1.36	1.23	1.92

trees. Random forest also provides a robust prediction but might not have the advantage in statistical inference compared to CoxBART.

9.3 Case Study

We have seen through multiple simulation examples that the Bayesian ensemble tree extension has its advantage when predicting patient-level survival curves. We analyze a generated dataset on time to event for "twined"-patients (one twin pair of patients have the same features X except for whether they have accepted the treatment and the resulted response). We use this study to demonstrate the application of the proposed methods and statistical inference from the predicted results.

In the case study, we assume we have collected historical data from a similar completed Phase III trial (i.e., historical data is mature survival data) and we have data from a completed phase II study where an exploratory endpoint is overall response (i.e., the survival data is not mature). The goal of the case study is to predict, given the historical data, what the mature survival curves from the Phase II study would look like and use this to assess whether or not the treatment has a sufficient survival benefit to move to a phase III study. Specifically, we assume we have observed $N_{historical} = 281$ pairs of twins and $N_{internal} = 69$ pairs of twins (for a total of $N_{historical} = 562, N_{internal} = 138$ subjects). We assume we have collected patients' information including their age, gender, smoking status, race, baseline tumor size, percentage change in tumor size and response after receiving certain

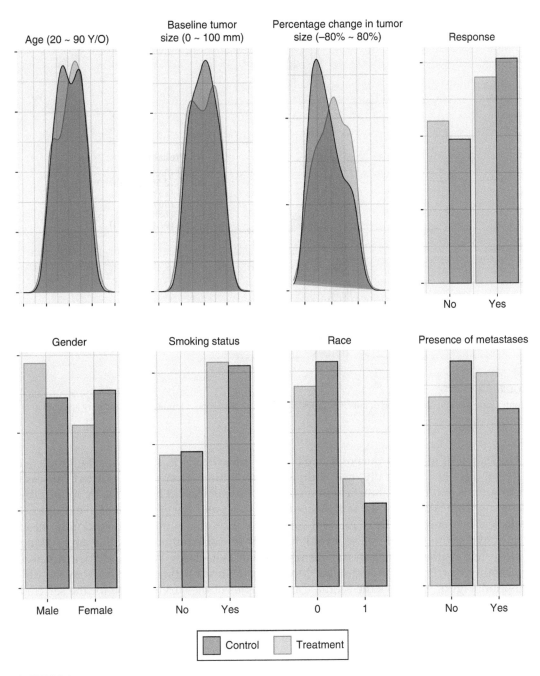

FIGURE 9.3
Covariate distribution of historical data.

treatment, and the presence of metastases. Figure 9.3 shows the distribution of empirical distributions of different covariates from historical data. After fitting the CoxBART model using the historical dataset, we predict the internal phase II patients' survival curves.

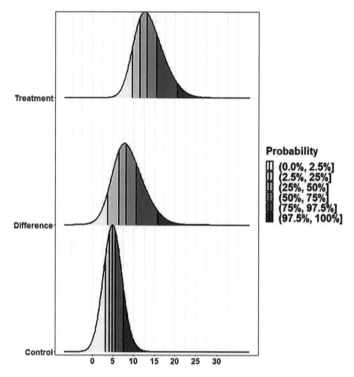

FIGURE 9.4

Monte Carlo sample distribution of survival times and difference in survival times for a randomly selected patient twin pair.

For statistical inference purposes, we conduct a Monte Carlo study over the predicted survival results. Specifically, we sample survival time from the predicted survival distributions and do the statistical inference over the empirical behaviors. By repeatedly sampling from 5000 posterior samples of each patient and the twin patient, we could get statistical inference over their survival curves. For example, suppose we randomly select pair of twins who are male, 32 years old, have a 67 mm size tumor at baseline, no smoking history, and neither of the patients has response or metastases. We predict their survival probability distribution and simulate Monte Carlo survival time samples from the distribution. Figure 9.4 shows the Monte Carlo samples of the survival time for the selected patient in the treatment group, his twin in the control group, and their survival difference. The patient in the treatment group has a significantly higher chance to survive longer compared to his twin brother in the control group, indicated by the treatment difference distribution having more than 97.5% of its mass above 0 months.

Ultimately, the question of interest in drug development related to how the drug shifts the distribution of survival times in the treatment arm relative to the control arm. The nature of this shift can be discerned by comparison of multiple quantiles between the treatment and control arms. As suggested by [35], it is of value to examine more than one quantile (e.g., median) and determine whether any differences observed are consistent across arms. We investigate the survival times and their difference at the survival quantiles of 10%, 25%, 50%, 75%, and 90% (i.e., using the sampled survival times from MCMC calculate each quantile for the control, treatment, and difference). Figure 9.5 shows the Monte Carlo

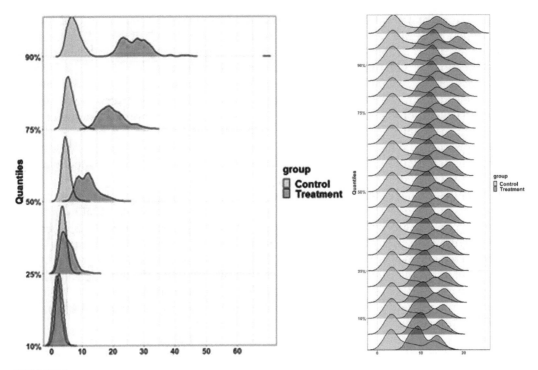

FIGURE 9.5

Monte Carlo sample distribution of the 10th, 25th, 50th, 75th, and 90th quantiles of simulated survival times. *Left:* For a randomly selected patient twin pair; *Right:* For the entirety of the treatment and control groups.

posterior samples for the different survival quantiles. The 10% and 25% survival quantiles are similar in the twins, but survival times are substantially longer in the treatment arm at the 50%, 75%, and 90% survival quantiles. This suggests that, for the twin pair, the impact of the treatment is to significantly increase survival. To further investigate the population survival quantiles, we repeat a similar Monte Carlo process but with all patients from the internal study in the treatment arm compared against all in the control arm. As shown in the right panel in Figure 9.5, when we consider the whole population in the treatment arm versus the control arm and plot the survival time quantiles, the treatment effect is also right-shifted. The overall predicted median survival time is 12.2 months for the control group and 22.0 months for the treatment group. Using these patient-level and summary distributions of the predicted mature survival times for the control and treatment arm of the internal trial, the company can make an informed decision whether this predicted difference in mature survival times is large enough to warrant further development.

9.4 Discussion

This work focuses on the comparison of a BART extension over survival problem with existing methods when analyzing survival data. It reviews different modeling approaches and compares them in terms of interpretative competence, prediction accuracy, and statistical inference. We introduced a nonparametric variant of Cox's proportional hazard model, which takes $h(t|x) = \lambda(t) \exp\{g(x)\}$ with the baseline hazard function $\lambda(t)$ modeled nonparametrically. Simulation studies are performed to judge the competence of the CoxBART estimator with the aforementioned models in regression scenarios. Compared to other semiparametric methods, such as the Cox linear model and the other parametric survival models that aim to model a particular functional relationship between the covariates and some survival outcomes, CoxBART offers a more flexible approach allowing nonparametric functional relationships. In regression scenarios the models perform closely when the proportional hazards assumption is met. However, the performance of the Cox linear model depreciates with respect to the other models when the proportional hazards assumption is violated.

Additionally, we have demonstrated how CoxBART can be applied to predict mature survival curves in a generated case study. This case study demonstrated that even when the internal phase II survival data is immature, by fitting the CoxBART method on similar but mature historical survival data one can obtain predicted mature survival curves. Using these predicted survival curves in the form of MCMC chains, it is possible to compare the treatment effect on the predicted mature survival times between the internal control and treatment arms. Further, since CoxBART is a Bayesian method, the full distribution of predicted survival times is available for all subjects allowing for the treatment effect to be explored at different survival quantiles.

In summary, our proposed CoxBART provides a decent alternative to the Cox Linear model and has an advantage in terms of statistical inference. The ensemble trees in BART bring the flexibility of a machine learning algorithm allowing for better capturing of complex relationships between the covariates and response.

References

[1] D. R. Cox, "Regression models and life-tables," *Journal of the Royal Statistical Society: Series B (Methodological)*, vol. 34, pp. 187–202, 1972.

[2] L. Breiman, J. Friedman, R. Olshen and C. Stone, "Cart," *Classification and Regression Trees; Wadsworth and Brooks/Cole: Monterey, CA, USA*, 1984.

[3] H. Ishwaran, U. B. Kogalur, E. H. Blackstone and M. S. Lauer, "Random survival forests," *The Annals of Applied Statistics*, vol. 2, pp. 841–860, 2008.

[4] J. D. a. P. R. L. Kalbfleisch, "Estimation of the average hazard ratio," *Biometrika*, vol. 68, pp. 105–112, 1981.

[5] J. P. a. M. M. L. Klein, "Semiparametric proportional hazards regression with fixed covariates," in *Survival Analysis*, Springer, pp. 243–293, 2003.

[6] W. Thompson Jr, "On the treatment of grouped observations in life studies," *Biometrics*, pp. 463–470, 1977.

[7] E. a. H. P. Arjas, "A note on the asymptotic normality in the Cox regression model," *The Annals of Statistics*, vol. 16, pp. 1133–1140, 1988.

[8] L. Fahrmeir, "Discrete survival-time models," *Wiley StatsRef: Statistics Reference Online*, 2014.

[9] L. Breiman, "Random forests," *Machine Learning*, vol. 45, pp. 5–32, 2001.

[10] R. A. Sparapani, B. R. Logan, R. E. McCulloch and P. W. Laud, "Nonparametric survival analysis using Bayesian additive regression trees (BART)," *Statistics in Medicine*, vol. 35, pp. 2741–2753, 2016.

[11] A. R. Linero, "A review of tree-based Bayesian methods," *Communications for Statistical Applications and Methods,* vol. 24, pp. 543–559, 2017.

[12] J. Hill, A. Linero and J. Murray, "Bayesian additive regression trees: a review and look forward," *Annual Review of Statistics and Its Application,* vol. 7, pp. 251–278, 2020.

[13] J. E. Starling, J. S. Murray, C. M. Carvalho, R. K. Bukowski, J. G. Scott and others, "Bart with targeted smoothing: An analysis of patient-specific stillbirth risk," *Annals of Applied Statistics,* vol. 14, pp. 28–50, 2020.

[14] H. A. Chipman, E. I. George and R. E. McCulloch, "Bayesian CART model search," *Journal of the American Statistical Association,* vol. 93, pp. 935–948, 1998.

[15] H. A. Chipman, E. I. George, R. E. McCulloch and others, "BART: Bayesian additive regression trees," *The Annals of Applied Statistics,* vol. 4, p. 266–298, 2010.

[16] J. Bleich and A. Kapelner, "Bayesian additive regression trees with parametric models of heteroskedasticity," *arXiv preprint arXiv:1402.5397,* 2014.

[17] P. R. Hahn and C. M. Carvalho, "Decoupling shrinkage and selection in Bayesian linear models: a posterior summary perspective," *Journal of the American Statistical Association,* vol. 110, pp. 435–448, 2015.

[18] R. E. McCulloch, C. Carvalho, and R. Hahn, "A general approach to variable selection using Bayesian nonparametric models," *Joint Statistical Meetings, Seattle,* vol. 8, 2015-08-09–2015-08-13.

[19] A. R. Linero, "Bayesian regression trees for high-dimensional prediction and variable selection," *Journal of the American Statistical Association,* vol. 113, pp. 626–636, 2018.

[20] A. R. Linero and Y. Yang, "Bayesian regression tree ensembles that adapt to smoothness and sparsity," *Journal of the Royal Statistical Society: Series B (Statistical Methodology),* vol. 80, pp. 1087–1110, 2018.

[21] P. Müller and R. Mitra, "Bayesian nonparametric inference–why and how," *Bayesian Analysis (Online),* vol. 8, 2013. https://projecteuclid.org/journals/bayesian-analysis/volume-8/issue-2/Bayesian-Nonparametric-Inference--Why-and-How/10.1214/13-BA811.full

[22] D. B. Dunson, "Bayesian nonparametric hierarchical modeling," *Biometrical Journal: Journal of Mathematical Methods in Biosciences,* vol. 51, pp. 273–284, 2009. https://onlinelibrary.wiley.com/doi/10.1002/bimj.200800183

[23] V. Bonato, V. Baladandayuthapani, B. M. Broom, E. P. Sulman, K. D. Aldape and K.-A. Do, "Bayesian ensemble methods for survival prediction in gene expression data," *Bioinformatics,* vol. 27, pp. 359–367, 2011.

[24] D. Oakes, "Bivariate survival models induced by frailties," *Journal of the American Statistical Association,* vol. 84, pp. 487–493, 1989.

[25] P. Hougaard, "Shared frailty models," in *Analysis of Multivariate Survival Data,* Springer, pp. 215–262, 2000.

[26] N. C. Henderson, T. A. Louis, G. L. Rosner and R. Varadhan, "Individualized treatment effects with censored data via fully nonparametric Bayesian accelerated failure time models," *Biostatistics,* vol. 21, pp. 50–68, 2020.

[27] Y. Li, A. R. Linero and J. S. Murray, "Adaptive Conditional Distribution Estimation with Bayesian Decision Tree Ensembles," *arXiv Preprint arXiv:2005.02490,* 2020.

[28] P. Basak, A. Linero, D. Sinha and S. Lipsitz, "Semiparametric analysis of clustered interval-censored survival data using soft Bayesian additive regression trees (SBART)," *Biometrics,* vol. 78, no. 3, pp. 880–893, 2021.

[29] T. Fernández, N. Rivera and Y. W. Teh, "Gaussian processes for survival analysis," *Advances in Neural Information Processing Systems,* vol. 29, pp. 5021–5029, 2016.

[30] M. De Iorio, W. O. Johnson, P. Müller and G. L. Rosner, "Bayesian nonparametric nonproportional hazards survival modeling," *Biometrics,* vol. 65, pp. 762–771, 2009.

[31] D. Sinha, J. G. Ibrahim and M.-H. Chen, "A Bayesian justification of Cox's partial likelihood," *Biometrika,* vol. 90, pp. 629–641, 2003.

[32] R. M. Neal, "Slice sampling," *The Annals of Statistics,* vol. 31, pp. 705–767, 2003.

[33] J. S. Murray, "Log-linear Bayesian additive regression trees for multinomial Logistic and count regression models," *Journal of the American Statistical Association*, vol. 116, no. 534, pp. 756–769, 2021.

[34] R. Etzioni, R. Gulati and D. Lin, "Measures of survival benefit in cancer drug development and their limitations," *Urologic Oncology: Seminars and Original Investigations*, vol. 33, no. 3, pp. 122–127, 2015.

10

Unleashing the Power of Digital Tools in Clinical Trials: A Systematic Review of Digital Measurement Considerations from Implementation Experience

Junjing Lin, Jianchang Lin, and Andy Chi

> *Style used to be an interaction between the human soul and tools that were limiting. In the digital era, it will have to come from the soul alone.*
>
> – **Jaron Lanier,** *Taking Stock* [1]

Introduction

As the line between clinical research and clinical care becomes increasingly blurry, personalized digital health products for measurement and intervention have shown to be beneficial to patients by improving quality of life, enabling early diagnosis, facilitating wider and more convenient access to healthcare resources, thereby extending overall patient benefit, even survival [2,3,4]. From sponsors' perspective, it can potentially enhance cost-effectiveness in conducting clinical research and improve disease management by including broader populations, decentralizing trial administration, and utilizing novel digital measurements. A more patient-centered, operationally efficient, and statistically robust approach toward digital health is imperative for advancing clinical research and patient care.

Even before the COVID-19 pandemic, patients with unmet medical needs have been among the most frail and vulnerable populations that suffer from chronic conditions and mental distress. Under the pandemic, especially before vaccination, these patients must cope with not only the burden of dealing with chronic illnesses but also the peril of being infected with COVID-19, a disease that can cause severe complications and has limited treatment options.

The concept of digital health has existed in US legislations since 1997 [6–13] and in FDA approval documents since 2012 [14]; 'mobile clinical trial' or 'decentralized clinical trial' has been widely discussed since 2017 [15]. The urgent need for continuing patient care without face-to-face contact under COVID-19 pushed the rapid and broad implementation of digital health, crossing the operational barriers over sponsors, providers, and regulators [16,17]. For instance, in April 2020, FDA published guidance on using digital health devices for treating psychiatric disorders during the pandemic [18], followed by the guidance on

DOI: 10.1201/9781003288640-10

noninvasive remote monitoring devices in June 2020 [19]. In September 2020, FDA further launched the Digital Health Center of Excellence [20].

As the world recovers from the pandemic, many digital health tools will remain advantageous in both clinical research and clinical care settings. Especially under more favorable regulatory environment, data generated from digital health tools will be increasingly used for regulatory decision-making in the coming years. In June 2020, European Medicines Agency (EMA) published the Q&A on qualification of digital technology–based methodologies to support approval of medicinal products [21]; in February 2021, FDA announced the Innovative Science and Technology Approaches for New Drugs (ISTAND) Pilot Program [22], to complement the existing drug development tool (DDT) qualification program to accelerate the evaluation of digital tools that may enable decentralized trials, develop novel endpoints, and assist patient assessments; in June 2021, EMA further published the guideline on computerized systems and electronic data in clinical trials [23] and posited that validation approaches should be risk proportionate, and that iterative and extensive validation may be needed to enable technology use to eventually support the pivotal data in an Marketing Authorization Application; in December 2021, FDA issued draft guidance 'Digital Health Technologies (DHTs) for Remote Data Acquisition in Clinical Investigations' [24] and highlighted the importance to validate the fit-for-purpose of a DHT to support its use and interpretability in the clinical investigations.

In light of the expanding and escalating adoption of digital health in clinical research setting, this chapter attempts to provide practical considerations on the basic tenets of design principle and program implementation when digital measurements are involved in clinical studies. The rest of the chapter is organized as follows: Section 2 aims to elucidate the subtle differences between digital measurements and digital endpoints; Section 3 focuses on operational and regulatory aspects of data collection tailored for digital measurements; Section 4 narrates a few design and statistical topics; and lastly, Section 5 provides additional remarks on design considerations.

10.1 Digital Measurements and Endpoints

Fundamental to the formulation of a design framework is the clarity to delineate the subtlety around the measurements and endpoints. Measurement is defined as the process of associating numbers with physical quantities and phenomena [25]. Measurement may be made solely by human senses, or by the aid of instruments and systems, which enables detection of quantities beyond the capabilities of the senses. The measurement systems can involve computational processing, where measurement signals are transformed mathematically, typically by various types of digital computers. The performance of measurement systems can be influenced by a range of intrinsic and extrinsic factors. The intrinsic factors are often described as the characteristics of the system, such as resolution and precision, as well as effects engendered in the measurement process, such as drift and hysteresis. Extrinsic factors are the ones that tend to obscure or alter the signals, including noise and interference, e.g., human errors. In light of this, it is conceivable that the central pillar of measurement theory concerns three elements, namely representation, error, and uniqueness, which are very much applicable in elucidating the crux of the digital measurements.

Representation. In clinical research, for digital measurements to be representative of clinical endpoints, the first and foremost criterion is being clinically meaningful. Clinically meaningful endpoints represent how a patient feels, functions, or survives [26,27]. In the context of clinical trials or interventional studies, endpoints must meet the requirements for study-specific scientific and regulatory objectives, accounting for the hierarchy of endpoint families relevant to the disease indication or process of interest. On the one hand, even within the same therapeutical area, endpoint considerations can be indication specific [29–32]; on the other hand, the hierarchy of endpoints imposes differential benchmarks for the 'meaningfulness', especially for regulatory purposes. For instance, a primary endpoint should be the measurement(s) capable of demonstrating the most clinically relevant and persuasive evidence directly pertinent to the primary objective of the study [28]. This means that the primary endpoint should reflect accepted standards and norms and, justified by earlier studies or published literature, can offer validated and reliable measures of treatment benefit in the targeted patient population. In this case, novel digital measurements, or common measurements captured with novel digital devices, may not be appropriate candidates for deriving a primary endpoint in a pivotal trial. Some example digital endpoints considered by different sponsors in studies of various phases can be found on the Digital Medicine Society website [33].

Error. The concept of error is essential to the understanding of uncertainty and the evaluations of the quality of digital measurements for constructing endpoints. The measurement error is generally unknown because the true value being measured is unknown. However, the uncertainty of the results of digital measurement process may be quantified and examined. To apprehend the desired qualifications of endpoints, it is imperative to shed light on common vocabulary that often lacks clarity in the recent literature: accuracy, precision, validity, reliability, repeatability, and reproducibility. *Accuracy*, a qualitative concept, is the closeness between the result of a measurement process and the true value ('reference', 'criterion', or 'gold standard' in practice) [34], whereas *precision* is the consistency of results from repeated measurement processes, regardless of the true value. Figure 10.1 presents an illustration of the concept accuracy vs. precision. Precision is not to be confused with *resolution*, which represents the smallest unit of measurements that a device can display [35]. *Validity*, conceptually akin to accuracy, indicates the degree to which a measurement process is assumed to measure vs. what it actually measures and includes three aspects: content validity, criterion validity, and construct validity [35]. Content validity usually involves subjective judgment regarding whether the desired concepts are covered by the measurement. Criterion validity is empirically based and depicts whether the measurement process can reflect actual performance, predict future performance, and distinguish characteristics vs. noncharacteristics. Construct validity, which relates to the conceptual basis captured by the measurement, is usually applied when there is no existing standard from which results can be compared. *Reliability* describes the extent to which the measurement process is consistent and can be illustrated in terms of internal consistency reliability, test-retest reliability, and interrater reliability [35]. The notion of reliability is similar to that of precision. *Repeatability*, or test-retest reliability, refers to the closeness of a particular result compared to the measurements rendered by the same process under same circumstances, e.g., exactly same procedure, observer, instrument, testing conditions, and location, etc., over a certain period of time [34]. In comparison, *reproducibility* is the closeness of agreement between the results of measurements of the same object carried out under changed conditions of the measurement process, such as principle, method, observer, instrument, reference standard,

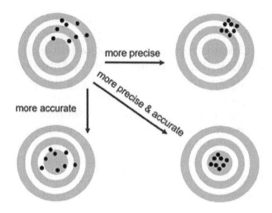

FIGURE 10.1
Illustration of accuracy vs. precision.

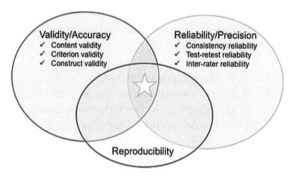

FIGURE 10.2
Illustration of the desirable 'error' properties of an endpoint.

location, conditions of use, or time [34]. Principally, for digital endpoints to be 'fit-for-purpose', they should be proven accurate/valid, precise/reliable, and reproducible, which requires rigorous validation processes [36,37]. Figure 10.2 shows an illustration of the desirable 'error' properties of an endpoint.

Uniqueness. Uniqueness concerns the degree to which the chosen representation is the only one viable for the object of interest. In the context of clinical studies, the concept of uniqueness calls for thorough deliberation of estimand, namely, the target of inference [38]. In general, there are multiple ways to quantify treatment effect. Treatment effect can be represented by survival benefit, adverse events of interest, quality of life measures, etc. For instance, for a specific quality of life measure, e.g. summary of items from Patient-Reported Outcomes Version of the Common Terminology Criteria for Adverse Events (PRO-CTCAE), different modalities, e.g. provisioned device vs. paper version, of data collection can impact the comparability or equivalence of the same questionnaires within or across patients [39,40]. If mixed-modality is generally not recommended but deviations are anticipated in a study, assessment of the comparability of the 'contaminated' data and additional sensitivity analyses may be needed. More discussions on this view will be presented in Section 4.

10.2 Operational and Regulatory Considerations

Now that the desirable properties of digital endpoints are conceptually elucidated, the vital aspects in day-to-day clinical operations and regulatory requirements that actualize the digital measurement process cannot be emphasized more.

10.2.1 Device Inclusion

Suppose that after vendor selection, a gamut of digital tools are available to be chosen for integration. From our implementation experience, two major factors that impact the decision are the value added and feasibility of execution. Specifically, the determination of value fundamentally depends on the study objectives and the scientific questions of interest. Once study objectives are in consensus with the study team, evaluations of how digital measurements can contribute to the study endpoints need to be made. Does the new way of measurement provide added value to having no measurement or what has been traditionally measured? Can the digital measurements be validated against a benchmark or an established endpoint? What is the level of evidence needed for the digital measurements to be employed as key endpoints or exploratory endpoints? Moreover, articulating the feasibility of digital tools with various integration options is multiplex. On the one hand, the perception of feasibility may shift from the study planning phase to study execution phase; on the other hand, program strategic priorities and study-level support are dynamic and subject to quick shift.

Figure 10.3 describes a hypothetical example of how the projection of value and feasibility can change when the study team updates knowledge by executing study startup activities. In this example, feasibility was first perceived as the capability of existing technology and patient acceptance. As the execution becomes more 'real', other factors, such as budget limit, timeline to integrate multiple digital tools, patient's burden of maintaining multiple devices, limitation of data integration process, etc., become dominant considerations. If the

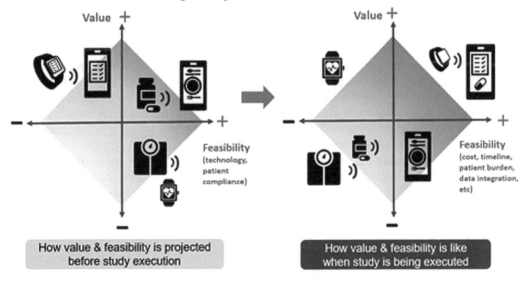

FIGURE 10.3
A hypothetical example of device inclusion decision.

value added by digital measurements is high, the tolerance for cost and timeline can be understandably higher, whereas if the value provided is relatively low, e.g., contributing to an exploratory endpoint with no prior regulatory consent, perhaps only the most efficient tools, i.e., least number of devices capable of collecting the desired data points and with short deployment timeframe, will be kept.

10.2.2 Local Standard and Regulatory Considerations

The capability and agility of adaptation to local standards and regulations is of vital importance to ensure smoothness of clinical operation when a global clinical study is executed. For instance, if a global study is designed to evaluate the impact of a common treatment for an adverse event, the differential standard of care in various regions will have an impact on the development of related digital tools and study documentation, including informed consent, training material, and eDiary specifications. In this case, it would be wise to plan ahead for the possible adjustment in terms of timeline and cost, and for the flexibility to incorporate changes without major structural revision. Another example is that certain digital procedures, e.g. eConsent, may not be viable to implement in some countries that impose restricted regulations on digital tools. For instance, as of the date when this book chapter is written, TeleVisit using iPhone cannot be physically delivered in China due to restrictions of the 'CallKit' functionality native to Apple devices [41]. If China is a key enrollment site for that study, a backup plan for enrollment or alternative informed consent procedure is recommended to be in place, and protocol language be flexible enough to cover such scenarios. To mitigate the risk of local 'surprises', local specialists can be involved in the review process; the selected vendors are encouraged to provide properly vetted solutions with scope and feasibility for all targeted countries; last but not least, careful preplanning and staying on top of global regulatory landscape is essential.

10.2.3 Integration Process

10.2.3.1 Timeline

No matter the study level or program level, meeting timeline constraints is an imperative element for claiming operational success in drug development. The incorporation of digital tools is anticipated to entail additional interdependent components when other study elements are still in limbo during the startup phase. Especially in the early stage, where introducing digital tools into routine clinical study is still relatively new for many parties, it is indispensable to build in extra problem-solving periods when crafting a study timeline. For instance, the review approval process may be lengthened to accommodate additional questions as some authorities and IRB/EC are unfamiliar with the digital solutions; last-minute changes in protocol or digital strategies that link to digital tool specification may result in considerable timeline delay in all components impacted; applications on digital devices may need to be approved several weeks prior to first site shipment; translation of digital content can take 12–14 weeks and more with increased complexity; user acceptance testing (UAT) can take several months or more; and digital requirement document needs to be developed prior to UAT. It is advisable to plan upfront, understand the interdependency among the processes, and set priorities and targeted timelines.

10.2.3.2 Data Flow and Data Standards

Behind the glamour of the growing functionalities that digital tools nowadays can provide, people less involved in day-to-day study operation and data management are often sanguine about the prospects of the ease of fetching data from multiple sources into clinical database, not to mention the granularity of data format and data monitoring requirement dependent upon the analysis goal and regulatory submission strategy. Before study execution, data captured in multiple digital devices are usually imagined to be connected to electronic data capture (EDC), if needed – all the data can be automatically uploaded to a centralized storage, which is ready for either real-time monitoring and analysis, or mapping to a sponsor EDC. However, during study execution, the deterrent effects from the limitations of device design, study conduct, patient compliance, or data management status quo on data transfer among devices, platforms, and EDC may be exposed. For instance, past failure in data quality from integrating eDiary with EDC, either due to poor compliance, gaps from data monitoring, or other technical challenges, can render hesitation to adopt integration under timeline constraints. Figure 10.4 and Figure 10.5

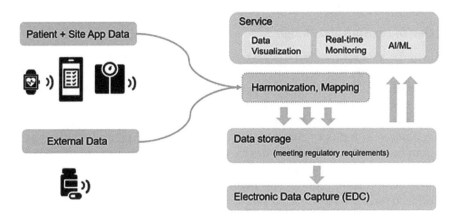

FIGURE 10.4
A hypothetical example of data flow during initial planning stage.

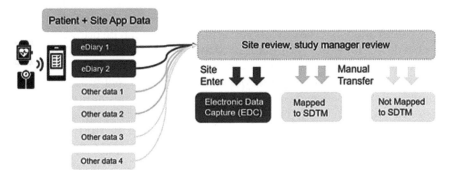

FIGURE 10.5
A hypothetical example of data flow during study execution stage.

showcase a hypothetical example where the plan of data flow is revised before and after study execution. In light of such situations, realistic arrangement of data capturing and mapping necessitates careful investigation of technical and operational status quo as well as developing a fallback plan. On the other hand, under the scenario where EDC integration is not pursued, processes must be in place to ensure sufficient data monitoring, checking, and cleaning to eventually meet the data quality and standard requirements. Especially in decentralized trials, the remote and passive data collection can range from 'via intermediates' to 'fully virtual' [42], leading to possibly little interference from trial participants, including patients and sponsor/site personnel, such that the usual data monitoring and checking supported by the intermediates such as EDC may be left out. Of note, the additional complexity of data monitoring, if done remotely, is also introduced by strict data protection rules in some regions [43]. Consequently, unambiguous goal of data standard and upfront determination of degree of 'virtuality' and the flow of critical data is recommended, particularly if the study data is to be submitted for new drug applications, abbreviated new drug applications, biologics license applications, or investigational new drug applications to the Center for Drug Evaluation and Research or the Center for Biologics Evaluation and Research [44,45].

10.2.3.3 Device Logistics and Design

The hurdle of device logistics and design elements concerns not only the explicit distribution plan, which entails foresight, but also the application prerequisite prior to delivery, as well as any diversion from blueprint postdelivery. First and foremost, the device logistics pivot on study design and schedule of events. If provisioned devices are scheduled to be incorporated into the study activities prior to enrollment, the demand for readiness of the devices in terms of numbers required, prior testing, and training at the sites is higher than the situation where the devices are only needed after enrollment. Note that applications usually need to be approved 2–3 weeks prior to first site shipment to permit preconfiguration and testing of devices before shipping, in current practice. On the other hand, if critical data are to be collected frequently with digital devices, the tolerance for the possibility of malfunctioning devices without a contingent plan is relatively low, e.g., when the computer system is under massive ransomware attack [46], backup devices may have to be delivered to patients at the outset; inventory and supply chain may allow in-time delivery should a device fail during the study; and alternative modality of capturing data may need to be approved in advance. Further, vigilance of device limitations is also crucial during the study planning phase so that the gap between what the devices are thought to supposedly collect and what the devices can actually collect can be bridged, which in turn influences the device logistics. For instance, for the same branded device, there is discrepancy between 'commercial grade' and 'medical grade'. In other words, the device functionalities, such as battery life, in daily situations can be quite different from those in a clinical study. Suppose a study is designed to capture daytime activities and sleep patterns, but the provisioned smartwatch only has 11-hour battery life. If the design fault is not caught before study execution, the patients may be disoriented during the study because of inconsistency between instructions and device functionality; the associated documentation would be rushed to be amended; devices can be too late to deploy updates; and the study may end up capturing neither daytime activities nor sleep patterns. Moreover, the device design and specifications merit careful concocted evaluation with the patient experience in mind. For example, for patients with small wrists, certain smart watches' bulky face and band may prevent patients from wearing them during certain daily activities. In order to capture patient experience, such as in an end-of-study satisfaction survey, question-naire developers shall be aware of their perception limitations and seek input from testers regarding the comprehensiveness or ambiguity in framing survey questions. Of note, from our experience, UAT for digital components can be time consuming and frustrating for some testers. UAT scripts are recommended to be written in a more user-friendly format and in less technical terms; ideal testers should have patient experience as well as site experience; and UAT meetings may be kicked off in person when situations allow, and daily touch points can be set up to obtain feedback from testers.

10.3 Design and Statistical Considerations

Statistical considerations are an integral part of study design: they facilitate the maneuver of study execution and yet can be perplexed or simplified by the study conduct. Among the multitude of relevant topics, this section will focus on a few essential ideas.

10.3.1 Study Objectives and Estimands

To address a scientific question of interest, an estimand describes the quantity to be estimated, which details the population, the endpoint, the method to account for inter-current event, and the population-level summary of the endpoint [38]. The ICH E9 (R1) addendum on estimands came into effect in the EU on July 30, 2020, and has been formally adopted by Health Canada since July 21, 2020 [47]. It provides a framework to translate study objectives into proper study design, data collection approach, and statistical meth-odologies for estimation and testing.

A salient feature of the estimand framework is the concept of intercurrent events [48]. Intercurrent events are events that occur post treatment initiation and either preclude observation of an endpoint-defining event or impact interpretation of endpoint [38]. In other words, intercurrent events can exert various degrees of influence on the quantifica-tion of treatment effect [49–52]. It is not surprising that intercurrent events were discussed in FDA's DHT guidance [24]. In the context of a study that incorporates digital tools, or a decentralized trial, prudence must be taken to anticipate the additional complexity of digital health–related intercurrent events. For instance, clarity on what constitutes com-pliance and whether such noncompliance is deemed an intercurrent event warrants fur-ther consideration. If in practice the compliance of using a digital tool is measured by the extent of missing data, the reason for missingness, which may sometimes be difficult to capture, can determine whether the noncompliance is related to an endpoint or is missing by random and will in turn impact the interpretation of compliance. A patient can be too sick to log in the data, which may be associated with an endpoint, or the digital device runs out of battery or a language is not available in the country where the device is provided, which is likely unrelated to the endpoint. The former scenario is an intercurrent event, whereas the latter scenario is not. Further, deciding whether on-study deviation is an inter-current event or not is not always trivial, namely, what deviations are acceptable in terms of maintaining usability of data as intended, or at least keeping the rest of the data intact? In reality, patients can miss entering eDiary due to misunderstanding of the completion timeline or because the device is not set up properly to send out reminders; a patient can enter data but switch the order of the assessment with other study procedures; or after a system-wide device outage, the site may substitute with a paper version during the outage, and continue using the paper version even when the outage is over, rendering inconsistent modalities of data collection from baseline vs. postbaseline within patients, or on various visits across patients. If these data are collected for a key endpoint, such data issues may be detrimental to study objectives, depending on whether an estimand was clearly defined and regulatory agency's buy-in. A thorough preplanning of such situations may enable additional data capture, fallback arrangement, or risk-based data monitoring, which can facilitate the interpretability of the data and endpoint derivation downstream. For issues that cannot be anticipated and purposefully captured, additional sensitivity analyses may be required to understand the impact of the potential intercurrent events.

10.3.2 Digital Measurement Types and Design Considerations

Most of the digital measurements can be classified into one of the two categories: digital biomarkers and electronic clinical outcome assessments (eCOAs), the digital counterparts of biomarkers and clinical outcome assessments (COAs), as described in the BEST (Biomarkers, EndpointS, and other Tools) Resource [53]. Formally, biomarkers are defined as characteristics (such as a physiologic, pathologic, or anatomic characteristic or measurement) that are objectively measured and evaluated as an indicator of normal biologic processes, pathologic processes, or biological responses to a therapeutic intervention [54]. Under the BEST Resource framework, the biomarkers are labeled by their intended usage: diagnostic, monitoring, pharmacodynamic/response, predictive, prognostic, safety, and susceptibility/risk, with a biomarker possibly fitting multiple categories, whereas COAs are defined as a measurement of a patient's symptoms, overall mental state, or the effects of a disease or condition on how the patient functions [54]. COAs are often categorized by the source of reporting, such as patient-reported outcome (PRO), observer-reported outcome (ObsRO), clinician-reported outcome (ClinRO), and performance outcome (PerfO) measures.

Measurement types vs. regulatory pathways. Before elaborating on the usage of particular digital measurements in a study, it would be beneficial to craft a strategy for integrating digital biomarkers and eCOA into a drug development process. One crucial consideration is the regulatory pathway, which guides how and when certain biomarkers can be incorporated into a development program and a study design. There are two major regulatory pathways for biomarker and COA: the first is through the Biomarker or COA Qualification Program [55,56]; the second is via drug approval process. Section 3011 of the 21st Century Cures Act [54] amended the Federal Food, Drug, and Cosmetic (FD&C) Act by appending a new section on qualification of drug development tools (DDTs). The purpose of qualifying a DDT is (1) to support or obtain approval or licensure of a drug or biological product under sec. 505 of FD&C Act, or sec. 351 of the Public Health Service (PHS) Act; or (2) to support the investigational use of a drug or biological product under sec. 505(i) of FD&C Act, or sec. 351(a)(3) of the PHS Act. In November 2020, FDA further published a guidance on the qualification process of DDT [57], where DDT is defined as methods, materials, or measures that can support drug development and regulatory review. This guidance does not clearly indicate the inclusion of digital biomarkers or eCOA, though BEST Resource considers digital biomarker as a subset of biomarkers. In the second pathway, nonqualified DDT may still be used in regulatory applications based on scientific reasoning and regulatory agreement. However, the benefits of undergoing qualification process include that once qualified, DDTs will be publicly available for use in any drug development program for the qualified COU and can generally be incorporated in IND, NDA, or BLA submissions without FDA's reconfirmation on its suitability. Additionally, in February 2021, FDA announced the Innovative Science and Technology Approaches for New Drugs (ISTAND) Pilot Program, designed to promote the development of novel DDT types, which are out of the scope of the existing DDT qualification program [22]. The ISTAND program covers tools that may help enable remote or decentralized trials and tools that utilize digital health technologies. No matter which pathways a program team decides to adopt, early engagement with regulatory agency to seek advice, especially for critical but nonqualified DDTs, may be necessary.

When a program team has a clearer understanding of the role of digital measurements in a drug development process, some further considerations on the following aspects may help direct the study design.

Measurement types vs. degree of decentralization. Under a specific context of use, evaluation needs to be carefully made on whether a digital measurement can be adequately valid and reliable to meet study requirements. For instance, considering the technological status quo, certain response biomarkers, e.g., for some dermatology indications, can probably be measured through digital tools, such as laptop camera with sufficient resolution, to support key disease assessment and so the study can more likely be designed in a more decentralized approach; whereas for imaging assessment that requires CT scan or MRI machines, the procedure should be done either on site or in a local clinic with proper machines as well as being able to meet other operational requirements. In this case, the study would be at best designed as a hybrid trial. Another example is safety and monitoring biomarker such as single 12-lead ECG. There are already existing ECG applications cleared by FDA for patient use or portable ECG machine for doctor or trained healthcare professional use [58,59]. If implementation cost is manageable for the study team, patients ideally should not be scheduled to come to the site just because of single ECG monitoring. Figure 10.6 displays a hypothetical example with a spectrum of data collection modes against the degree of the trial decentralization.

Measurement types vs. usage as surrogate endpoints. Unlike endpoint, surrogate endpoint does not directly measure the clinical benefit of primary interest but is supposed to predict that clinical benefit based on evidence from a variety of sources. Depending on the levels of clinical validation, surrogate endpoints can be classified into three types: validated surrogate endpoint, reasonably likely surrogate endpoint, and candidate surrogate endpoint. Reasonably likely surrogate endpoints are supported by strong scientific rationale, but the data available is not adequate to prove that they are a validated surrogate endpoint. For biomarker or COA to be qualified as validated surrogate endpoint, data from randomized clinical trials are generally required to show that surrogate endpoint is predictive of the clinical endpoint of interest, in combination with unambiguous understanding of epidemiologic, pathophysiologic, therapeutic, or other scientific mechanism. But in areas of unmet medical needs, FDA is open to early consultation and flexible and feasible approaches to studying and reviewing such drugs, including the use of innovative study design and novel endpoints [60]. And reasonably likely surrogate endpoints are more likely to be acceptable to support accelerated approval than traditional approval, to provide seriously ill patients with more promising treatments. Among the digital measurement types, digital versions of the response and predictive biomarkers have high potential to be used

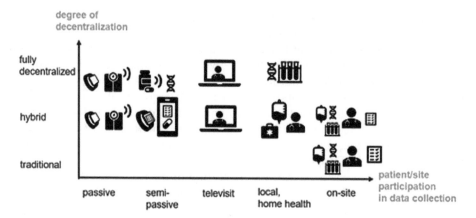

FIGURE 10.6

A hypothetical example of how data collection modes vary with different degrees of trial decentralization.
Passive: little patient/site interference; semipassive: requires patient action or actively enter but no action
from site; televisit: does not require patient to visit the site, or health professional to visit patient; local/home
health: requires patient go to local clinic or health professional to visit patients; on-site: patients are required to
visit the site enrolled.

as reasonably likely surrogate endpoints in disease areas of highly unmet needs. Statistical
methods for evaluating and reporting surrogate endpoints have been an ongoing topic of
discussion in the literature [61–64].

10.3.3 Statistical Considerations

Compared to traditional clinical assessments that are often done by human and collected
via case report forms, digital measurements often come from a 'black box' or preprocessed
by computer algorithms. A deeper understanding of the digital data-generating mechanism may be necessary to evaluate the data limitation and appropriateness of the analysis method, which may also impact the study design and conduct. For instance, an
actigraphy device or physical activity monitor typically collects three-dimensional time
series data through a microelectromechanical system that captures accelerations relative
to the Earth's gravitational field [65]. It may go unnoticed that each device has its own
frame of reference and can be aggregated at different temporal resolutions. If the digital
measurements are to be compared among patients in a study, ensuring the comparability
of these digital measurements may require technical knowledge and careful planning of
device options (e.g., Bring-Your-Own device vs. uniform provisioned device), deciding
how the device should be worn, and how the data should be aggregated, among other
operational considerations.

Moreover, depending on the digital measurement complexity, volume, and heterogeneity, existing analysis methodologies that work under traditional clinical trials may require
a modification or a revamp. Using actigraphy data as an example again, as such data are
not typically collected in a traditional trial, activity summaries derived from this source
may require further validation before clinically meaningful conclusions can be drawn. For
instance, suppose the research interest is to study how health status is associated with the
activity level. How to use statistical method to label a time interval as 'active' for a patient,
or to classify a patient as 'active'? What data should be input to perform the classification,

raw accelerometry data, or higher resolution summaries such as step counts? How to account for cross-patient heterogeneity? Can the conclusion be drawn on an individual level or population level? Existing statistical methods may not be established to provide straightforward answers to these questions.

On one hand, when the research questions are more of predictive vs. explanatory nature, artificial intelligence (AI) or machine learning (ML) methods are playing an unprecedented role due to the advancement of cloud and GPU-based computing power and capability of ingesting and learning from an assemblage of data. Benjamens et al. (2020) [66] reviewed 29 FDA-approved AI/ML-based medical technologies for applications in several therapeutic areas from 2016 to 2020. For the approvals under radiology/oncology, the algorithms are utilized for different cancer diagnosis, including breast, liver, and lung cancer; for the approvals under neurology as first or second medical specialty, the function of the algorithms vary from diagnosis of sleeping disorders to that of stroke detection, acute intracranial hemorrhage triage, and MRI brain interpretation.

On the other hand, data sharing effort across industry and advanced data platform technologies, e.g., cloud, blockchain, etc., proffer the opportunity for more efficient clinical data sharing and integration, thus facilitating regulatory review. The creation of the cloud-based data-sharing platform Accumulus Synergy in 2020 is an example where a coalition of big pharma makes consorted effort to break the logjam of unnecessary complexity and inefficiency in regulatory submission and review process [67]; Semantic Web technologies and Life Sciences Lined Open Data cloud enable web-scale semantic processing and integration of data and knowledge from multiple sources in different biomedical domains [68]; and blockchain, traditionally used for managing cryptocurrency records, can be applied to create more secure and interoperable infrastructure to manage electronic health records [69].

10.4 Discussions

With the efflorescence of digital health technologies in clinical research, this chapter strives to continue a constructive dialogue in the understanding and implementation of digital measurements to ameliorate the possible qualm of naivete, the overcoming of which could lead to tremendous advancement in the way we conduct clinical research. This has been an ongoing focus of clinical research effort: Alzheimer's Drug Discovery Foundation launched Diagnostics Accelerator program in July 2018 to accelerate novel biomarker development for Alzheimer's and related dementias [70]; 2019 Lung Cancer Treatment Focused Research Grant program awarded Drs. Rendle and Takvorian for a project to evaluate the impact of digital intervention, an AI-enabled 'chat bot', on adherence to oral targeted therapies [70]; Brigham and Women's Hospital is developing 'imPROvE Breast Cancer Care Next Generation Patient-Reported Outcomes System' [72]; Memorial Sloan-Kettering Cancer Center developed 'MyMSK Recovery Tracker' [74]; and in August 2020, Northwestern University received grant from National Institute of Mental Health to advance digital mental health research [73].

Besides what are highlighted in this paper, ethical considerations ensuing from digital measurements are indispensable when premediating study design and implementation. As mentioned in the Belmont Report [75], the ethical tenets guiding the conduct of biomedical and behavioral research involving human subjects are respect for persons, beneficence, and justice. For instance, the principle of respect for persons is often manifest in the process of informed consent, where patients are given the chance to opt for what may or may not happen to them. The standards or possibilities for 'true' informed consent can get even more perplexed when no clear verdict can be reached on what contents are considered sufficient and comprehensible (e.g., an exhaust list of data privacy agreements, functionality specifications for multiple devices, etc.), or what decisions are deemed voluntary (e.g., "black-box" AI-assisted device that enable passive data collection, clinical data aggregation and disease management). Additional discussions on these aspects can be found in the recent literature [1,76,77].

In spite of many challenges, digital health technologies will be increasingly prevalent in clinical research. To support successful study design and conduct, it is imperative to strategize operations and stay on top of the global regulatory landscape. As data and experience accumulate, more evidence will emerge to qualify the use of digital endpoints for supporting regulatory decision-making, sound understanding of the science, and thus advancing clinical research and clinical care.

References

1. Lanier J. Taking stock. Updated January 1, 1998. Accessed February 18, 2021. www.wired.com/1998/01/lanier/
2. Basch E, Deal AM, Dueck AC, et al. Overall survival results of a trial assessing patient-reported outcomes for symptom monitoring during routine cancer treatment. JAMA. 2017: 318(2): 197–198. doi:10.1001/jama.2017.7156
3. Denis F, Lethrosne C, Pourel N, et al. Randomized trial comparing a web-mediated follow-up with routine surveillance in lung cancer patients. J Natl Cancer Inst. 2017: 109(9). doi:10.1093/jnci/djx029
4. Denis F, Basch E, Septans AL, et al. Two-year survival comparing web-based symptom monitoring vs routine surveillance following treatment for lung cancer. JAMA. 2019: 321(3): 306–307. doi:10.1001/jama.2018.18085
5. U.S. Food & Drug Administration. Know your treatment options for COVID-19. Updated March 11, 2021. Accessed March 18, 2021. www.fda.gov/consumers/consumer-updates/know-your-treatment-options-covid-19
6. Balance Budget Act of 1997. Updated 1997. Assessed February 18, 2021. www.congress.gov/bill/105th-congress/house-bill/2015
7. US Congress. Benefits Improvement and Protection Act of 2000. Updated 2020. Accessed February 18, 2021. www.congress.gov/bill/106th-congress/house-bill/5661
8. US Congress. Bipartisan Budget Act of 2018. www.congress.gov/bill/115th-congress/house-bill/1892/text
9. US Congress. Health Information Technology for Economic and Clinical Health Act of 2009. Updated 2009. Accessed February 18, 2021. www.healthit.gov/sites/default/files/hitech_act_excerpt_from_arra_with_index.pdf.
10. US Congress. Compilation of Patient Protection and Affordable Care Act. Updated May 2010. Accessed February 18, 2021. http://housedocs.house.gov/energycommerce/ppacacon.pdf.
11. US Congress. Medicare Access and CHIP Reauthorization Act of 2015. Updated 2015. Accessed February 18, 2021. www.congress.gov/bill/114th-congress/house-bill/2/text
12. US Congress. Bipartisan Budget Act of 2018. Updated 2018. Accessed February 18, 2021. www.congress.gov/bill/115th-congress/house-bill/1892/text

13. US Congress. Physician Fee Schedule of 2019. Updated 2019. Accessed February 18, 2021. www.cms.gov/Medicare/Medicare-Fee-for-Service-Payment/PhysicianFeeSched

14. U.S. Food and Drug Administration. Evaluation of Automatic Class III Designation (De Novo) for Proteus Personal Monitor Including Ingestion Event Marker. Updated May 2012. Accessed February 18, 2021. www.accessdata.fda.gov/cdrh_docs/reviews/k113070.pdf

15. Clinical Trials Transformation Initiative. Program: Digital Health Trials. Accessed February 18, 2021. www.ctti-clinicaltrials.org/programs/mobile-clinical-trials

16. Kadakia K, Patel B and Shah A. Advancing digital health: FDA innovation during COVID-19. npj Digit. Med. 2020;3:161. doi: 10.1038/s41746-020-00371-7

17. U.S. Food and Drug Administration. digital health policies and public health solutions for COVID-19. Updated March 2020. Accessed March 2, 2021. www.fda.gov/medical-devices/coronavirus-covid-19-and-medical-devices/digital-health-policies-and-public-health-solutions-covid-19

18. U.S. Food and Drug Administration. Enforcement policy for digital health devices for treating psychiatric disorders during the Coronavirus disease 2019 (COVID-19) public health emergency. Updated April 2020. Accessed March 2, 2021. www.fda.gov/media/136939/download

19. U.S. Food and Drug Administration. Enforcement policy for non-invasive remote monitoring devices used to support patient monitoring during the Coronavirus disease 2019 (COVID-19) public health emergency (revised). Updated October 2021. Accessed March 2, 2021. www.fda.gov/news-events/press-announcements/fda-launches-digital-health-center-excellence

20. U.S. Food and Drug Administration. FDA launches the Digital Health Center of Excellence. Updated September 2020. Accessed March 2, 2021. www.fda.gov/media/136290/download

21. European Medicines Agency. Questions and answers: qualification of digital technology-based methodologies to support approval of medicinal products. Updated June 2020. Accessed February 18, 2021. www.ema.europa.eu/en/documents/other/questions-answers-qualification-digital-technology-based-methodologies-support-approval-medicinal_en.pdf

22. U.S. Food and Drug Administration. Innovative Science and Technology Approaches for New Drugs (ISTAND) pilot program. Updated February 2021. Accessed March 2, 2021. www.fda.gov/drugs/drug-development-tool-ddt-qualification-programs/innovative-science-and-technology-approaches-new-drugs-istand-pilot-program

23. European Medicines Agency. Guideline on computerised systems and electronic data in 5 clinical trials. Updated June 2021. Accessed December 31, 2022. www.ema.europa.eu/en/documents/regulatory-procedural-guideline/draft-guideline-computerised-systems-electronic-data-clinical-trials_en.pdf

24. U.S. Food and Drug Administration. Digital health technologies for remote data acquisition in clinical investigations. Updated January 2022. Accessed December 31, 2022. www.fda.gov/media/155022/download

25. Encyclopedia Britannica website. Measurement. Updated 4 February 2020. Accessed February 18, 2021. www.britannica.com/technology/measurement

26. European Network for Health Technology Assessment website. Endpoints used for Relative Effectiveness Assessment Clinical Endpoints. Updated November 2015. Accessed February 18, 2021. https://eunethta.eu/wp-content/uploads/2018/01/WP7-SG3-GL-clin_endpoints_amend2015.pdf

27. Sullivan EJ. Clinical trial endpoints. Updated November 2013. Accessed February 18, 2021. www.fda.gov/media/87594/download

28. European Medicines Agency. ICH Topic E 9 statistical principles for clinical trials. Updated January 1998. Accessed February 18, 2021. www.ema.europa.eu/documents/scientific-guideline/ich-e-9-statistical-principles-clinical-trials-step-5_en.pdf

29. U.S. Food and Drug Administration. Clinical trial endpoints for the approval of cancer drugs and biologics guidance for industry. Updated December 2018. Accessed February 18, 2021. www.fda.gov/media/71195/download

30. U.S. Food and Drug Administration. clinical trial endpoints for the approval of non-small cell lung cancer drugs and biologics guidance for industry. Updated April 2015. Accessed February 18, 2021. www.fda.gov/media/116860/download

31. U.S. Food and Drug Administration. Nonmetastatic, castration-resistant prostate cancer: Considerations for metastasis-free survival endpoint in clinical trials. Updated November 2018. Accessed February 18, 2021. www.fda.gov/media/117792/download

32. U.S. Food and Drug Administration. Pathological complete response in neoadjuvant treatment of high-risk early-stage breast cancer: use as an endpoint to support accelerated approval. Updated July 2020. Accessed February 18, 2021. www.fda.gov/media/83507/download

33. Digital Medicine Society (DiMe). DiMe's library of digital endpoints. Updated January 17, 2021. Accessed February 18, 2021. www.dimesociety.org/index.php/knowledge-center/library-of-digital-endpoints

34. National Institute for Standards and Technology. Guidelines for evaluating and expressing the uncertainty of NIST measurement results. Updated December 2007. Accessed February 18, 2021. http://physics.nist.gov/Pubs/guidelines/contents.html

35. TrajkoviC G. Measurement: accuracy and precision, reliability and validity. In: Kirch W. (eds) *Encyclopedia of Public Health*. Springer, Dordrecht. 2008. doi: 10.1007/978-1-4020-5614-7_2081

36. Goldsack JC, Coravos A, Bakker JP, et al. Verification, analytical validation, and clinical validation (V3): the foundation of determining fit-for-purpose for Biometric Monitoring Technologies (BioMeTs). *npj Digit. Med.* 2020: 3: 55. doi: 10.1038/s41746-020-0260-4

37. Godfrey A, Vandendriessche B, Bakker JP, Fitzer-Attas C, Gujar N, Hobbs M, et al. Fit-for-purpose biometric monitoring technologies: leveraging the laboratory biomarker experience. *Clin Transl Sci*, 2021: 14: 62–74. doi:10.1038/s41746-020-0260-4

38. European Medicines Agency. ICH Topic E9 (R1) Addendum on estimands and sensitivity analysis in clinical trials to the guideline on statistical principles for clinical trials. Updated February 2020. Accessed February 18, 2021. www.ema.europa.eu/documents/scientific-guideline/ich-e9-r1-addendum-estimands-sensitivity-analysis-clinical-trials-guideline-statistical-principles_en.pdf

39. Coons SJ, Gwaltney CJ, Hays RD, Lundy JJ, Sloan JA, Revicki DA, et al. Recommendations on evidence needed to support measurement equivalence between electronic and paper-based patient-reported outcome (PRO) measures: ISPOR ePRO Good Research Practices Task Force report. *Value in Health*. 2009: Jun: 12(4): 419–29. doi: 10.1111/j.1524-4733.2008.00470.x

40. Eremenco S, Coons SJ, Paty J, Coyne K, Bennett AV, McEntegart D. PRO data collection in clinical trials using mixed modes: report of the ISPOR PRO mixed modes good research practices task force. *Value in Health*. 2014: Jul: 17(5): 501–16. doi: 10.1016/j.jval.2014.06.005

41. Apple Developer Forum. Disabling Callkit for China apps. Assessed February 15, 2021. https://developer.apple.com/forums/thread/103083#320740

42. Khozin S and Coravos A. Decentralized trials in the age of real-world evidence and inclusivity in clinical investigations. *Clin Pharmacol Ther*. 2019: 106:25–27. doi: 10.1002/cpt.1441

43. European Commission. Data protection in the EU. Assessed February 18, 2021. https://ec.europa.eu/info/law/law-topic/data-protection/data-protection-eu_en

44. U.S. Food and Drug Administration. Providing regulatory submissions in electronic format – standardized study data. Updated October 2020. Accessed February 18, 2021. www.fda.gov/media/82716/download

45. U.S. Food and Drug Administration. Data standards in the drug lifecycle. Updated December 2016. Accessed February 18, 2021. https://accessdata.fda.gov/scripts/cder/data-standards/

46. Terry M. Clinical trial software company hit by massive ransomware attach. *Biospace*. Updated October 2020. Accessed February 18, 2021. www.biospace.com/article/clinical-trial-software-company-eresearchtechnology-hit-by-ransomware-attack/

47. Government of Canada. Notice – release of ICH E9(R1): defining the appropriate estimand for a clinical trial/ sensitivity analyses. Updated July 21, 2020. Accessed February 18, 2021.

www.canada.ca/en/health-canada/services/drugs-health-products/drug-products/appli cations-submissions/guidance-documents/international-conference-harmonisation/effic acy/notice-ich-e9-r1-defining-appropriate-estimand-clinical-trial-sensitivity-analysis.html

48. Jin M, Liu G. Estimand framework: delineating what to be estimated with clinical questions of interest in clinical trials. *Contemp Clin Trials*. 2020: Sep: 96:106093. doi:10.1016/j. cct.2020.106093
49. Lipkovich I, Ratitch B and Mallinckrodt CH. Causal inference and estimands in clinical trials. *Statistics in Biopharmaceutical Research*. 2020: 12(1): 54–67. doi:10.1080/19466315.2019.1697739
50. Ratitch B, Bell J, Mallinckrodt C, et al. Choosing estimands in clinical trials: Putting the ICH E9(R1) into practice. *Therapeutic Innovation & Regulatory Science*. April 2019. doi:10.1177/2168479019838827
51. Qu Y, Fu H, Luo J and Ruberg SJ. A general framework for treatment effect estimators considering patient adherence. *Statistics in Biopharmaceutical Research*. 2020: 12(1): 1–18. doi: 10.1080/19466315.2019.1700157
52. Bornkamp B, Rufibach K, Lin J, Liu Y., Mehrotra DV, Roychoudhury S, et al. Principal stratum strategy: potential role in drug development. *Pharmaceutical Statistics*. 2021: 1–15. doi: 10.1002/pst.2104
53. FDA-NIH Biomarker Working Group. BEST (Biomarkers, EndpointS, and other Tools) resource. Silver Spring (MD): Food and Drug Administration (US). Last updated January 25, 2021. Accessed March 2, 2021. www.ncbi.nlm.nih.gov/books/NBK326791/pdf/Bookshel f_NBK326791.pdf
54. U.S. Congress. 21st Century Cures Act. Last updated December 2016. Accessed March 2, 2021. www.congress.gov/114/bills/hr34/BILLS-114hr34enr.pdf
55. U.S. Food and Drug Administration. Biomarker qualification program. Accessed March 2. 2021. www.fda.gov/drugs/drug-development-tool-ddt-qualification-programs/biomar ker-qualification-program
56. U.S. Food and Drug Administration. Clinical Outcome Assessment (COA) qualification program. Accessed March 2. 2023. www.fda.gov/drugs/drug-development-tool-ddt-qualif ication-programs/clinical-outcome-assessment-coa-qualification-program
57. U.S. Food and Drug Administration. Qualification process for drug development tools guidance for industry and FDA staff. Updated November 2020. Accessed March 2, 2021. www.fda.gov/media/133511/download
58. U.S. Food and Drug Administration. K180157S001 Appendix 2 510 (k) summary. Updated May 2018. Accessed March 2, 2021. www.accessdata.fda.gov/cdrh_docs/pdf18/K180 157.pdf
59. U.S. Food and Drug Administration. K171360 510 (k) summary. Updated January 2018. Accessed March 2, 2021. www.accessdata.fda.gov/cdrh_docs/pdf17/K171360.pdf
60. U.S. Food and Drug Administration. PDUFA reauthorization performance goals and procedures fiscal years 2018 through 2022. Updated 2018. Accessed March 2, 2021. www.fda. gov/media/99140/download
61. Prentice RL. Surrogate endpoints in clinical trials: definition and operational criteria. *Statist Med*. 1989: 8: 431–440. doi: 10.1002/sim.4780080407
62. Weir CJ and Walley RJ. Statistical evaluation of biomarkers as surrogate endpoints: a litera-ture review. *Statist Med*. 2006: 25: 183–203. doi:10.1002/sim.2319
63. Gilbert PB, Qin L and Self SG. Evaluating a surrogate endpoint at three levels, with applica-tion to vaccine development. *Statist Med*. 2008: 27: 4758–4778. doi:10.1002/sim.3122
64. Xie W, Halabi S, Tierney JF, Sydes MR, Collette L, Dignam JJ, et al. A systematic review and recommendation for reporting of surrogate endpoint evaluation using meta-analyses. *JNCI Cancer Spectrum*. 2019: 3(1). doi:10.1093/jncics/pkz002
65. Karas M, Bai J, Strączkiewicz M, Harezlak J, Glynn NW, Harris T, et al. Accelerometry data in health research: challenges and opportunities. *Stat Biosci*. 2019: 11: 210–237. doi:10.1007/ s12561-018-9227-2

66. Benjamens S, Dhunnoo P and Meskó B. The state of artificial intelligence-based FDA-approved medical devices and algorithms: an online database. *npj Digit. Med.* 2020: 3: 118. doi: 10.1038/s41746-020-00324-0

67. Bioworld. Accumulus' collaborators plan to streamline data sharing and communications. Updated Jan 2021. Assessed March 2021. www.bioworld.com/articles/502727-accumulus-collaborators-plan-to-streamline-data-sharing-and-communications.

68. Kamdar MR, Fernández JD, Polleres A, Tudorache T. and Musen MA. Enabling web-scale data integration in biomedicine through Linked Open Data. *npj Digit. Med.* 2019: 2: 90. doi: 10.1038/s41746-019-0162-5

69. Vazirani AA, O'Donoghue O, Brindley D, and Meinert E. Blockchain vehicles for efficient medical record management. *npj Digit. Med.* 2020: 3: 1. doi:10.1038/s41746-019-0211-0

70. Alzheimer's Drug Discovery Foundation. diagnostics accelerator: digital biomarkers. Assessed Mar 2, 2021. www.alzdiscovery.org/research-and-grants/funding-opportunities/digital-biomarkers

71. Lung Cancer Research Foundation. 2019 Lung cancer treatment focused research grant program. Updated 2019. Accessed March 2, 2021. www.lungcancerresearchfoundation.org/research/our-investigators/previously-funded-research/2019-lung-cancer-treatment-focused-research-grant-program-university-of-pennsylvania-katharine-rendle-phd-msw-mph/

72. Pusic A. Patient-facing digital applications: engaging and supporting cancer patients. Updated July 2020. Accessed March 2, 2021. www.nationalacademies.org/event/07-13-2020/docs/D52D553FB37CBC6B73AA40437EDDE4E787C322C6DAE7

73. Northwestern University. NIMH ALACRITY center grant seeks to change depression treatment paradigm. Updated August 2020. Accessed Mar 2, 2021. www.nucats.northwestern.edu/news/2020/alacrity-center-grant.html

74. Memorial Sloan Kettering Cancer Center. MyMSK recovery tracker. Updated November 2020. Accessed March 2, 2021. www.mskcc.org/cancer-care/patient-education/mymsk-recovery-tracker

75. U.S. Department of Health & Human Services. The Belmont Report. Updated January 2018. Assessed March 2, 2021. www.hhs.gov/ohrp/regulations-and-policy/belmont-report/read-the-belmont-report/index.html

76. Coravos A, Goldsack JC, Karlin DR, Nebeker C, Perakslis E, Zimmerman N, et al. Digital medicine: a primer on measurement. *Digit Biomark.* 2019: May 9: 3(2): 31–71. doi:10.1159/000500413

77. Nebeker C, Torous J, and Bartlett Ellis RJ. Building the case for actionable ethics in digital health research supported by artificial intelligence. *BMC Med.* 2019: 17: 137. doi:10.1186/s12916-019-1377-7

78. Nebeker C, Bartlett Ellis RJ, and Torous J. Development of a decision-making checklist tool to support technology selection in digital health research. *Translational Behavioral Medicine.* 2020: 10(4): 1004–1015. doi:10.1093/tbm/ibz074.

11

Use of Surrogate Endpoints in Clinical Development

Liwen Wu, Qing Li, and Jianchang Lin

11.1 Surrogate Endpoints in Clinical Trials

The ultimate goal of clinical trials is to establish evidence of clinical efficacy and safety on the investigational agents compared to standard of care or placebo controls.

This is traditionally done using clinical endpoints that are directly related to the disease condition and progression, such as overall survival or progression-free survival. However, these endpoints may require lengthy follow-up periods and many patients to achieve precision in the statistical estimate of treatment effects, which can be either too difficult or too expensive to measure. In the past decades, there has been increasing interest in using short-term surrogate endpoints that can serve as proxy of the primary clinical endpoint, to make key decisions in the drug development process. For example, in newly diagnosed Philadelphia Chromosome–Positive Acute Lymphoblastic Leukemia (ALL), Minimal Residual Disease (MRD)–negative Complete Response (CR) can be used as a surrogate endpoint for Event-Free-Survival (EFS) to avoid confounding effects due to treatment switching when analyzing survival data (Berry et al. 2017). Similarly, in patients with newly diagnosed multiple myeloma, the postinduction CR rates and MRD are considered important predictors for PFS and OS (Harousseau et al. 2010; Munshi et al. 2017). These endpoints are considered "indirect" measurements of treatment effects and can be collected or observed in a relatively shorter period of time as compared to their standard, or primary, clinical endpoint counterpart.

A surrogate endpoint should be justified by requiring the treatment effect which could predict the effect on the primary endpoint. This relationship should be stronger than simply having two correlated endpoints (Fleming and DeMets 1996). Surrogate endpoint is formally defined as "a response variable for which a test of the null hypothesis of no relationship to the treatment groups under comparison is also a valid test of the corresponding null hypothesis based on the true endpoint" (Prentice 1989). In other words, the validity is examined by whether the treatment effect on the primary endpoint is fully captured by the surrogate endpoint, which has been considered a very stringent criterion. In practice, a comprehensive understanding of the causal pathway of the disease's natural history as well as both the on-target and off-target mechanisms of action of the investigational agents may be sufficient to justify the selection of surrogate endpoints (Fleming and Powers 2012). Additionally, systematic reviews or metaanalysis by using finished clinical

DOI: 10.1201/9781003288640-11

191

trial–level study data and patient-level study data can also be utilized to explore the relationship between surrogate and the primary endpoints.

Following this approach, many studies have investigated the feasibility of substituting the primary endpoints with surrogates and how to model the treatment effects from them (Freedman, Graubard, and Schatzkin 1992; Buyse and Molenberghs 1998; Buyse et al. 2000). Fleming et al. (1994) explored another area where they considered the surrogate endpoint as "auxiliary variable" and included its information in an augmented likelihood estimator together with the primary endpoint. This approach, instead of replacing the primary endpoint completely, requires a weaker assumption on the correlation structure between endpoints.

For serious and life-threatening diseases, FDA constituted the Accelerated Approval (AA) pathway to provide patients with earlier access to promising treatment and speed up drug approval based on surrogate endpoints (Fashoyin-Aje et al. 2022). However, sponsors are still required to conduct confirmatory trials to verify potential clinical benefits in terms of long-term clinical endpoints and obtain traditional approval. An AA indication may be withdrawn if the confirmatory trials fail to demonstrate clinical benefit, for example, Melflufen for multiple myeloma (Olivier and Prasad 2022). There are many reasons that could be attributed to the uncertainty between AA and full approval, including the choice of endpoints, study designs, intended and unintended cross-over effects, study populations, and the disease's natural history. New options are being proposed to reduce the uncertainty, for example, the "Single Trial Model," which combines an initial starting phase based on surrogate endpoint that could support AA at an interim assessment and then continues into a broader phase for full approval (FOCR 2022).

In this chapter, we will discuss two general frameworks to utilize surrogate endpoint information to accelerate drug development: (1) use surrogate endpoint to make interim decision in an adaptive 2-in-1 design and (2) incorporate surrogate endpoint in estimating interim conditional power that can be adopted in various adaptive design settings. Both methods are newer ways of incorporating different endpoints into development strategy and reflect emerging needs and challenges in improving patient's access to new treatments and mitigating the risks and uncertainties associated with the rapidly changing drug development landscape. We will also include several case studies to illustrate how to utilize surrogate endpoint information with these methods.

11.2 Utilizing Surrogate Endpoint in Adaptive Design

11.2.1 2-in-1 Designs and Extensions

2-in-1 design (Chen et al. 2018) is becoming popular in oncology drug development, as it allows for the flexibility of using different endpoints at different decision points, allowing for a seamless transition from phase 2 to phase 3. This design framework is a good example of using surrogate endpoint to facilitate adaptive decisions in a drug development strategy and also reflects the needs of the FDA's initiative, "Project FrontRunner," that encourages using an earlier surrogate endpoint to support accelerated approval with conversion to standard approval with long-term endpoint from the same randomized study (FOCR 2022). This design is particularly useful for diseases that have long natural history, such as those that require longer observational periods for survival outcome to mature, with well-established surrogate endpoints, and in settings where the development landscape shows opportunities to demonstrate convincing and clinically meaningful improvement.

Starting with a small phase 2 study, based on interim observed data, sponsors may either seamlessly advance to a full-scale confirmatory phase 3 trial with a predetermined maximum number of subjects, or remain in phase 2 development, akin to a Go/No-Go decision between phase 2 and phase 3 development. The interim decision of whether to expand to phase 3 study can be made based on the same primary endpoint to be used at the final analysis, or some earlier endpoints that could inform clinical benefits, i.e., surrogate endpoint.

Let X, Y, and Z denote the test statistics at the interim analysis, the final analysis at the end of the phase 2 study, and the final analysis at the end of the phase 3 study, respectively. The design can be cast in a dichotomized decision framework. If the interim analysis based on X, which is usually an earlier surrogate endpoint, shows promising treatment effect, i.e., X > c, the trial expands to large-scale phase 3 confirmatory study. Otherwise, if X < c, the trial remains a phase 2 study with a smaller sample size. The interim decision threshold, c, is a key design parameter to be specified before the conduct of the study. Chen et al. (2018) proved that, under a generally held correlation assumption, $\rho_{XY} > \rho_{XZ}$, the overall type I error of such a design is controlled conservatively at the nominal level, so no multiplicity adjustment is necessary.

There are many extensions proposed from the original Chen's 2-in-1 design. Chen, Li, and Deng (2020) generalized it to scenarios with multiple interim decisions (K-in-1 design) and multiple endpoints. Jin and Zhang (2021) incorporated treatment or dose selection into a 2-in-1 design framework. Li et al. (2022) proposed a flexible 2-in-1 design, where the final sample size can also be adjusted at the interim analysis to mitigate the risk of uncertainty/variability of treatment effect at the designing stage and provide sufficient power at the end of the study.

11.2.2 The Modified Conditional Power (MCP) Approach

A more general school of adaptive designs utilizes some interim decision tools to make clinical trial modifications, such as claiming early stopping for efficacy or futility, selecting subgroups/treatment arms, and adjusting final sample size of the study. Conditional power has been commonly used in these settings (Mehta and Pocock 2011). However, in adaptive designs where interim analysis is planned early in the study, conditional power based on immature data from the primary endpoint might be biased (Lin, Bunn, and Liu 2019). To take full advantage of the data observed at the interim, Li et al. (2021) proposed a modified conditional power approach that incorporates the information collected from both surrogate endpoint and primary endpoint to estimate the interim conditional power.

Denote the treatment effect for surrogate endpoint X as $\theta^{s,X}$ and that for the primary endpoint as Z for the corresponding group of patients s. It is assumed that there exists some prior knowledge about the relationship between the two endpoints, $f{:}\hat{\theta}^{s,X} \to \hat{Z}^{(s)}$, which could be represented in a linear form $f\left(\hat{\theta}^{s,X}\right) = a + b{*}\hat{\theta}^{s,X}$ as shown in Figure 11.1, and a and b are two constant values estimated from prior information. This kind of prior knowledge can be obtained from existing clinical trials, published data, real-world data (RWD), or meta-analyses. For example, in patients with advanced NSCLC, researchers built a linear regression model between trial-level ORR odds ratio and PFS hazard ratio and found a strong association, based on data collected from 15 studies (Blumenthal et al. 2015).

Supposing the test statistic $\hat{Z}_1^{(s)}$ for the primary endpoint and the treatment effect $\hat{\theta}^{s,X}$ for the surrogate endpoint are observed at the interim readouts, their information can be combined in a weighted average fashion. Let $t = n_1/n_2$ (n_1 is the sample size at interim; n_2

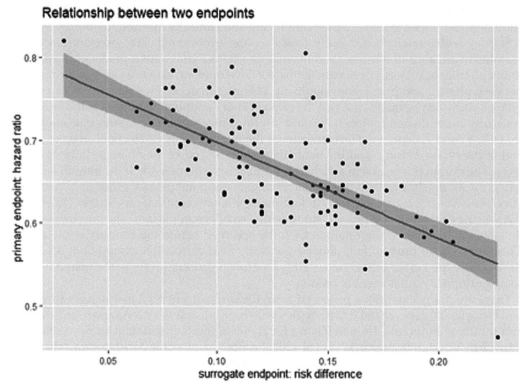

FIGURE 11.1
Relationship between primary endpoint and surrogate endpoint.

is the sample size at final analysis) represent the information fraction at the interim analysis; the modified CP can be calculated as follows:

$$CP_s^{(1)}\left(\hat{Z}_1^{(s)},\tilde{n}_2\right)=1-\Phi\left(\frac{Z_\alpha\sqrt{n_2}-\hat{Z}_1^{(s)}\sqrt{n_1}}{\sqrt{\tilde{n}_2}}-\frac{\sqrt{\tilde{n}_2}}{\sqrt{n_1}}\left(\hat{Z}_1^{(s)}t+f\left(\hat{\theta}^{s,X}\right)(1-t)\right)\right),\qquad(1)$$

$$CP_s^{(2)}\left(\hat{Z}_1^{(s)},\tilde{n}_2\right)=1-\Phi\left(\frac{Z_\alpha\sqrt{n_2}-\hat{Z}_1^{(s)}\sqrt{n_1}}{\sqrt{\tilde{n}_2}}-\frac{\sqrt{\tilde{n}_2}}{\sqrt{n_1}}\left(\frac{\hat{Z}_1^{(s)}f\left(\hat{\theta}^{s,X}\right)}{\hat{Z}_1^{(s)}(1-t)+f\left(\hat{\theta}^{s,X}\right)t}\right)\right),\qquad(2)$$

$$CP_s^{(3)}\left(\hat{Z}_1^{(s)},\tilde{n}_2\right)=1-\Phi\left(\frac{Z_\alpha\sqrt{n_2}-\hat{Z}_1^{(s)}\sqrt{n_1}}{\sqrt{\tilde{n}_2}}-\frac{\sqrt{\tilde{n}_2}}{\sqrt{n_1}}\left(\frac{\hat{Z}_1^{(s)}f\left(\hat{\theta}^{s,X}\right)}{\hat{Z}_1^{(s)}(1-F_c(t))+f\left(\hat{\theta}^{s,X}\right)F_c(t)}\right)\right),\qquad(3)$$

for $s=S$, where $f\left(\hat{\theta}^{s,X}\right)$ represents a predicted primary treatment effect by plugging the observed $\hat{\theta}^{s,X}$ in a known historical model, and $F_c(t)$ is the cumulative density function of the survival time for the control group at information fraction t. These equations represent three different weighting strategies to incorporate the directly observed treatment effect and the predicted treatment effect based on the surrogate endpoint The first one is a direct weighted average of these two counterparts based on the information proportion t, at the interim analysis, while the other two are derived based on a semiparametric analysis of the primary and surrogate survival endpoints (Li et al. 2021; Yang and Prentice 2005).

11.2.3 Type I error considerations

One key consideration when utilizing multiple endpoints in a trial design is the statistical integrity, i.e., the control of overall type I error. In general, if a surrogate endpoint is used to substitute a primary clinical endpoint for decision making at the end of the study, no type I error inflation is expected, because there is still one chance to reject the null hypothesis based on the surrogate endpoint observed. However, if a surrogate endpoint is used to guide interim adaptation, type I error may be inflated. An example is the subgroup enrichment design discussed by Jenkins, Stone, and Jennison (2011), where OS serves as the primary endpoint and correlated PFS is used for subgroup selection at the interim. Multiplicity adjustment techniques, such as closure testing principle, alpha splitting, and the graphic approach, can be applied to control the overall type I error under such settings. Special cases are present in the context of 2-in-1 designs, where the overall type I error may be deflated given a mild correlation assumption between the endpoints (Chen et al. 2018). Adaptive 2-in-1 designs can also take advantage of such assumptions and show type I error control by adding constraints on interim decision criteria (Li et al. 2022). When the surrogate endpoint information is used in the modified conditional power approach discussed in this section, since the final analysis is still based only on the primary endpoint, no multiplicity adjustment is required. If other interim adaptation is planned based on MCP, e.g., subgroup or treatment arm selection, similar type I error considerations apply as discussed in the previous case, where interim adaptation is planned based on surrogate endpoint only.

11.3 MCP Applied to Different Settings

11.3.1 Delayed Treatment Effect

When the MCP method was first proposed by Li et al. (2021), it was designed to tackle challenges brought by capturing delayed treatment effect in a clinical trial, particularly in the adaptive design setting. It is not uncommon to observe delayed treatment effects in oncology and hematology studies due to the mechanism of certain drugs. The challenge becomes more problematic if the treatment effect is evaluated based on long-term clinical endpoints, such as overall survival and progression-free survival. A recent example is observed in the randomized phase 3 trial to evaluate the effect of Pembrolizumab versus Chemotherapy for patients with non–small cell lung cancer (NSCLC), where the primary endpoint was progression-free survival (Reck et al. 2016). The late separation of Kaplan-Meier (KM) curves not only poses doubt on the proportional hazard assumption required by the standard Cox model–based analysis but also puts early interim analysis at risk, since, under such a setting, researchers may falsely stop a trial if the interim decision is based on the traditional conditional power estimate that assumes future unobserved data follows the same trend as current observations. Without considering the surrogate endpoint in the interim decision, the interim analysis is usually planned at a later stage of the clinical trial in the trial design stage.

In order to facilitate a stable and early interim decision making, MCP could be employed to improve interim decision making, if a short-term surrogate endpoint is observed at the interim with more accuracy than the primary endpoint, and if the treatment effect in terms of the surrogate endpoint could "predict" that in the primary endpoint. Li et al. (2021) demonstrated via simulation that a moderately or highly correlated surrogate endpoint leads to better interim decisions and overall power gain at the end of the study. This approach is more advantageous when the duration of the delayed treatment effect is longer, whereas the traditional method to project treatment effect trend using only the primary endpoint may fall short of useful information at the interim analysis.

11.3.2 Subgroup Enrichment Design

Another area of application for the MCP method is the adaptive subgroup enrichment design setting as shown in Figure 11.2. With broadening and deepening knowledge about the biological nature and molecular basis of disease procession, more and more disease-specific biomarkers have been investigated during drug development. For example, human epidermal growth factor receptor (EGFR) tyrosine kinase inhibitors show clinical benefits in NSCLC patients with EGFR mutation but not the others (Ohashi et al. 2013). In multiple myeloma, patients within the high-risk cytogenetic subgroup respond better to monoclonal antibodies than those in the standard-risk group (Sonneveld et al. 2016). To mitigate the risk of phase 3 failure, there has been an increased interest to conduct late-phase confirmatory trials with subgroup enrichment feature, where trials may start with all-comers, but the enrollment is limited to only specific subgroups after the interim readout. In such a setting, the traditional conditional estimate for the target subgroup may be biased or inaccurate if the interim analysis is planned early in the study and/or if the subgroup is a small proportion of the full population (Lin, Bunn, and Liu 2019). Wu et al. (2022) extended the MCP approach to adaptive subgroup enrichment designs. The addition of surrogate endpoint information at the interim leads to more informed and correct population selections and overall power gain at the end of the trial.

11.3.3 Platform Trial

A platform trial is a randomized study that combines multiple substudies and objectives together under one single master protocol, which allows simultaneous comparison of multiple investigational doses/agents/therapy to a common control group. It has become popular to facilitate efficient drug development, particularly under recent FDA initiatives

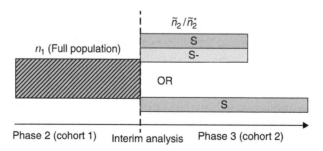

FIGURE 11.2
Seamless Phase 2/3 enrichment design using MCP.

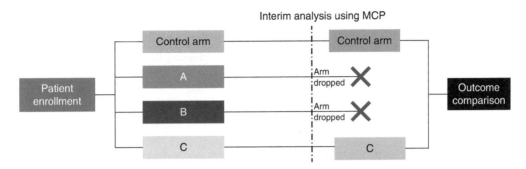

FIGURE 11.3
Platform trial using MCP method.

like Project Optimus, where multiple dosage groups are compared to select the optimal dose. However, a critical challenge for confirmatory platform trial is immature data for interim decisions, such as treatment arm selection and sample size determination. Zhong et al. (2022) extended the MCP method to such a setting to improve decision making as shown in Figure 11.3. With surrogate endpoint information incorporated into the interim decision making, this method also reflects the thinking behind Project FrontRunner (FOCR 2022), another recent initiative from FDA that was introduced earlier in this chapter.

11.4 Case Studies

In this section, we present three case studies to illustrate how the methods introduced in the previous section apply to real-world decision-making processes.

11.4.1 A 2-in-1 Design with Sample Size Adaptation for Multiple Myeloma

In Li et al. (2022), authors gave a multiple myeloma case study to demonstrate the utility and benefits of using surrogate endpoint in a flexible 2-in-1 design. In this case study, the sponsor wants to explore the option of a seamless phase 2/3 design for late-phase development of a promising investigational treatment combination in patients with relapsed and refractory multiple myeloma (RRMM). To expedite the development while also remaining fully flexible in terms of the overall development strategy, the sponsor decides to adopt a similar framework of the 2-in-1 design (Chen et al. 2018). At a planned interim analysis, if the investigational therapy demonstrates promising treatment effect compared with the standard-of-care control arm, the sponsor will expand the trial to enroll more patients in a confirmatory setting, i.e., as a phase 3 study, and perform the final analysis with total information collected from both stages. Alternatively, if the investigational therapy doesn't meet the expansion criteria, the sponsor wants to remain in phase 2 development with a smaller fixed sample size, which allows more time to collect evidence of the clinical benefits and decide whether a large-scale confirmatory trial is warranted or not in the future. The primary endpoint of the phase 3 study is set to be overall survival (OS), and that of the phase 2 study is set to be progression-free survival (PFS). Both are common endpoints to demonstrate efficacy in late-phase RRMM studies. The interim analysis is planned early in the

TABLE 11.1

Interim decision rule for the multiple myeloma case study with flexible 2-in-1 design.

Interim Scenario	Interim Decision	Primary Endpoint for Final Analysis	Final Event Size
$X \leq 2.206$	Remain in phase 2 development	PFS	58
$X > 2.206$	Expand to phase 3 confirmatory setting	OS	120–270

study, so an earlier intermediate endpoint and the key secondary endpoint of the study, objective response rate (ORR), is used to facilitate a more informed decision at the interim, given that both PFS and OS may be immature. In RRMM studies, superior ORR has been proven to be a good proxy of survival benefit.

To ensure sufficient power at the end of the study, a sample size reestimation procedure is also planned at the interim analysis. This procedure is based on the phase 3 primary endpoint, OS, and the log-rank test to be performed at the end of the study. Based on the interim observed hazard ratio, the total number of OS events is expected to be between 180 and 330, which is required to detect a range of optimistic to moderate hazard ratios (0.617–0.7) with 90% power. If the study remains in phase 2 development, a total of 118 PFS events are required to achieve 90% power to detect a 0.55 hazard ratio. The interim analysis is triggered after 60 OS events have been observed, corresponding to a 0.33 information fraction. At the interim analysis, a standardized test statistic X is calculated for the key secondary endpoint ORR and compared to a decision threshold. Table 11.1 summarizes the interim decision rule of the proposed design.

This decision threshold in Table 11.1 is decided based on a clinically meaningful difference in the target patient population and was calibrated by extensive simulation (for details about the setting, please refer to Li et al. (2022)). The sponsor also sets a maximum sample size of 500 patients, based on budget, enrollment, and other operational constraints.

The trial starts with the phase 2 stage and equally allocates 120 patients between the investigational combination therapy and the control arm. The interim analysis is triggered after observing 60 OS events, and it is 21 months after the study starts. The interim observed ORR difference is 0.227, and the standardized testing statistic is 3.157, so the interim decision is expanding to phase 3 trial. The observed hazard ratio of OS at the interim look is 0.664, and the conditional power is 81.3% (<90%). Following a conditional power–based event size reestimation rule, the final event size increases from 120 to 227 events. After observing all the OS events after 52 months, the final observed hazard ratio of OS is 0.749, with log-rank test statistic of 2.173 (p value = 0.015). The trial concluded with significant evidence of the treatment effect of the investigational treatment over the control (Figure 11.4).

11.4.2 Subgroup Enrichment Design Using Surrogate Endpoint: A Multiple Myeloma Example

Wu et al. (2022) proposed a new adaptive subgroup enrichment design that incorporates surrogate information in the conditional power calculation at interim decision making while allowing sample size reestimation (SSR). They illustrated the study design using an adaptive seamless phase 2/3 randomized study with a subgroup enrichment feature for multiple myeloma (MM) disease patients.

In a phase I study, a high complete response (CR) rate is observed in the safety expansion and dose-optimizing cohorts. Specifically, the CR rate is higher than expected in

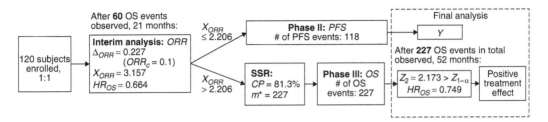

FIGURE 11.4
Decision path for multiple myeloma case study with flexible 2-in-1 design.

the high-risk cytogenetic subgroup patients. However, with the limited sample size, researchers are not sure whether the higher CR rate is random or not. Therefore, the subgroup enrichment feature is planned for selecting the right population for this new drug combination. In order to make an informed Go/No-Go decision at the end of the phase 2 stage with limited sample size, the interim analyses are planned to utilize all critical efficacy information including both primary endpoint PFS and key secondary endpoint CR. At the interim analyses, researchers need to make the decisions of (1) whether to go to phase 3 trials; (2) how many patients and events are needed for phase 3 trials; and (3) whether to enroll high-risk patients only or entire populations. According to similar studies in the MM field, patients with a higher probability of CR are likely to have better PFS time (Harousseau et al. 2010). Thus, the numerical correlation between risk difference (treatment-control) and the log-rank test statistic of PFS is assumed to be about −0.6 in this example (Avet-Loiseau et al. 2020; Daniele et al. 2022).

In this study, totally 300 patients will be enrolled in this seamless phase 2/3 randomized clinical trial. Assuming an exponential distribution for PFS, a minimum of 160 PFS events is required to detect an optimistic hazard ratio of 0.6 with approximately 90% power using a one-sided log-rank test at 0.025 level. Under similar assumptions, a maximum of 224 PFS events are needed to detect a hazard ratio of 0.66 for a more realistic scenario. Therefore, the total number of PFS events for the final analysis ranges from 160 events to 224 events depending on the different assumptions. It is also assumed that 8 patients per month will be enrolled in the phase II stage and 15 patients per month will be enrolled in the phase III stage separately. Considering an estimated 52-month study duration, roughly 300 patients are needed to generate 160 to 224 events based on maintaining 90% power to test the primary endpoint PFS at one-sided alpha level 0.025. The primary endpoint of this study is PFS and the key secondary endpoint is CR rate. The analysis for phase II part will be performed when approximately 40 PFS events are observed in the ITT population. The criteria and all possible interim decisions based on modified CP are shown in Table 11.2.

Suppose at the interim analysis, because the PFS data is not mature, a hazard ratio of 0.98 in the full population is observed and 1.15 is observed in the cytogenetic subgroup. The corresponding log-rank statistics are −0.05 and 0.27, respectively, and the corresponding CP for the full population and the cytogenetic subgroup are both below 0.05. According to the interim decision rule in Table 11.2, the interim decision will be stopping the trial due to futility.

However, the interim decision could be changed if surrogate endpoint CR is considered in the interim analysis. Suppose at the interim analysis, the observed CR difference for the full population is about 0.19 and that for the high-risk subgroup is about 0.38. Applying the assumed historical linear model, the predicted log-rank test statistics are 0.09 and −1.73

TABLE 11.2

Interim decision of subgroup enrichment design MM example.

Interim Criteria	Zone	Phase 3 Population	Final Event Size
$CP_{All} \geq 0.9$	Favorable	Full population	160
$0.9 > CP_{All} \geq 0.4$	Promising	Full population	Adaptive, (160,224)
$0.4 > CP_{All} \geq 0.05$ &$CP_{Sub} \geq 0.5$	Enrichment	Cytogenetic subgroup	Adaptive, (160,224)
$0.4 > CP_{All} \geq 0.05$ &$0.5 > CP_{Sub} \geq 0.05$	Unfavorable	Full population	160
$CP_{All} < 0.05$& $CP_{Sub} < 0.05$	Futility	-	-

for the full population and subgroup, respectively. Using the first weighted function (Wu et al. 2022), the modified CP is now 0.66 for the cytogenetic high-risk subgroup and below 0.05 for the full population. Thus, the interim decision goes to the enrichment zone, and the corresponding reestimated event size for the subgroup becomes 168. The trial will continue enrolling and enter the phase 3 stage with an expanded event size but only recruit high-risk cytogenetic subgroup. After observing 168 events in this subgroup, a final analysis is conducted. With the extended event size and study duration, the final estimate of the hazard ratio is about 0.68 in the subgroup (p = 0.006), demonstrating a significant treatment effect in the high cytogenetic subgroup. In summary, the modified conditional power using surrogate endpoint design provides an opportunity to rescue a promising drug for the subgroup patients even if the primary endpoint data at interim analysis is not mature enough.

11.4.3 Seamless Phase II/III Design Incorporating Dose Optimization: NSCLC Example

Traditionally in oncology study, the maximum tolerated dose (MTD) from phase I study will be used as the recommended dose for phase II and phase III clinical trials (Ananthakrishnan et al. 2017). This dose-response relationship was built based on systemic chemotherapies because higher chemotherapy doses will often lead to bigger tumor size reductions. However, with the rapid development of new oncology therapy options such as target therapy, immunotherapy, and cell therapy, this assumption may not be valid anymore (FOCR 2021). For example, immunotherapy calls for the patients' own immune system to fight against cancer instead of directly killing the cancer tumors directly; thus it will take some time for patients' body to react and observe the actual treatment effect. In this scenario, if the dose is too high, the patients may drop the study drug earlier due to AE and thus miss the effective treatment because of the short treatment duration. In this case study, targeted therapy A is a novel drug for a rare mutation non–small cell lung cancer (NSCLC) disease. In a phase 1/2 dose-escalation and safety expansion study, researchers have found promising safety profiles and a higher ORR in the later-line treatment. At the same time, researchers plan to initial clinical trials in first-line settings to potentially benefit patients earlier. However, due to the limited sample size in the Phase I trial, the recommended Phase II/III doses cannot be determined in the first-line setting. In order to select the best doses for the study, this study is further exploring three doses in the phase II part. Therefore, an adaptive platform seamless phase II/III study with a dose selection feature is planned to select the right dose for this new drug in the first-line setting and accelerate the development. To make an informed Go/No-Go decision at the phase 2 stage with limited sample size, the interim decision is planned to utilize the MCP approach to include both primary endpoint PFS and key secondary endpoint ORR. According to previous studies with the same indication, patients with a higher probability of response to ORR tend to have better PFS (Reck et al. 2016). The numerical correlation between risk difference (treatment-control) and log-rank test statistic is assumed to be about –0.6 in this case study.

In this study, a total of 320 patients (80 for each different dose arm and 80 for control) will be enrolled at the Phase II stage and 280 patients (140 for control and 140 for the selected dose arm) will be enrolled at the phase III stage in this confirmatory clinical trial as illustrated. Assuming an exponential distribution for primary endpoint PFS, a minimum of 190 PFS events is required to detect an optimistic hazard ratio of 0.6 with approximately 90% power using a one-sided log-rank test at alpha level 0.025. Under similar assumptions of type 1 and type 2 error rates, a maximum of 240 PFS events is needed to detect a hazard ratio of 0.66. Therefore, the total number of PFS events for the final analysis will range from 190 events to 240 events. Assuming 15 patients will be enrolled per month during both phase II and phase III stages, with an approximate 50-month study duration, the total sample size of 600 is calculated based on maintaining 90% power to test the primary endpoint PFS at one-sided alpha level 0.025.

The primary endpoint of this study is PFS and the key secondary endpoint is ORR. The objective of the phase II part is to check for futility, to determine the PFS event size, and to select the best dose to be used in the subsequent phase III stage. The analysis for the end of phase II will be performed when approximately 40 PFS events are observed in the ITT population. The criteria and all possible interim decisions based on modified CP are shown in Table 11.3.

Assuming the medium dose arm C is the superior arm with a hazard ratio of 0.6 compared to the control group, the hazard ratios for low dose arm A and high dose arm B are 0.9 and 0.8, respectively. Suppose that at the interim analysis, due to immature information from the PFS data, we observe a hazard ratio of 1.06 in the low dose arm A, 0.81 in the high dose arm B, and 0.87 in the medium dose arm C. The corresponding log-rank statistics are 0.19, –0.67, and –0.42, respectively, and the corresponding CP are 0.0001, 0.24, and 0.10. Based on the interim decision rule in Table 3, continuing the high dose arm B with 190 event size will be selected. Thus, this trial will be continued with arm B. At the final analysis, the estimated hazard ratio is 0.87 (p = 0.26); thus we fail to conclude that arm B is significantly superior.

However, the decision would be very different if the surrogate endpoint ORR is considered during interim analysis. Suppose at the interim analysis, the ORR difference for arm A, arm B, and arm C versus control is 0.1, 0.2, and 0.3, respectively. By an assumed historical linear model, the predicted log-rank test statistics are 0.08, –0.16, and –0.9 for the three doses arms, respectively. If the weighted function 1 in Zhong et al. (2022) is

TABLE 11.3

Interim decision of dose optimization NSCLC case study.

CP	Zone	Decision
$CP \geq 0.9$	Favorable	Do not increase sample size
$0.9 > CP \geq 0.5$	Promising	Increase sample size, continue enrollment
$0.05 < CP < 0.5$	Unfavorable	Do not increase sample size
$CP \leq 0.05$	Futility	Terminate the arm

used, the modified CP are 0.25, 0.001, and 0.87 for arm A, arm B, and arm C, respectively. Thus, the interim decision is to choose the medium dose arm C, and the corresponding reestimated event size for arm C becomes 240. The trial continues into the Phase 3 stage with an expanded event size of 240. After observing 240 events in arm C, the final analysis is conducted. With the extended event size and study duration, the final estimate of the hazard ratio is about 0.62 (p = 0.001), which shows a statistically significant treatment effect for the medium-dose arm. In summary, the improved design provides an opportunity to select the most effective dose for a novel nonchemotherapy.

References

Ananthakrishnan, Revathi, Stephanie Green, Mark Chang, Gheorghe Doros, Joseph Massaro, and Michael LaValley. 2017. "Systematic comparison of the statistical operating characteristics of various phase I oncology designs." *Contemporary Clinical Trials Communications* 5: 34–48.

Avet-Loiseau, Hervé, Heinz Ludwig, Ola Landgren, Bruno Paiva, Chris Morris, Hui Yang, Kefei Zhou, Sunhee Ro, and Maria-Victoria Mateos. 2020. "Minimal residual disease status as a surrogate endpoint for progression-free survival in newly diagnosed multiple myeloma studies: a meta-analysis." *Clinical Lymphoma Myeloma and Leukemia* 20 (1): e30–e37.

Berry, Donald A, Shouhao Zhou, Howard Higley, Lata Mukundan, Shuangshuang Fu, Gregory H Reaman, Brent L Wood, Gary J Kelloff, J Milburn Jessup, and Jerald P Radich. 2017. "Association of minimal residual disease with clinical outcome in pediatric and adult acute lymphoblastic leukemia: a meta-analysis." *JAMA Oncology* 3 (7): e170580–e170580.

Blumenthal, Gideon M, Stella W Karuri, Hui Zhang, Lijun Zhang, Sean Khozin, Dickran Kazandjian, Shenghui Tang, Rajeshwari Sridhara, Patricia Keegan, and Richard Pazdur. 2015. "Overall response rate, progression-free survival, and overall survival with targeted and standard therapies in advanced non–small-cell lung cancer: US Food and Drug Administration trial-level and patient-level analyses." *Journal of Clinical Oncology* 33 (9): 1008.

Buyse, Marc and Geert Molenberghs. 1998. "Criteria for the validation of surrogate endpoints in randomized experiments." *Biometrics* 1014–1029.

Buyse, Marc, Geert Molenberghs, Tomasz Burzykowski, Didier Renard, and Helena Geys. 2000. "The validation of surrogate endpoints in meta-analyses of randomized experiments." *Biostatistics* 1 (1): 49–67.

Chen, Cong, Keaven Anderson, Devan V Mehrotra, Eric H Rubin, and Archie Tse. 2018. "A 2-in-1 adaptive phase 2/3 design for expedited oncology drug development." *Contemporary Clinical Trials* 64: 238–242.

Chen, Cong, Wen Li, and Qiqi Deng. 2020. "Extensions of the 2-in-1 adaptive design." *Contemporary Clinical Trials* 95: 106053.

Daniele, Patrick, Carla Mamolo, Joseph C Cappelleri, Timothy Bell, Alexander Neuhof, Gabriel Tremblay, Mihaela Musat, and Anna Forsythe. 2022. "Response rates and minimal residual disease outcomes as potential surrogates for progression-free survival in newly diagnosed multiple myeloma." *PLoS One* 17 (5): e0267979.

Fashoyin-Aje, Lola A, Gautam U Mehta, Julia A Beaver, and Richard Pazdur. 2022. "The on-and off-ramps of oncology accelerated approval." *The New England Journal of Medicine* 387 (16): 1439–1442.

Fleming, Thomas R, and David L DeMets. 1996. "Surrogate end points in clinical trials: are we being misled?" *Annals of Internal Medicine* 125 (7): 605–613.

Fleming, Thomas R, and John H Powers. 2012. "Biomarkers and surrogate endpoints in clinical trials." *Statistics in Medicine* 31 (25): 2973–2984.

Fleming, Thomas R, Ross L Prentice, Margaret S Pepe, and David Glidden. 1994. "Surrogate and auxiliary endpoints in clinical trials, with potential applications in cancer and AIDS research." *Statistics in Medicine* 13 (9): 955–968.

FOCR. 2021. "Optimizing dosing in oncology drug development." Friends of Cancer Research Annual Meeting 2021, https://friendsofcancerresearch.org/publications/.

FOCR. 2022. "Accelerating investigation of new therapies in earlier metastatic treatment settings." Friends of Cancer Research Annual Meeting 2022, https://friendsofcancerresearch.org/publications/.

Freedman, Laurence S, Barry I Graubard, and Arthur Schatzkin. 1992. "Statistical validation of intermediate endpoints for chronic diseases." *Statistics in Medicine* 11 (2): 167–178.

Harousseau, Jean-Luc, Antonio Palumbo, Paul G Richardson, Rudolf Schlag, Meletios A Dimopoulos, Ofer Shpilberg, Martin Kropff, Alain Kentos, Michele Cavo, and Anatoly Golenkov. 2010. "Superior outcomes associated with complete response in newly diagnosed multiple myeloma patients treated with nonintensive therapy: analysis of the phase 3 VISTA study of bortezomib plus melphalan-prednisone versus melphalan-prednisone." *Blood, the Journal of the American Society of Hematology* 116 (19): 3743–3750.

Jenkins, Martin, Andrew Stone, and Christopher Jennison. 2011. "An adaptive seamless phase II/III design for oncology trials with subpopulation selection using correlated survival endpoints." *Pharmaceutical Statistics* 10 (4): 347–356.

Jin, Man, and Pingye Zhang. 2022. "A seamless adaptive 2-in-1 design expanding a phase 2 trial for treatment or dose selection into a phase 3 trial." *Statistics in Biopharmaceutical Research* 14 (3): 334–341.

Li, Qing, Jianchang Lin, Mengya Liu, Liwen Wu, and Yingying Liu. 2022. "Using surrogate endpoints in adaptive designs with delayed treatment effect." *Statistics in Biopharmaceutical Research* 14 (4): 661–670.

Li, Runjia, Liwen Wu, Rachael Liu, and Jianchang Lin. 2022. "Flexible seamless 2-in-1 design with sample size adaptation." *arXiv Preprint arXiv:2212.11433*.

Lin, Jianchang, Veronica Bunn, and Rachael Liu. 2019. "Practical considerations for subgroups quantification, selection and adaptive enrichment in confirmatory trials." *Statistics in Biopharmaceutical Research* 11 (4): 407–418.

Mehta, Cyrus R, and Stuart J Pocock. 2011. "Adaptive increase in sample size when interim results are promising: a practical guide with examples." *Statistics in Medicine* 30 (28): 3267–3284.

Munshi, Nikhil C, Herve Avet-Loiseau, Andy C Rawstron, Roger G Owen, J Anthony Child, Anjan Thakurta, Paul Sherrington, Mehmet Kemal Samur, Anna Georgieva, and Kenneth C Anderson. 2017. "Association of minimal residual disease with superior survival outcomes in patients with multiple myeloma: a meta-analysis." *JAMA oncology* 3 (1): 28–35.

Ohashi, Kadoaki, Yosef E Maruvka, Franziska Michor, and William Pao. 2013. "Epidermal growth factor receptor tyrosine kinase inhibitor–resistant disease." *Journal of Clinical Oncology* 31 (8):1070.

Olivier, Timothée, and Vinay Prasad. 2022. "The approval and withdrawal of melphalan flufenamide (melflufen): Implications for the state of the FDA." *Translational Oncology* 18:101374.

Prentice, Ross L. 1989. "Surrogate endpoints in clinical trials: definition and operational criteria." *Statistics in Medicine* 8 (4): 431–440.

Reck, Martin, Delvys Rodríguez-Abreu, Andrew G Robinson, Rina Hui, Tibor Csőszi, Andrea Fülöp, Maya Gottfried, Nir Peled, Ali Tafreshi, and Sinead Cuffe. 2016. "Pembrolizumab versus chemotherapy for PD-L1–positive non–small-cell lung cancer." *The New England Journal of Medicine* 375: 1823–1833.

Sonneveld, Pieter, Hervé Avet-Loiseau, Sagar Lonial, Saad Usmani, David Siegel, Kenneth C Anderson, Wee-Joo Chng, Philippe Moreau, Michel Attal, and Robert A Kyle. 2016. "Treatment of multiple myeloma with high-risk cytogenetics: a consensus of the International Myeloma Working Group." *Blood, the Journal of the American Society of Hematology* 127 (24): 2955–2962.

Wu, Liwen, Qing Li, Mengya Liu, and Jianchang Lin. 2022. "Incorporating surrogate information for adaptive subgroup enrichment design with sample size re-estimation." *Statistics in Biopharmaceutical Research* 14 (4): 493–504.

Yang, Song, and Ross Prentice. 2005. "Semiparametric analysis of short-term and long-term hazard ratios with two-sample survival data." *Biometrika* 92 (1): 1–17.

Zhong, Chengxue, Qing Li, Liwen Wu, and Jianchang Lin. 2022. "Using surrogate information to improve confirmatory platform trial with sample size re-estimation." *Journal of Biopharmaceutical Statistics* 32 (4): 547–566.

12

Advanced Clinical Trial Design that Utilizes Real-World Evidence

Qing Li, Yingying Liu, and Debarshi Dey

Introduction

Randomized clinical trials have been considered the gold standard for evaluating the efficacy and safety of the treatment since the bias of unmeasured confounders is reduced through the randomization process (Meldrum 2000). On the other hand, conducting randomized clinical trials also faces many challenges. Enrolling a large number of subjects in randomized clinical trials will take a long time and cost a lot, which may be an obstacle for many sponsors with limited resources. Moreover, sometimes it is not ethical to conduct randomized clinical trials for some rare and life-threatening diseases. Last but not least, if there are multiple drug candidates, it is not possible to compare all the drugs versus the other drugs through randomized clinical trials. With the limitations of traditional randomized clinical trials, regulatory agencies, clinicians, and statisticians are actively evaluating alternative methods to overcome the limitations. In December 2018, FDA published a new strategic framework for FDA's Real-World Evidence program (FDA 2018a). In Dec 2021, FDA published the draft guidance on Considerations for the Use of Real-World Data and Real-World Evidence to Support Regulatory Decision-Making for Drug and Biological Products. Moreover, FDA published guidance for different types of RWD including electronic health records (FDA 2018b, FDA 2021a), medical claim data (FDA 2021a), and registries (FDA 2021b). In 2022, FDA also published the final guidance of Data Standards for Drug and Biological Product Submissions Containing Real-World Data to clearly define the data standards and documents used for regulatory decisions (FDA 2022a). In February 2022, FDA published the draft guidance of Considerations for the Design and Conduct of Externally Controlled Trials for Drug and Biological Products (FDA 2022b). This guidance provides a definition of externally controlled trials (ECTs) and outlines different types of ECTs such as historical controls, natural history controls, external concurrent controls, and synthetic controls. The guidance suggests that sponsors and applicants should carefully evaluate the suitability of ECTs based on the scientific and regulatory context, data quality and availability, and potential biases and limitations. It also provides recommendations for the design and conduct of ECTs, including control data sources selection and characterization, eligibility criteria for study subjects, endpoints and assessments, statistical methods for analysis, and measures to reduce bias and ensure data quality. The guidance discusses regulatory considerations for using ECTs to support drug and biological product development and approval, such as the need for preapproval consultation with the FDA, criteria for determining whether ECTs can provide substantial evidence of effectiveness, and the potential impact of ECTs on labeling and postmarketing requirements.

Agencies across the world also published much guidance regarding the RWE (NMPA 2020, Arlett et al. 2022, Flynn et al. 2022, Nishioka et al. 2022). At the same time, researchers outside regulatory agencies are also working on this critical topic. Bolislis et al. 2020 summarized and analyzed data from 27 cases for which real-world data (RWD) were applied in regulatory approval. Yang and Yu (2021) systematically summarized and provided an overview of how the RWE is used in the entire drug development and evaluation. Li et al. (2021) reviewed and summarized how to use external groups in clinical development with RWE and historical data through multiple case studies. Specifically, Li et al. (2020) discussed the practical considerations of utilizing propensity score methods in clinical development when the RWE is used.

At the same time, with the rapid development of the RWE field, there are multiple advanced designs and methodologies proposed. In this chapter, we discuss some advanced designs and methodologies used for analyzing RWE. In part I, the platform RWE study design using a case study will be discussed. In part II, the hybrid RWE study design methods used to combine RWD and clinical trial data will be discussed. In the end, we will summarize the challenges and opportunities of new RWE methodologies.

12.1 Platform RWE Study Design with a DLBCL Case Study

The literature on real-world evidence (RWE) often compares the treatment effect of only one investigational drug against another synthetic control group (Bolislis et al. 2020, Li et al. 2021). However, in fast-developing therapeutic areas like oncology, there are multiple new drugs available for a given indication. Therefore, comparing the efficacy and safety profiles among multiple regiments of interest will be advantageous for researchers, clinicians, and payers to better understand the comparative effectiveness of different options. A platform RWE study design as shown in Figure 1 has the potential to address this scientific question. In a platform RWE study, an investigational regimen of interest can be compared with multiple standards of care, placebos, active controls, or other treatments (see Figure 12.1). This platform RWE requires a substantial amount of high-quality RWD to support the analysis. The data sources for the treatment and control arms can vary, with the treatment arm data potentially coming from single-arm clinical trials

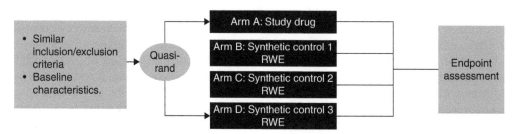

FIGURE 12.1
Platform RWE study design.

and control group data sourced from different RWE sources, such as historical trials, electronic health records, or health claim data. To account for the heterogeneity of data across different arms, it is important to select patients with similar inclusion and exclusion criteria, baseline characteristics, administration of treatment, index date definitions, and outcome measurements. Additionally, statistical modeling, such as propensity score methods, should be applied to reduce confounding bias, which arises from the lack of direct randomization. After the confounding bias is reduced through statistical modeling, one can compare the treatment effect.

Specially for the propensity score models, the simplified notations are as follows:

- Let i denote the i th subject in the dataset
- Let Z_i denote the treatment assignment: $Z_i = 1$ if subject i was in the treated group; $Z_i = 0$ if subject i is in the synthetic control group j
- Let X_i denote the observed baseline covariates for subject i
- Let Y_i denote the outcome for subject i: $Y_i(1)$ is the outcome for subject i if the subject was assigned to the treated group; $Y_i(j)$ is the outcome for subject i if he or she was assigned to the control group j.

The propensity scores are often estimated through a logistic regression: use Z_i as the dependent variable and X_i as the independent variables to fit the logistics regression for each synthetic control j, then the predicted probability $e(X_i) = \Pr(Z_i = 1|X_i) = 1/(1 + e^{-X_i\beta})$ is the estimated propensity score for each subject.

The procedure for conducting the Platform RWE study is summarized as follows:

1. Propensity score is estimated through a logistic regression with identified prognostic variables in the model
2. Perform propensity score matching stratification or IPTW for the treated arm versus the selected synthetic control arm
3. Check the baseline covariates balance through propensity score distribution and standardized difference
4. Estimate the treatment effect for the treated arm versus the selected synthetic control arm using the existing propensity score method
5. Repeat the above process for all synthetic control arms of interests
6. Adjust p value due to multiplicity as needed

12.1.1 Case Study of a Platform RWE Design: A DLBCL Case Study

Lymphoma disease is classified into two subtypes: non-Hodgkin lymphoma and Hodgkin lymphoma. Among non-Hodgkin lymphomas, diffuse large B-cell lymphoma (DLBCL) is the most commonly occurring form (Li et al. 2018). After the R-CHOP (rituximab, cyclophosphamide, doxorubicin, vincristine, and prednisone) first-line chemotherapy, there are still roughly 30% of patients experiencing a relapsed/refractory (R/R) of DLBCL disease (Sarkozy et al 2019, Crump et al. 2017). With the rapid development of lymphoma drugs, there are multiple available treatment options for R/R DLBCL treatments including Lenalidomide monotherapy (L), tafasitamab plus lenalidomide combo therapy (TL), bendamustine and rituximab (BR), and rituximab plus gemcitabine and oxaliplatin (R-GemOx) (NCCN 2021). The FDA granted accelerated approval of tafasitamab in July 2020 for patients with R/R DLBCL not eligible for autologous stem cell transplant (ASCT) based on the findings of the L-MIND study (FDA 2020). To assess the contribution of Tafasitamab when added to lenalidomide, the RE-MIND (NCT04150328) trial was conducted (Zinzani et al. 2021); however, the study only provided an indirect comparison between TL and L alone. In response, RE-MIND2 (NCT04697160), a retrospective observational cohort study, was also conducted to generate a historical control of routinely administered therapies, to compare with the tafasitamab + lenalidomide combination from the L-MIND trial. The primary analysis results of RE-MIND2 were reported in 2022 (Nowakowski et al. 2022).

The present study employs a platform RWE design that encompasses multiple treatment arms to provide a comprehensive evaluation of the comparative effectiveness of tafasitamab with respect to other potential treatments for relapsed/refractory diffuse large B-cell lymphoma (DLBCL). The study collected retrospective data from patients diagnosed with DLBCL between 2010 and 2020 from various academic hospitals, public hospitals, and private practices across Europe, North America, and the Asia-Pacific region. The data contained information regarding systemic therapies for R/R DLBCL, including bendamustine and rituximab (BR), R-GemOx, rituximab plus lenalidomide (R2), Pola-BR, CAR-T therapies, and others. The data were collected using electronic data capture methods, including the Medidata RAVE electronic case report form and the Cardinal Health electronic survey tool. To resemble the patient population of the L-MIND study, the inclusion and exclusion criteria of the RE-MIND2 study, which included factors such as patient population, lines of therapy, and disease history, were employed. Additionally, important individual-level baseline characteristics were also documented (as presented in Table 12.1).

After the data source was determined, the cohorts of interest should be planned. The treatment cohorts of interest with available data by the time of publication (Nowakowski et al. 2022) include (1) pooled systemic therapies cohort, (2) BR, and (3) R-GemOx. Statistical modeling was performed to create propensity score matched sets for each cohort, and nine critical baseline covariates were identified for the propensity score models, based on clinical relevance. These covariates were: age, Ann Arbor Stage, refractoriness to last line therapy, number of prior lines of therapy, history of primary refractoriness, prior ASCT, elevated lactate dehydrogenase (LDH), neutropenia, and anemia. The propensity scores were estimated using logistic regression with the nine identified covariates, and propensity score matching methods (nearest neighbor) were used to link patients with similar baseline characteristics across different groups. The absolute standardized difference was also calculated to assess the balance of the selected baseline covariates.

As shown in Figure 4.2, 3454 patients were enrolled in the RE-MIND2 study based on the inclusion criteria. After applying the eligibility and matching criteria, 961, 282, and 235 patients remained eligible for propensity score matching from the systemic therapies, BR, and R-GemOx cohorts, respectively. The number of eligible patients from the treated arm TL was reduced from 81 to 76 after the same criteria were applied. The nearest neighbor propensity score matching procedure was then applied, resulting in 76, 75, and 74 matched pairs in the systemic therapies, BR, and R-GemOx cohorts, respectively. The absolute standardized difference for each covariate was found to be below 0.2 for all three arms, with a range of 0 to 0.08 for the systemic therapies cohorts and 0 to 0.19 for the BR and R-GemOx cohorts. This indicates that the baseline covariates were well balanced between the treated and control arms.

The primary endpoint of this study is overall survival (OS), which is defined as the time from the index date (start of a given therapy) until death due to any cause. Secondary endpoints include objective response rate (ORR), complete response (CR) rate, duration of response (DOR), event-free survival (EFS), progression-free survival (PFS), time to next treatment (TTNT), and treatment discontinuation due to AEs. Due to the content limitations,

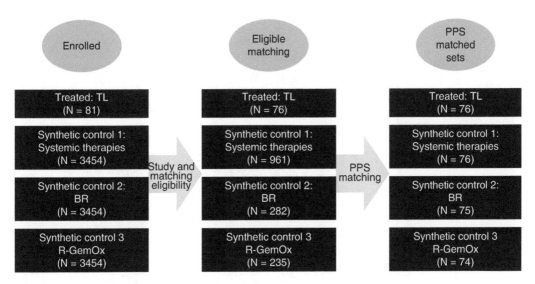

FIGURE 12.2
Matching flow of the DLBCL case study.

this chapter will only present the results of primary endpoints and some selected secondary endpoints as shown in Table 12.2. For a complete definition of endpoints, as well as results from primary and sensitivity analyses, the reader is referred to the original publication (Nowakowski et al. 2022).

The median OS in the pooled systemic therapies, BR, and R-GemOx cohorts were 11.6, 9.9, and 11.0 months, respectively, while in the PL cohort the median OS was 34.1, 31.6, and 31.6 months. Statistically significant differences in OS were observed between the PL cohort and each of the three synthetic control groups. The hazard ratio (HR) between PL and systemic therapies was 0.553, with a 95% confidence interval (CI) of 0.358–0.855 and a p value of 0.0068. The HR between PL and BR was 0.418, with a 95% CI of 0.272–0.644 and a p value of <0.0001. The HR between PL and R-GemOx was 0.467, with a 95% CI of 0.305–0.714 and a p value of 0.0003. The ORR difference between TL and systemic therapies, BR, and R-GemOx, are 18.42%, 12.00%, and 22.91%, respectively. Among them, ORR was significantly higher for TL cohorts compared with systemic therapies and R-GemOx cohort. The ORR difference between TL and systemic therapies, BR, and R-GemOx, were 17.11%, 10.67%, and 16.22%, respectively. Similarly, CR was significantly higher for TL cohorts compared with systemic therapies and R-GemOx cohort. DOR for the treated group was 26.1, which was much higher compared to all three synthetic control groups (6.6, 9.2, and 9.5). PFS results are also statistically significant when comparing the TL cohort with all three synthetic control arms.

12.2 Hybrid RWE Study Design

Despite the well-known advantages of RCTs, for some severe ultrarare diseases, after an efficacious drug is available on the market, it could become unethical to randomize subjects to a placebo when developing a new dose regimen or therapy. Therefore, to conduct a

TABLE 12.1

Demographics and baseline characteristics of matched TL compared with systemic therapies, BR and R-GemOx.

		Systemic			BR			R-GemOx		
		TL	Sys	Stand Diff	TL	BR	Stand Diff	TL	R-GemOx	Stand Diff
Age	<70 years	33 (43.4%)	31 (40.8%)	0.05	33 (44.0%)	33 (44.0%)	0.00	31 (41.9%)	26 (35.1%)	0.14
	>70 years	43 (56.6%)	45 (59.2%)		42 (56.0%)	42 (56.0%)		43 (58.1%)	48 (64.9%)	
Ann Arbor Stage	I + II	19 (25.0%)	19 (25.0%)	0.00	18 (24.0%)	19 (25.3%)	0.03	18 (24.3%)	15 (20.3%)	0.10
	III + IV	57 (75.0%)	57 (75.0%)		57 (76.0%)	56 (74.7%)		56 (75.7%)	59 (79.7%)	
Refractoriness to last prior therapy	Yes	34 (44.7%)	35 (46.1%)	0.03	33 (44.0%)	32 (42.7%)	0.03	33 (44.6%)	29 (39.2%)	0.11
	No	42 (55.3%)	41 (53.9%)		42 (56.0%)	43 (57.3%)		41 (55.4%)	45 (60.8%)	
No. of prior systemic trt lines	1	39 (51.3%)	39 (51.3%)	0.00	39 (52.0%)	39 (52.0%)	0.00	39 (52.7%)	41 (55.4%)	0.05
	2 & 3	37 (48.7%)	37 (48.7%)		36 (48.0%)	36 (48.0%)		35 (47.3%)	33 (44.6%)	
History of primary refractoriness	Yes	14 (18.4%)	12 (15.8%)	0.07	14 (18.7%)	19 (25.3%)	0.16	14 (18.9%)	14 (18.9%)	0.00
	No	62 (81.6%)	64 (84.2%)		61 (81.3%)	56 (74.7%)		60 (81.1%)	60 (81.1%)	
Prior ASCT	Yes	9 (11.8%)	10 (13.2%)	0.04	9 (12.0%)	14 (18.7%)	0.19	8 (10.8%)	8 (10.8%)	0.00
	No	67 (88.2%)	66 (86.8%)		66 (88.0%)	61 (81.3%)		66 (89.2%)	66 (89.2%)	
Elevated LDH	LDH > ULN	41 (53.9%)	44 (57.9%)	0.08	41 (54.7%)	37 (49.3%)	0.11	41 (55.4%)	48 (64.9%)	0.19
	LDH < ULN	35 (46.1%)	32 (42.1%)		34 (45.3%)	38 (50.7%)		33 (44.6%)	26 (35.1%)	
Neutropenia	ANC < $1.5 * 10^9$/L	2 (2.6%)	2 (2.6%)	0.00	2 (2.7%)	4 (5.3%)	0.14	2 (2.7%)	5 (6.8%)	0.19
	ANC >= $1.5 * 10^9$/L	74 (97.4%)	74 (97.4%)		73 (97.3%)	71 (94.7%)		72 (97.3%)	69 (93.2%)	
Anemia	Hgb < 10 g/dL	6 (7.9%)	5 (6.6%)	0.05	6 (8.0%)	5 (6.7%)	0.05	6 (8.1%)	5 (6.8%)	0.05
	Hgb > 10 g/dL	70 (92.1%)	71 (93.4%)		69 (92.0%)	70 (93.3%)		68 (91.9%)	69 (93.2%)	

TABLE 12.2

Results of primary and selected secondary endpoints of TL compared with systemic therapies, BR, and R-GemOx.

	Systemic Therapies		BR		R-GemOx	
	TL (N = 76)	Systemic therapies (N = 76)	TL (N = 75)	BR (N = 75)	TL (N = 74)	BR (N = 74)
OS median (months)	34.1	11.6	31.6	9.9	31.6	11.0
(95% CI)	(18.3–NR)	(8.8–16.1)	(18.3–NR)	(5.3–13.7)	(18.3–NR)	(7.9–16.8)
HR with 95% CI	0.553	(0.358–0.855)	0.418	(0.272–0.644)	0.467	(0.305–0.714)
P value	0.0068		<0.0001		0.0003	
ORR, n (%)	51 (67.1)	37 (48.7)	50 (66.7)	41 (54.7)	51 (68.9)	34 (45.9)
ORR difference in %	18.42		12.00		22.91	
95% CI	(1.905–34.204)		(–4.657– 28.173)		(6.285–38.722)	
P value	0.0323		0.1810		0.0076	
CR, n (%)	29 (38.2)	16 (21.1)	29 (38.7)	21 (28.0)	29 (39.2)	17 (23.0)
CR difference in %	17.11		10.67		16.22	
95% CI	(0.579–32.952)		(–5.987 to 26.891)		(–0.548 to 32.318)	
P value	0.0324		0.2252		0.050	
DOR, median (months)	26.1	6.6	26.1	9.2	26.1	9.5
95% CI	(13.9–NR)	(4.4–11.8)	(13.9–NR)	(5.3–12.5)	(13.9–NR)	(5.5–13.2)
PFS median (months)	12.1	5.8	12.1	7.9	14.1	5.1
(95% CI)	(5.9–22.5)	(3.1–6.4)	(5.5–22.5)	(4.3–11.3)	(6.3–28.0)	(3.5–9.5)
HR with 95% CI	0.424	(0.278–0.647)	0.527	(0.344–0.809)	0.433	(0.288–0.653)
P value	<0.0001		0.0028		<0.0001	

clinical trial for this new therapy, the only option is to randomize subjects between a new experimental treatment arm and an active control arm using the approved regimen. Provided the ultrarare disease population, it could be almost impossible to recruit enough patients to demonstrate the superiority of the new therapy over the approved regimen. In cases like this, if data from the pivotal trial of the approved regimen is available, then it becomes a natural option as a pool of historical data to help augment the concurrent control arm for a boost in power. However, the comparability of the historical and current data needs to be assessed before pooling to ensure that minimal bias is introduced by the use of historical data. Viele et al. (2014) introduced an intuitive frequentist approach called "test-then-pool," which pools the historical data with the concurrent control data only if the hypothesis of equality cannot be rejected at a significance level α. The "test-then-pool" method aims to borrow all information from the historical control data pool when deemed appropriate, while some Bayesian methods like power prior can support dynamic borrowing, which discounts the historical information if there is heterogeneity between the historical control and concurrent data. Wang et al. (2019) also proposed to use the propensity score method (Rosenbaum and Rubin, 1983) to stratify subjects from the historical control pool and apply power prior to each propensity score stratum for Bayesian inference.

If the desire is to select a subset of subjects from the historical control pool to construct a historical control arm with those who share more similarity in baseline covariates as those in the current trial, then the propensity score matching approach can be utilized. This is a popular method in observational studies to ensure covariate balance between groups and reduce confounding bias (Rosenbaum, 2010). The matching design has the following advantages (Lu, 2021): (1) it is a nonparametric way to balance covariate distributions and is thus more robust; (2) it resembles the randomization design, so it ensures the statistical inference for randomized design can be applied to the matched data and it is interpretable to clinicians and patients; and (3) it is more objective as the matching process does not involve the outcome. Liu et al. (2022) introduced two hybrid RWE study designs that are based on propensity score matching. These two designs balance key observed baseline covariates and ensure comparability of the outcomes between the historical and concurrent control arms, hence providing protection against unmeasured confounders.

12.2.1 First Hybrid RWE Study Design – Conditional Borrowing

There has always been concern that using historical data could introduce unpredictable confounding even if it was generated from a previous trial done by the same sponsor as the current trial, with the same inclusion/exclusion criteria and mostly the same investigators. So, the first hybrid RWE study design – conditional borrowing was proposed to control unmeasured confounding and minimize unpredictable biases. Assume the current trial randomizes the study population (RP) into a treatment arm (TA) and a concurrent control arm (CC). The conditional borrowing design has the following steps:

1. Construct the historical control (HC) candidate by matching the historical control pool (HCP) data with the current trial data (or equivalently the randomized population: RP = TA + CC) based on key baseline covariates using the propensity score method.
2. Assess the covariate balance between the HC candidate and the RP using the absolute standardized difference for mean (ASD) and/or the log-ratio of standard deviations

3. If the covariates between the HC candidate and the RP are balanced, then check the comparability between the HC candidate and the concurrent control arm (CC) based on a prespecified closeness criterion for the outcome variable.

If the HC passes both the covariate balance and the outcome comparability checks, then the subjects from HC will be pooled with those in the CC arm to construct the augmented control arm (CA = HC + CC) and formal testing will be performed between the treatment arm (TA) and the augmented control arm CA. Otherwise, borrowing data from the historical control pool (HCP) will very likely introduce bias because either the key baseline covariates cannot be well balanced between the historical control (HC) and the current trial (RP) through matching or the outcomes between the historical control (HC) and the concurrent control (CC) differs substantially due to some unmeasured confounders that are not controlled through matching. The closeness criteria can be based on the distance between the HC mean and CC mean measured in the unit of standard errors of the means if the outcome variable is continuous. Equivalently, the comparability can be assessed using the confidence intervals for the proportions or median survival time if the response variable is binary or time-to-event, respectively. Figure 12.3 helps illustrate the conditional borrowing steps described above.

To maintain the study integrity, the matching process involves only the baseline covariates, and the comparability criteria that determine the outcome closeness between the two sources of control should be agreed upon among all stakeholders prior to conducting the matching. For larger concurrent trials where a good baseline covariate balance between TA and CC can be achieved through randomization, the propensity score matching can also be done between the historical control pool (HCP) and the concurrent control (CC) arm. However, the proposal to use the entire current trial population RP for the propensity score matching step has the advantage that this step can be performed before unblinding so that the HC candidate can be determined before the treatment arms are revealed and the outcomes are assigned to TA and CC.

Simulation studies have been conducted to study the overall Type I error, power profile, and borrowing rate by varying the concurrent control (CC) outcome mean around the outcome mean of the historical control pool (HCP). Figure 12.4 presents the two-sided Type I error profile, borrowing rate (empirical probability of borrowing), and power of conditional borrowing.

For the conditional borrowing, Type I error rate is controlled at the significance level α when the CC mean is the same as the HCP mean but begins to increase when the CC mean

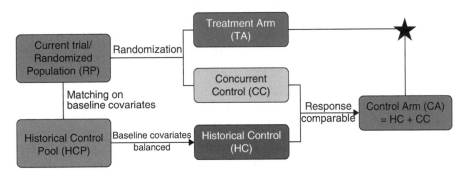

FIGURE 12.3
Illustration of conditional borrowing.

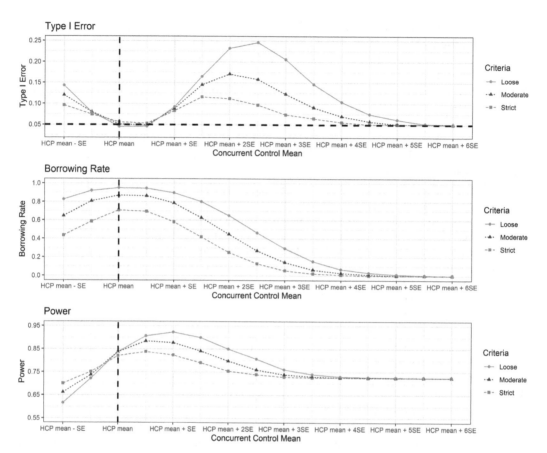

FIGURE 12.4

Type I error rate, borrowing rate, and power for conditional borrowing.

diverges from the HCP mean. The Type I error inflation is bounded with the magnitude of the inflation depending on the strictness of the outcome closeness criteria. With a two-sided test, Type I error is inflated when the CC mean differs from the HCP mean on both sides, but inflation when the CC mean is less than the HCP mean can be avoided by using a one-sided test. The borrowing rate is at its maximum when the CC mean equals the HCP mean and gradually drops down to zero as the difference between the CC mean and the HCP mean increases. These results suggest that when the distribution of the current control data is the same as the historical data, the conditional borrowing method increases the power without inflating Type I error, and it is able to detect the overall distributional shift of CC from HCP and automatically adjust the probability of borrowing.

12.2.2 Second Hybrid RWE Study Design – Intermediate-outcome Assisted Borrowing

In the context of conditional borrowing design, the feasibility of borrowing historical data can only be determined after the final unblinding. However, there may be situations where such determination needs to occur before the primary endpoint is available at the final analysis. The second hybrid RWE study design – intermediate outcome-assisted borrowing

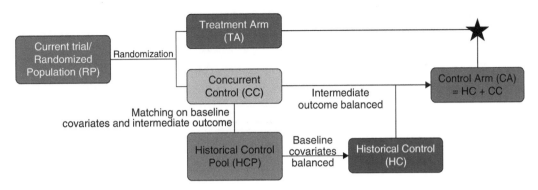

FIGURE 12.5
Illustration of intermediate outcome-assisted borrowing.

can control for unmeasured biases in the absence of the primary endpoint. This approach incorporates one or more intermediate outcomes in the propensity score matching process, with these intermediate outcomes potentially being the primary endpoint evaluated at an earlier time point or some biomarker/surrogate endpoints that reflect the treatment effect earlier and are known to have moderate/high correlation with the primary endpoint. This approach utilizes the early movement of the intermediate outcome measures related to clinical benefit and actively controls for any unmeasured confounding through matching on these endpoints. Since intermediate outcomes are measured posttreatment, matching needs to occur only between the historical control pool and the concurrent control arm and any treatment arm data needs to be restricted from the one performing the matching. The postmatching balance of the intermediate outcomes needs to be carefully checked together with other baseline covariates before pooling the two control arms so that comparability can be ensured. Acceptable balance criterion for the intermediate outcomes which could be the same as or even more stringent than that for the baseline covariates needs to be prespecified to avoid subjectivity. Figure 12.5 helps illustrate the intermediate outcome-assisted borrowing steps described above.

The results of the intermediate outcome-assisted borrowing are presented in Figure 12.6. The absolute standardized difference for mean (ASD) threshold of 0.25 is used for good balance for all the baseline covariates (Stuart, 2010), and an ASD of 0.1 is applied to impose a better balance for the intermediate outcome (Austin, 2009; Mamdani et al., 2005; Normand et al., 2001). The Type I error for the intermediate outcome-assisted borrowing is only under reasonable control when the correlation between the intermediate outcome and the primary endpoint is high, and the curves under the high-correlation scenario are similar in shape to those for the conditional borrowing method. This suggests that a good intermediate outcome can also provide information on the similarity between the historical and concurrent control data and guide researchers toward a more informed decision.

12.2.3 A Rare Hematological Disease Case Study

A case study is presented here to illustrate the implementation of the methods introduced above. This is a randomized study of a rare hematological disease with a design feature to potentially borrow from RWD. The primary endpoint is progression-free survival (PFS), and the secondary endpoint is objective response rate (ORR). Given the limited patient population and slow recruitment rate, the study only expects to enroll with a 2:1

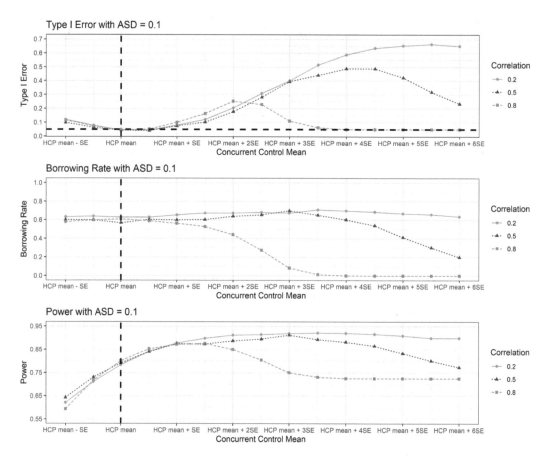

FIGURE 12.6

Type I error rate, borrowing rate, and power for intermediate outcome-assisted borrowing.

randomization ratio between the experimental treatment and standard of care (SOC). However, to achieve 80% power at a significance level of 0.05, 115 events will be required to detect a hazard ratio of 0.6 with the assumption that the PFS distribution is exponential. So, the study team identified 100 patients treated with SOC from suitable RWD sources based on comparable inclusion and exclusion criteria, prior treatment, disease type, and endpoint availability and hope to borrow 30 patients from the historical data to augment the control group and increase the power.

The median progression-free survival time is used for the outcome comparability check for the conditional borrowing design. Propensity score matching is performed using important baseline covariates identified through literature review. Following matching, the balance of all variables used in the matching is checked using the absolute standardized difference for mean (ASD) of 0.25, and the 68% confidence interval (CI) is constructed for the median PFS of the historical control. If the median PFS of the concurrent control falls within this CI, then it is feasible to borrow from the historical control. For outcome-assisted borrowing, ORR is used as the intermediate outcome as it is highly correlated with the primary survival endpoint and has been commonly used as the surrogate endpoint to support accelerated approval in oncology trials (FDA, 2018). Figure 12.7 presents the Kaplan-Meier curves for the current study of 90 patients and the historical control pool with 100 patients.

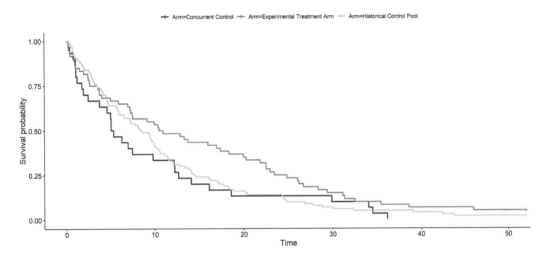

FIGURE 12.7
Kaplan-Meier curves for the current study and the historical control data pool.

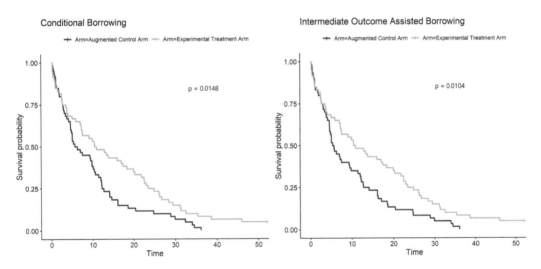

FIGURE 12.8
Kaplan-Meier curves after borrowing from historical data.

The hazard ratio (HR) for the current study is 0.655 with a p value of 0.065. If the conditional borrowing design is applied, the median PFS of the two control arms satisfy the comparability criteria specified above and it is feasible to borrow from the historical control pool. The matched historical control arm satisfies the covariate balance check and the resulting HR between the experimental treatment arm and the augmented control arm of SOC is 0.629 with a p value of 0.0148. Else, if the intermediate outcome-assisted borrowing design is used, all the baseline covariates pass the postmatching balance check with ASD of 0.25 and the ASD of the ORR is less than 0.1. Although not required by the algorithm, a further comparability check on the primary PFS endpoint also confirms that the median PFS of the concurrent control is within the 68% CI of the median PFS of the historical control and it is safe to pool the matched historical control arm with the concurrent control. The resulting HR is 0.6141 with a p value of 0.0104. This case study is a good example of an underpowered study that borrowing a subset from the RWD that is similar to the concurrent control could help increase the probability of trial success.

12.3 Summary

In this chapter, we explored the application of advanced clinical trial designs using real-world evidence (RWE). We presented a case study of diffuse large B-cell lymphoma (DLBCL) to demonstrate the use of platform RWE design and a case study of a rare hematological disease to illustrate the hybrid RWE design. These advanced designs surpass the conventional RWE clinical trial designs, which primarily focus on comparing a single-arm study with a synthetic control arm derived from real-world data (RWD). While the methodologies for these advanced designs are relatively simple to implement in drug development and evaluation, their application faces several technical and operational challenges.

First, both the platform RWE design and the hybrid RWE study design demand higher data quality compared to traditional RWE studies, as they involve multiple arms from both treatment and control arms from clinical trials and RWD. Therefore, a systematic data collection and cleaning platform is necessary to ensure consistently high data quality across all arms. Additionally, the hybrid control trial requires randomization of the current trial, making it imperative to establish a comprehensive blinding plan during the matching process to protect the study's integrity.

In conclusion, the rapid growth of RWD presents numerous opportunities for the development and application of advanced RWE methodologies. However, these new methods also raise the bar for technical and operational requirements for RWE researchers, demanding close cross-functional collaboration between RWD platform, clinical operations, statisticians, data scientists, clinicians, regulatory agencies, and the development of a reliable protocol and statistical analysis plan.

References

Arlett, P., Kjær, J., Broich, K., & Cooke, E. (2022). Real-world evidence in EU medicines regulation: enabling use and establishing value. *Clinical Pharmacology and Therapeutics, 111*(1), 21.

Austin, P. C. (2009). Balance diagnostics for comparing the distribution of baseline covariates between treatment groups in propensity-score matched samples. *Statistics in Medicine, 28*(25), 3083–3107.

Bolislis, W. R., Fay, M., & Kühler, T. C. (2020). Use of real-world data for new drug applications and line extensions. *Clinical Therapeutics, 42*(5), 926–938.

Crump, M., Neelapu, S. S., Farooq, U., Van Den Neste, E., Kuruvilla, J., Westin, J., ... & Gisselbrecht, C. (2017). Outcomes in refractory diffuse large B-cell lymphoma: results from the international SCHOLAR-1 study. *Blood, the Journal of the American Society of Hematology, 130*(16), 1800–1808.

Flynn, R., Plueschke, K., Quinten, C., Strassmann, V., Duijnhoven, R. G., Gordillo-Marañon, M. et al. (2022). Marketing authorization applications made to the European medicines agency in 2018–2019: What was the contribution of real-world evidence?. *Clinical Pharmacology & Therapeutics, 111*(1), 90–97.

Food and Drug Administration [FDA]. (2018a). Framework for FDA's Real-World Evidence Program, 2018. www.fda.gov/media/120060/download

Food and Drug Administration [FDA]. (2018b). Use of Electronic Health Record Data in Clinical Investigations Guidance for Industry, 2018. www.fda.gov/media/97567/download

Food and Drug Administration [FDA]. (2020). Multi-discipline Review: Application Number: 761163Orig1s000, 2020. www.accessdata.fda.gov/drugsatfda_docs/nda/2020/7611 63Orig1s000MultidisciplineR.pdf

Food and Drug Administration [FDA]. (2021a). Real-World Data: Assessing Electronic Health Records and Medical Claims Data to Support Regulatory Decision-Making for Drug and Biological Products Draft Guidance for Industry, 2021. www.fda.gov/media/152503/download

Food and Drug Administration [FDA]. (2021b). Real-World Data: Assessing Registries to Support Regulatory Decision-Making for Drug and Biological Products Guidance for Industry Draft Guidance for Industry, 2021. www.fda.gov/media/154449/download

Food and Drug Administration [FDA]. (2022a). Submitting Documents Using Real-World Data and Real-World Evidence to FDA for Drug and Biological Products Guidance for Industry, 2022. www.fda.gov/media/124795/download

Food and Drug Administration [FDA]. (2022b). Considerations for the Design and Conduct of Externally Controlled Trials for Drug and Biological Products Guidance for Industry, 2022. www.fda.gov/media/164960/download

Li, Q., Chen, G., Lin, J., Chi, A., & Davies, S. (2021). External control using RWE and historical data in clinical development. In H. Yang, & B. Yu (Eds.), *Real-World Evidence in Drug Development and Evaluation* (pp. 71–100). Chapman and Hall/CRC.

Li, Q., Lin, J., Chi, A., & Davies, S. (2020). Practical considerations of utilizing propensity score methods in clinical development using real-world and historical data. *Contemporary Clinical Trials, 97*, 106–123.

Li, S., Young, K. H., & Medeiros, L. J. (2018). *Diffuse large B-cell lymphoma. Pathology, 50*(1), 74–87.

Liu, Y., Lu, B., Foster, R., Zhang, Y., Zhong, Z. J., Chen, M., & Sun, P. (2022): Matching design for augmenting the control arm of a randomized controlled trial using real-world data. *Journal of Biopharmaceutical Statistics, 32*(1), 124–140.

Lu, B. (2021). Causal inference for observational studies/real-world data. In H. Yang & B. Yu (Eds.), *Real-world Evidence in Drug Development and Evaluation* (pp. 129–148). CRC Press.

Mamdani, M., Sykora, K., Li, P., Normand, S. L., Streiner, D. L., Austin, P. C., Rochon, P. A., & Anderson, G. M. (2005). Reader's guide to critical appraisal of cohort studies: 2. Assessing potential for confounding. *BMJ, 330*(7497), 960–962.

Meldrum, M. L. (2000). A brief history of the randomized controlled trial: From oranges and lemons to the gold standard. *Hematology/Oncology Clinics of North America, 14*(4), 745–760.

National Comprehensive Cancer Network (NCCN). (2021). NCCN clinical practice guidelines in oncology: B-cell lymphomas v4.2021.

National Medical Products Administration (NMPA). (2020). Guidelines for Real-World Evidence to Support Drug Development and Review (Interim), 2020. https://redica.com/wp-cont ent/uploads/NMPA_-Attachment_-_Guiding-Principles-of-Real-World-Data-Used-to-Gener ate-Real-World-Evidence-Trial.pdf

Nishioka, K., Makimura, T., Ishiguro, A., Nonaka, T., Yamaguchi, M., & Uyama, Y. (2022). Evolving acceptance and use of RWE for regulatory decision making on the benefit/risk assessment of a drug in Japan. *Clinical Pharmacology & Therapeutics, 111*(1), 35–43.

Normand, S. T., Landrum, M. B., Guadagnoli, E., Ayanian, J. Z., Ryan, T. J., Cleary, P. D., & McNeil, B. J. (2001). Validating recommendations for coronary angiography following acute myocardial infarction in the elderly: A matched analysis using propensity scores. *Journal of Clinical Epidemiology, 54*(5), 387–398.

Nowakowski, G. S., Yoon, D. H., Peters, A., Mondello, P., Joffe, E., Fleury, I., ... Salles, G. (2022). Improved efficacy of Tafasitamab plus lenalidomide versus systemic therapies for relapsed/

refractory DLBCL: RE-MIND2, an observational retrospective matched cohort study. *Clinical Cancer Research: An Official Journal of the American Association for Cancer Research, 28*(18), 4003–4017.

Rosenbaum, P. R. (2010). *Design of Observational Studies*. Springer.

Rosenbaum, P. R., & Rubin, D. B. (1983). The central role of the propensity score in observational studies for causal effects. *Biometrika, 70*(1), 41–55.

Sarkozy, C., & Sehn, L. H. (2019). New drugs for the management of relapsed or refractory diffuse large B-cell lymphoma. *Ann Lymphoma, 3*(10), 19.

Stuart, E. A. (2010). Matching methods for causal inference: A review and a look forward. *Statistical Science, 25*, 1–21.

Viele, K., Berry, S., Neuenschwander, B., Amzal, B., Chen, F., Enas, N., Hobbs, B., Ibrahim, J. G., Kinnersley, N., Lindborg, S., et al. (2014). Use of historical control data for assessing treatment effects in clinical trials. *Pharmaceutical Statistics, 13*(1), 41–54.

Wang, C., Li, H., Chen, W., Lu, N., Tiwari, R., Xu, Y., & Yue, L. Q. (2019). Propensity score-integrated power prior approach for incorporating real-world evidence in single-arm clinical studies. *Journal of Biopharmaceutical Statistics, 29*(5), 731–748.

Yang, H., & Yu, B. (Eds.). (2021). *Real-world Evidence in Drug Development and Evaluation*. CRC Press.

Zinzani, P. L., Rodgers, T., Marino, D., Frezzato, M., Barbui, A. M., Castellino, C., Meli, E., Fowler, N. H., Salles, G., Feinberg, B., Kurukulasuriya, N. C., Tillmanns, S., Parche, S., Dey, D., Fingerle-Rowson, G., Ambarkhane, S., Winderlich, M., & Nowakowski, G. S. (2021). RE-MIND: Comparing Tafasitamab + Lenalidomide (L-MIND) with a real-world lenalidomide monotherapy cohort in relapsed or refractory diffuse large B-cell lymphoma. *Clinical Cancer Research: An Official Journal of the American Association for Cancer Research, 27*(22), 6124–6134. https://doi.org/10.1158/1078-0432.CCR-21-1471

13

Case Studies in Statistical Safety Monitoring

Jordan J. Elm and Renee L. Martin

It is quite common for a junior clinical investigator to write a proposal for a pilot study with a specific aim of "demonstrating safety" for their intervention of interest. In truth, it is quite difficult to demonstrate that a study intervention is safe, especially in a small sample. In statistical terms, this aim translates to a null hypothesis that the intervention is equally safe to control. However, failure to reject this null hypothesis, a p value greater than 0.05, does not prove that the null hypothesis is true or imply that the intervention is safe. The best possible result would be able to state that no safety concerns were identified.

The development of a statistical plan for safety monitoring starts with a detailed discussion of the safety objectives. Well-designed safety objectives will focus on identifying potential harms rather than trying to prove that a new intervention is safe. This requires careful consideration of the safety events or outcomes of special interest and how they will be measured, presented, and statistically tested. However, unlike efficacy hypotheses, safety hypotheses cannot always be prespecified due to unexpected adverse events. The assessment of safety is ongoing during the clinical trial life-cycle and is not simply a phase I or phase II trial objective. Sometimes safety concerns are not detected until the intervention comes to market.

In this chapter we begin with an exploration of safety issues across the lifespan of drug development: phases 1, 2, and 3. Next, we introduce key considerations for developing a safety monitoring plan, collection of safety data, and statistical aspects. A variety of graphical approaches to safety monitoring are provided. Throughout the chapter we present real-world trials to frame the lesson points.

13.1 Safety Issues in Early and Late Phase Trials

13.1.1 Early Phase

Phase I or dose finding trials, such as the "3 + 3" design, Up-and-Down, or Continual Reassessment Method (CRM) designs, are designed to identify the maximum tolerated dose (MTD) based on dose-limiting toxicities (DLTs). The Continual Reassessment Method provides enhanced ability to find the MTD compared to the 3 + 3 design.[1] These designs work well when the intervention toxicities are expected at a relatively high frequency, such as 1 out of 3 subjects or 1 out of 5 subjects.

For example, Selim et al. employed a CRM design to identify the MTD of deferoxamine in intracerebral hemorrhage (ICH).[2] The study was designed to identify the MTD as the dose of deferoxamine associated with a 0.4 probability of dose-limiting toxicity, derived from the serious adverse event rate in placebo patients of recently completed ICH trials. After 20 participants were enrolled and treated according to the algorithm, the prespecified convergence criterion was met, yielding an estimated MTD of 62 mg/kg/day. DLTs were observed in two of six participants treated at the MTD.

Next, a phase 2 trial was initiated to evaluate the futility of 62 mg/kg/day.[3] After 42 subjects had been randomized, the Data and Safety Monitoring Board (DSMB) identified an increased risk of acute respiratory distress syndrome (ARDS) in the deferoxamine arm (6/21, or 28.6%), and the trial was terminated. Although the MTD threshold was 40%, this was for a broader definition of toxicity than just ARDS. Selim et al. revised the protocol in an effort to improve the safety profile, resulting in the iDEF trial: an evaluation of the futility of 32 mg/kg/day over 3 days, in a patient population excluding those at high risk of ARDS. ARDS was observed in only 1.4% of the iDEF deferoxamine arm.[4]

This case provides an example of the challenges of identifying and responding to safety concerns in early-phase trials. In hindsight, had the phase I trial continued to enroll subjects at the MTD in order to obtain more safety data before moving it into phase 2, perhaps the increase in ARDS event rate might have been identified sooner. On the other hand, although there was a statistically significant imbalance observed in ARDS in the phase 2 trial, there were only 21 subjects randomized to the 62 mg/kg/day deferoxamine arm, and this was an unexpected event. One may contemplate whether the DSMB should have allowed the trial to continue enrolling at the higher dose (62 mg/kg/day) to ascertain whether this was a spurious finding. It is not uncommon that the MTD identified in phase I is too high a dose, and a phase 2 trial may best be designed to explore more than one dose with this scenario in mind.

13.1.2 Late Phase

Safety issues can emerge in later phase studies as well. Based on results from the Albumin in Acute Stroke (ALIAS) Pilot clinical trial, the ALIAS study was designed to assess the effect of 2 g/kg of 25% human albumin infused intravenously within 5 hours of ischemic stroke.[5,6] The primary outcome was a composite of the 90-day modified Rankin Scale and National Institute of Health Stroke Scale (NIHSS). In the ALIAS Pilot study it was established that this dosing regimen would lead to an approximate 12–14% risk of mild to moderate pulmonary edema or congestive heart failure.[5] However, unanticipated safety issues with mortality began to arise during the onset of the study, and after 434 subjects were randomized the study was halted due to increased mortality in the albumin-treated arm of the study. After an extensive, unblinded review of the data, it was determined that the expected events of both congestive heart failure and pulmonary edema could be easily managed with diuretic therapy and were not directly associated with increased early mortality. Thus, using more stringent eligibility criteria and increased monitoring of fluids along with increased safety monitoring, the ALIAS study was restarted as ALIAS Part 2.[6]

13.2 Designing an Appropriate Safety Monitoring Plan

13.2.1 Know What Is Expected

The key steps to consider when developing a safety monitoring plan are presented in Table 13.1. The first step is to know what is anticipated just due to the disease and what might additionally be expected with the intervention under study. This will depend on what is already known about the drug from prior studies and whether this is a new or repurposed product. There may be events that we can anticipate based on the drug's target or mechanism of action. For products with an investigators' brochure or label, this provides a starting point for expected events rates, but one should be mindful of what is anticipated due to the disease alone and whether the new population could have a different baseline rate. Epidemiological or natural history data or the control group from another trial of similar patients can be used to estimate the anticipated rate in the control group. Once the control rate is estimated, we must consider how much of an increase would give cause for concern. This clinically worrisome increase can be used to define safety stopping rules. An example of this may be a relative risk exceeding 2 or 3 or an absolute increase of some magnitude (e.g. 5%, 10%). In abstract terms, most people might agree that a relative risk of 2 is worrisome and 3 is cause for alarm but consider that, with a very low control rate (1%), it is possible to have a RR of this magnitude with a very small absolute difference (1% versus 2% is RR of 2). Clearly this requires consideration of the risk/benefit ratio, and this will be a disease-dependent choice.

The POINT trial of dual antiplatelet therapy versus aspirin observed just such an increase in the rate of major hemorrhage (1% aspirin versus 2% dual), but this was offset by the decrease in major ischemic events (5% dual versus 6.5% aspirin).[7] Oncology trials often accept a high toxicity rate for short-term use of life-saving therapies. For progressive diseases such as Parkinson's disease, if we can delay neurodegeneration then we may accept other potentially harmful events. For example, several trials have tested drugs with known safety issues for use in other indications such as sirolimus in multiple system atrophy and pioglitazone and nilotinib in Parkinson's disease.[8,9,10]

13.2.2 Measuring Safety: Prospective versus Passive Collection

In many clinical trials the collection of adverse events is passive. The subject is asked, "What unusual symptoms or medical problems have you experienced since last visit?" All adverse events regardless of relatedness are reported per the protocol. Those events

TABLE 13.1

Considerations when developing a safety plan.

1. Anticipate potential harms
2. Define safety outcomes
3. Determine expected rates (drug/control group)
4. Define clinically worrisome increase
5. Consider the sample size/type I error rate
6. Define statistical approach to monitoring
7. Be cautious of unexpected events

can then be centrally coded according to a medical dictionary [e.g., Medical Dictionary for Regulatory Activities (MedDRA)]. Coded adverse events (AEs) are then grouped by body system and preferred term. Frequencies by treatment group are reviewed by the DSMB to assess for worrisome increases. However, this practice is imperfect because a single event may be reported multiple times as individual signs and symptoms rather than the diagnosis. The classification by body system is often too broad to closely monitor a concerning mechanism of action. Similar types of events may be coded as different preferred terms making it harder to detect safety issues, for example, Nausea/Vomiting/Dyspepsia or Skin reaction/Rash.[11] Training sites to consistently report the diagnosis rather than signs and symptoms, grouping related terms in frequency tables, and using composites of major safety events are recommended to avoid missing a safety signal.

Prospectively collecting safety events by posing a specific interview question to the subject leads to better ascertainment than with passive collection described above and avoids many of the issues with coding as well.[12] However, this is only possible for anticipated events. Some trials will employ a team of experts to uniformly assess events across all subjects to determine whether each event meets the trial definition of an outcome. This can help standardize event ascertainment in a blinded fashion and is generally performed by a team of specialists known as Central Adjudicators. A well-defined operational definition is still critical at the point of data collection, since adjudications are often dependent on what gets reported by the site. See Table 13.2 for a sample of the operational definitions of the safety events of interest from the POINT trial Case Report Form.[13,14]

A poorly conceived safety monitoring plan may focus exclusively on reporting serious adverse events (SAEs). An adverse event is an SAE if it meets the Food and Drug Administration (FDA) definition. In brief, an SAE results in any of the following outcomes: death, life-threatening, hospitalization, disability/permanent damage, congenital anomaly/birth defect, or requiring medical/surgical intervention to prevent one of the outcomes listed in this definition.[15] It is important to note that related events may not always result in an SAE; thus, focusing only on the frequency of SAEs may make it harder to observe increased safety event rates. The FDA and IRBs have reporting guidelines for SAEs, but it is difficult for these groups to determine causality because they are neither treating the subjects nor able to perform aggregated analyses. Indeed, the FDA revised their reporting guidelines in 2011 due to overreporting which was hindering the ability to detect safety concerns. They have provided recommendations for assessing relatedness and possible causality.[11,15]

13.2.3 Who Is Reviewing the Safety of an Ongoing Trial?

The site investigator sees subject-level data but only at their site. The Medical Monitor reviews events one at a time as they occur, often without reference to the cumulative person time. The FDA, European Medicines Agency (EMA), and Central Institutional Review Board (CIRB) receive reports of the select events that meet their reporting requirements either in real time or annually in aggregate. Typically, the DSMB is the only independent scientific group to view summaries of event rates by treatment group during the trial, and thus they are key to detecting safety concerns midcourse. Initially, DSMBs are often fully unblinded or "partially blinded" with tables showing treatment codes (A or B) rather than the names. In the latter case, DSMBs should be free to fully unblind when appropriate to complete their charge. The frequency of reporting to the DSMB and schedule of meetings is study dependent and based on the level of risk to the study participants. At a minimum,

TABLE 13.2

Example of operational definitions of key safety outcomes (excerpt from the POINT trial Adverse Event Case Report Form).

- **Symptomatic intracerebral hemorrhage:** Any extravascular blood in the brain parenchyma, judged to be nontraumatic, and not in the area of an acute/subacute ischemic infarct, associated with and identified as the predominant cause of new neurologic symptoms (including headache) or death. In the case of a mixed intracranial hemorrhage [Intracerebral Hemorrhage (ICH), Subarachnoid Hemorrhage (SAH, Subdural Hemorrhage (SDH), and/or Intraventricular Hemorrhage (IVH)], the event should be classified according to the primary site of hemorrhage by the judgment of the clinician. For example, if a patient has a large ICH with a small amount of SAH, and the ICH is felt to be the primary site of bleeding, this should be classified as ICH. Criteria: Evidence of hemorrhage in the brain parenchyma demonstrated by head imaging, surgery, or autopsy, which is not in the same territory of an underlying acute or subacute ischemic stroke, and is judged to be associated with any new neurologic symptoms (including headache) or leading to death.

- **Asymptomatic intracerebral hemorrhage:** An acute extravasation of blood into the brain parenchyma, judged to be nontraumatic, and not in an area of an acute/subacute ischemic infarct, without associated neurologic symptoms or leading to death. In the case of a mixed intracranial hemorrhage (ICH, SAH, SDH and/or IVH), the event should be classified according to the primary site of hemorrhage by the judgment of the clinician. For example, if a patient has a large ICH with a small amount of SAH, and the ICH is felt to be the primary site of bleeding, this should be classified as ICH. Criteria: evidence of hemorrhage in the brain parenchyma demonstrated by head imaging, surgery, or autopsy, which is not in the same territory of an underlying acute or subacute ischemic stroke, and is not judged to be associated with any new neurologic symptoms or leading to death.

- **Other symptomatic intracranial hemorrhage:** Any extravascular blood within the cranium judged to be nontraumatic, and the predominant cause of the clinical deterioration or that led to death. Other Intracranial Hemorrhage is defined as an acute extravasation of blood into the subarachnoid space, epidural space, subdural space or intraventricular space with associated symptoms (including headache). In the case of a mixed intracranial hemorrhage (ICH, SAH, SDH and/or IVH), the event should be classified according to the primary site of hemorrhage by the judgment of the clinician. For example, if a patient has a large ICH with a small amount of SAH, and the ICH is felt to be the primary site of bleeding, this should be classified as ICH. Criteria: Evidence of hemorrhage in the subarachnoid space, epidural space, or subdural space demonstrated by head imaging, surgery, or autopsy.

- **Other asymptomatic intracranial hemorrhage:** An acute extravasation of blood into the subarachnoid space, epidural space, subdural space or intraventricular space without associated symptoms, and judged to be nontraumatic. In the case of a mixed intracranial hemorrhage (ICH, SAH, SDH and/or IVH), the event should be classified according to the primary site of hemorrhage by the judgment of the clinician. For example, if a patient has a large ICH with a small amount of SAH, and the ICH is felt to be the primary site of bleeding, this should be classified as ICH. Criteria: Evidence of hemorrhage in the subarachnoid space, epidural space, or subdural space demonstrated by head imaging, surgery, or autopsy.

- **Major hemorrhage other than intracranial hemorrhage (life-threatening or non-life-threatening):** A hemorrhagic event, judged to be nontraumatic, that results in intraocular bleeding causing loss of vision, the need for a transfusion of two or more units of red cells or the equivalent amount of whole blood, or the need for hospitalization or prolongation of existing hospitalization. This may include bleeding events related to surgical procedures but not those related to accidental trauma. Life-threatening hemorrhagic events will be defined as those that are fatal or require use of intravenous inotropic medication to maintain blood pressure, interventional treatment (including surgical, endoscopic or endovascular interventions), or transfusion of four or more units of red cells or the equivalent amount of whole blood. Non-life-threatening hemorrhagic events will be defined as those classified as major hemorrhagic events but not as life-threatening.

- **Minor hemorrhage other than intracranial hemorrhage:** All hemorrhagic events leading to interruption or discontinuation of the study drug but not classifiable as major hemorrhagic events. This may include bleeding events related to surgical procedures but not those related to accidental trauma.

DSMBs should receive semiannual reports throughout trial enrollment corresponding with semiannual meetings of the committee.

13.3 Statistical Considerations

A well-designed trial should prespecify a formal plan for how safety data will be monitored during the trial. This is sometimes designated as a Safety Monitoring Plan or DSMB Monitoring Plan. This study document should clearly describe the details of interim safety monitoring including what data will be monitored, the timing and frequency of safety data reviews, and criteria that will guide early termination for safety. It should also include procedures for reporting serious adverse events to the DSMB/FDA/CIRB. The safety analysis population should include only those subjects who received the study intervention. Unlike the intent-to-treat analysis, crossovers should be analyzed according to the treatment received. The denominator should take into account not just the number of patients but also the time in which subjects were on the intervention (person-years or risk set).

Detection of harms, rather than "proving safety," is a better objective for trials in all phases. Some trials have prespecified adverse events of special interest that they want to closely monitor in addition to all adverse events. For these cases, the safety plan should include a section that defines the expected rates of these special events to provide a framework for the DSMB members.

13.3.1 Monitoring for Safety

Consider a trial with a treatment known to increase risk such as an antithrombotic drug for ischemic stroke. The mechanism of action of the drug may produce hemorrhage, but some increased risk of hemorrhage is acceptable if the drug is efficacious. The relevant question of interest is whether the increased risk is above an agreed-upon threshold. This threshold, typically the expected rate on the control arm, or perhaps a slightly higher acceptable rate, should be determined prior to the trial start. If the expected rate of major hemorrhage on the control arm was 5% and if the treatment rate was 10%, this would be considered a serious safety concern. How should this be monitored?

To test the hypothesis that the proportion of major hemorrhage in treatment group H_0: $p < 0.05$ versus H_A: $p > 0.05$, a one-sample chi-squared test with 0.05 one-sided significance level will have 80% power to reject the null hypothesis that the proportion of hemorrhage is 0.05 at the alternative proportion of 0.10 when the sample size is 150 in the treatment group. Clearly, we would want to identify the harm before 150 subjects were enrolled if there was a true safety concern.

Ongoing monitoring for safety should occur frequently. The timing should depend on the risk but could be monthly, quarterly, semiannually, enrollment driven (e.g., every 10 patients), or after every event. Early-phase and exploratory studies where risks may be more uncertain need more frequent monitoring.

For the above example, the DSMB could formally monitor the primary safety event every 30 patients (or monthly) by looking at the probability that the event of interest for the treatment group exceeds the expected control rate (5%). If, for a given arm, the probability that the event rate exceeds the expected rate is "too high," for example, greater than

TABLE 13.3

Monitoring of primary safety outcome using Bayesian posterior probability.

	Frequency of Event	N Enrolled	% Subjects	Probability That Event Rate Is >5%*
First DSMB Report				
Treatment Group A	1	15	7%	0.49
Treatment Group B	2	15	13%	0.82
Second DSMB Report				
Treatment Group A	2	30	7%	0.57
Treatment Group B	4	30	13%	0.93
Third DSMB Report				
Treatment Group A	2	45	4%	0.36
Treatment Group B	6	45	13%	0.97**

* Bayesian posterior probability assuming a weighted beta (0.05*W, 0.95*W) prior with W = 5 subjects.

** The (posterior) probability that the event rate is greater than 5% in group B is 97%. The DSMB may recommend terminating enrollment.

95%, then enrollment may be stopped or paused. The DSMB may review detailed patient profiles to determine whether there are additional clinical considerations.

Table 13.3 shows an example of this as presented at the first, second, and third DSMB meeting. We see that the event rate is 13% in group B each time, but by the third meeting, enough data has been accrued that there is 97% certainty that the true event rate is greater than the expected rate of 5%. This approach is similar to a one-sample frequentist test at 0.05 level (one-sided) but has a more direct interpretation, although the prior could affect this. In this example, we set the prior to be consistent with the expected rate of 5% by weighting this with only 5 subjects' worth of data to make it relatively noninformative. A lower weight, for example, 1 or 3 subjects' worth of data, may result in earlier detection of harm, whereas a higher weight would downplay early signals of harm.

13.3.2 Example of Formal Safety Stopping Rule

An example of monitoring for specific adverse events was in the SHINE trial.[16] The SHINE trial was designed to compare intensive glucose monitoring to standard sliding scale monitoring in ischemic stroke patients with high blood pressure at admission or known diagnosis of type II diabetes.[17] The primary efficacy outcome was a 90-day functional outcome measured by the modified Rankin scale. In addition to collecting all adverse events for the 90-day study period, the trial investigators wanted to closely monitor the intensive arm for severe hypoglycemia (<40 mg/dL) events during treatment as well as all-cause death within 90 days. Based on previous literature, the investigators expected zero severe hypoglycemia events in the standard arm and an expected rate of all-cause death in the standard arm of 14%. They did not want to see more than a 4% rate of severe hypoglycemia in the intensive arm (absolute risk difference of 4%) and wanted no difference (absolute risk difference of 0%) in all-cause mortality. Prior to study enrollment, the investigators shared this information with the DSMB in the Safety Monitoring Plan and concluded that stopping for harm would be considered by the DSMB if at any time the lower limit of a 95% confidence interval on the risk difference of the proportion of severe hypoglycemia events between the two treatment arms exceeded 4%, or if the lower limit of a 95% confidence interval on the unadjusted relative risk of all-cause death exceeded 1. Table 13.4 was

TABLE 13.4

Simulated number of events for stopping criteria.

	Severe Hypoglycemia Events			
N per Group	Total subjects with Event in Control Arm (%)	Total subjects with Event in Exp Arm (%)	Risk Difference (Δ)	Lower Limit of 95% Cl for Δ
50	0(0)	7(14)	14	4.4
50	1(2)	9(18)	16	4.7
100	0(0)	10(10)	10	4.1
100	2(2)	14(14)	12	4.7
200	0(0))	16(8)	8	4.2
200	4(2)	22(11)	9	4.2
500	0(0)	31(6.2)	6.2	4.1
500	10(2)	45(9)	7	4.2
700	0(0)	41(6)	6	4.1
700	14(2)	59(8.4)	6.4	4.1

provided in the Safety Plan with simulated scenarios of the number of events for this to occur during enrollment.

13.3.3 Powering for Safety Analyses

Most small trials are not designed to detect differences in safety outcomes between groups as the sample size needed to detect small differences is not feasible. Small- to medium-sized studies will likely be underpowered for head-to-head two-group comparisons of a primary safety outcome. Figure 13.1 A shows the minimum detectable difference at 80% power (one-sided alpha of 0.05) with n = 50 per group in a two-sample test of proportions. For example, if the expected event rate in the control is 5%, then there is 80% power to detect a difference if the true treatment event rate is 24%, an absolute increase of 19% or RR of nearly 5. It is hard to envision any scenario in which that much increase would be acceptable. Similarly, with a one-sample test (Figure 13.1 B) if the expected event rate in the control is 5%, then there is 80% power to detect a difference if the true treatment event rate is 20%, an absolute increase of 15% or RR of nearly 4.

13.3.4 Type I Error Rate for Safety Analyses

It is well known that multiple "looks" at the data will increase the likelihood of finding a statistically significant difference even if none exists. Yet in the setting of safety monitoring we are trying to quantify risks, so multiplicity is less of a concern. Thus, while inflation of the type I error rate should be a consideration, we do not want to be too conservative. For example, applying a uniform p value of 0.01 for all safety analyses may alleviate multiplicity concerns without strongly controlling the familywise error rate. Focusing on estimation rather than hypothesis testing can also be adopted and, as discussed above, may help us to identify harms for which we are underpowered.

For large trials group sequential or alpha-spending function approaches may be used to protect the type I error rate from repeated testing for an expected safety outcome. These can be useful for protecting the trial from stopping early based upon a "random high," particularly very early in the trial. Trials that stop early tend to have an exaggerated estimate

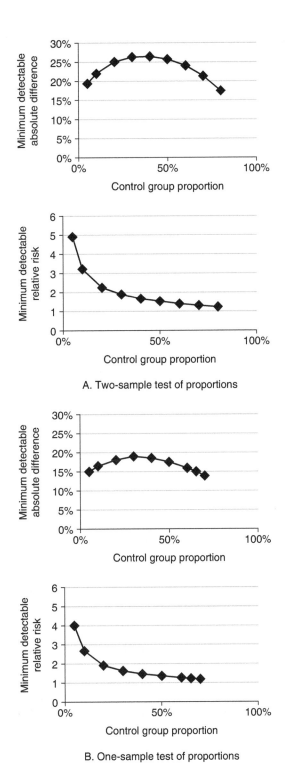

FIGURE 13.1
Minimum detectable difference for power = 80%, alpha = 0.05 1-sided, N = 50/group. A. Two-sample test of proportions. B. One-sample test of proportions.

of the true treatment effect. In this case, the error is that the trial would be stopped based on a safety difference that does not actually exist, presumably in the absence of an efficacy signal. While certainly the trial should be stopped if interim data suggest the trial poses an unreasonable risk to participants, safety monitoring requires a combination of statistical and clinical input.

13.4 Graphical Approaches to Presenting Safety Data

Graphical displays of adverse event data can be a useful alternative to extensive data listings when reporting safety data to the DSMB during a trial. These figures may make it easier to identify unexpected safety signals.

13.4.1 Volcano Plots and Forest Plots

Volcano plots are one way to graphically display adverse event data. Figure 13.2 illustrates an example of a volcano plot of adverse events classified into preferred terms using the MedDRA coding dictionary. Such a graphical display shows several important features of safety data simultaneously. The individual bubbles represent classified adverse events, the bubble size indicates the total number of events occurring in the trial, the x-axis indicates the difference in proportion of events between treatment arms (risk difference), and the y-axis indicates the unadjusted p-value (on the $-\log_{10}$ scale) from the comparison of the difference in proportions of the specific adverse event between the two treatment arms. The $-\log_{10}$ scale is used in order to create a more readable graphic that avoids adverse events with extreme differences between treatment arms being crowded in one location of the graph. A y-axis value of 1 is equivalent to a p value of 0.10. As the bubbles rise on the y-axis, this indicates smaller p values and more extreme differences between treatment arms for the relevant event. There can be variations made to this plot, including plotting the risk or odds ratio on the x-axis, adjusting the p values for multiplicity, and plotting the raw p value on the y-axis in a reversed order of largest to smallest. Programming code is available in SAS, R, and Stata to produce volcano plots.[18,19]

   An alternative to the volcano plot for displaying safety data is the forest plot. This type of graphic is commonly used for the presentation of metaanalyses where the results from individual trials with the same or common clinical endpoint are displayed. Figure 13.3 below illustrates the use of the forest plot to display safety data. The x-axis displays the risk difference and 95% confidence interval for each MedDRA-classified adverse event on the y-axis. The odds ratio, hazard ratio, or relative risk can be substituted for the risk difference on the x-axis. This visual of safety data provides a simplified view of safety events that may be occurring more in one treatment arm than the other and provides an easy way to identify statistically significant potential signals of harm when the confidence interval excludes the vertical reference line (0 in the case of the risk difference).

13.4.2 Heat Maps

Some safety data is measured quantitatively, but summarizing it ordinally may be better for detecting safety concerns. For quantitative measures like laboratory values, vital signs, and ECGs, safety monitoring should focus on examination of extreme observations rather

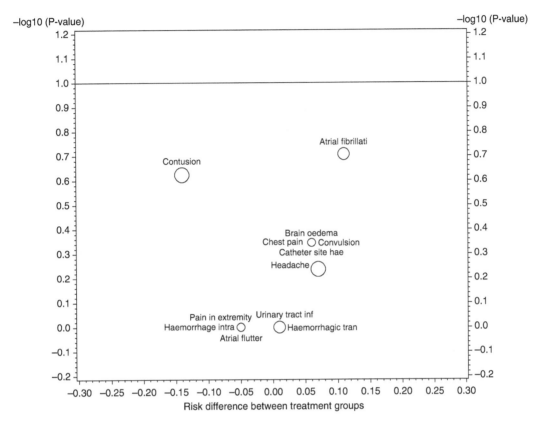

FIGURE 13.2
Volcano plot example.

than group means. Some studies will use a central laboratory which provide normal/low/high reference limits and alert values. In the absence of standardized reference ranges, sample quantiles (5th, 95th) or a clinically defined benchmark may be used. By converting the quantitative data to categorical variables by using the centralized definitions of "low," "normal," "high," and "high alert," shift tables or heat maps can be used to track changes from baseline. A heat map is an easy way to monitor longitudinal, ordinal data, without summarizing the data.

The NET-PD LS-1 trial randomized patients to creatine versus placebo; thus an increase in laboratory creatinine levels was expected. In the NET-PD LS-1 trial[20] a box and whisker plot of creatinine reveals a small increase in group means, but outliers are hard to distinguish (Figure 13.4A). In contrast, by graphing the categorical data as a heat map, it becomes sharply obvious that most patients in the creatine-treated group experience increases in creatinine at the first visit (Figure 13.4B).

13.4.3 Individual Patient-Level Profiles

To protect the blind in the NET-PD LS-1 trial, the central laboratory did not return an enrolled subject's creatinine result back to the site investigator unless the subject's level was greater than an alert value. The protocol defined a subject-level "stopping rule" such that if a subject's creatinine was greater than 2, then the site investigator would be notified.

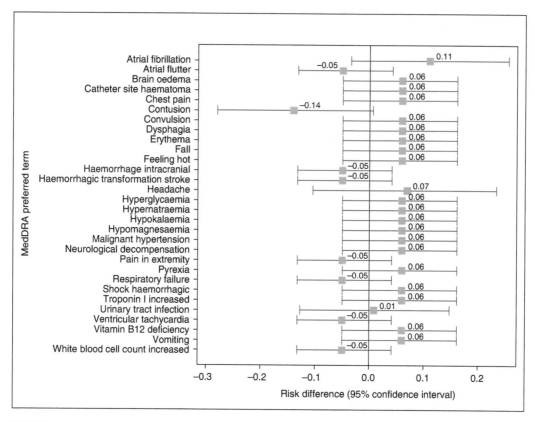

FIGURE 13.3
Forest plot example.

If this occurred, the subject must stop taking study drug but would continue to be followed up. Early in the course of the trial, there were a small number of subjects (7 out of 500) who experienced alert values, all of which occurred in the same treatment group.

Anticipated or expected adverse events are things that can be planned, but how should unexpected adverse events be monitored? A sentinel event should trigger enhanced monitoring activity. The importance of unexpected events depends on the frequency and severity of the risk relative to the potential benefit.

In the NET-PD LS-1 trial, the early safety data triggered a series of additional safety monitoring activities including the addition of a nephrologist to the DSMB, additional subject level stopping criteria (e.g., doubling from baseline), unscheduled collection of labs, monitoring within gender and age groups, and weighing the potential risk of elevated creatinine levels preventing the ability to diagnose true renal problems. Figure 13.5 gives an example of a patient profile that was provided to the DSMB for any subject who experienced a creatinine alert value.

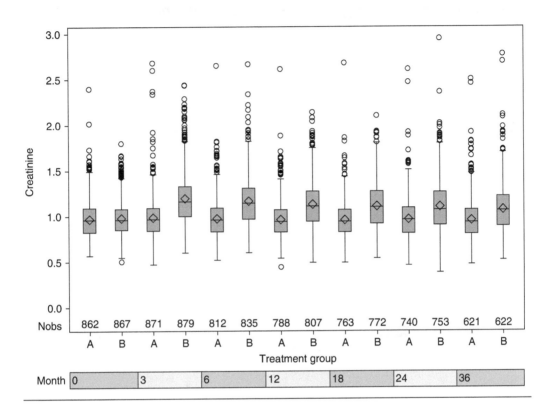

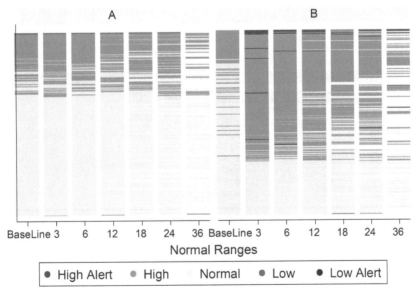

FIGURE 13.4
A and B. Box and Whisker plot versus Heat Map of Creatinine Labs in the LS-1 trial.

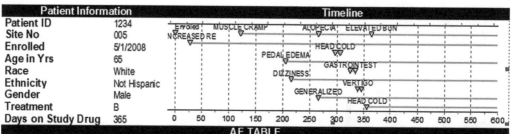

AE Term	Days from Enrollment to AE Start	Days from Enrollment to AE Stop	Severity	Related to Study	SAE
RESTLESS LEG	33		Mild	Probably Not	No
MUSCLE CRAMPS	131		Moderate	Probably Not	No
PEDAL EDEMA	210		Mild	Probably Not	No
DIZZINESS	220		Mild	Probably Not	No
ACHES	269		Mild	Probably Not	No
ALOPECIA	268		Mild	Probably Not	No
HEAD COLD	302	311	Mild	Definitely Not	No
VIRUS	329	338	Mild	Definitely Not	No
VERTIGO	342	349	Moderate	Probably Not	No
ELEVATED BUN	365		Mild	Probably Not	No

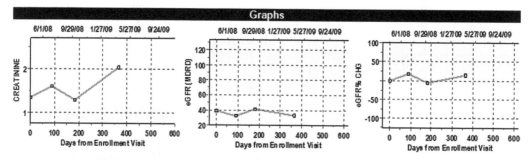

Shaded portion of graphs reflects normal range.

Lab Test	Days from Enroll	Lab Result
BILIRUBIN (URINE)	0	Negative
BILIRUBIN (URINE)	89	Negative
BILIRUBIN (URINE)	182	Negative
GLUCOSURIA	0	Negative
GLUCOSURIA	89	Negative
GLUCOSURIA	182	Negative
HEMATURIA	0	Negative
HEMATURIA	89	Negative
HEMATURIA	182	Negative
KETONURIA	0	Negative
KETONURIA	89	Negative
KETONURIA	182	Negative

FIGURE 13.5

Example of patient profile (release 2.0 Statistical Solutions www.statsol.ie).

13.5 Summary

The detection of safety concerns and decisions around them are a continual part of all phases of clinical trials and require careful planning and monitoring. In summary, it is important to know what is expected with the experimental intervention, to know what is anticipated from the disease, to prespecify safety events of special interest, and to consider the intervention's risk versus benefit. We can improve detection of safety events by being consistent with data collection such as by reporting diagnoses rather than signs and symptoms and by using a medical coding dictionary. Adverse event tables should group closely related events, and where possible we should use composites for key safety events in order to increase power. We should be reasonable if adjusting for multiple comparisons so as not to miss detecting a safety concern. In general, stopping rules should be used as guidelines rather than mandatory. The final decision to stop a trial should be based on a combination of clinical and statistical considerations. Unexpected serious adverse events that are potentially related to the intervention should prompt increased monitoring of similar events by the DSMB. We have shown several examples in which unexpected events resulted in a change in monitoring activities or the study protocol.

References

1   Wheeler GM, Mander AP, Bedding A, et al. How to design a dose-finding study using the continual reassessment method. *BMC Med Res Methodol*. 2019; 19:18. https://doi.org/10.1186/s12874-018-0638-z

2   Selim M, Yeatts S, Goldstein JN, Gomes J, Greenberg S, Morgenstern LB, Schlaug G, Torbey M, Waldman B, Xi G, Palesch Y; Deferoxamine mesylate in intracerebral hemorrhage investigators. Safety and tolerability of deferoxamine mesylate in patients with acute intracerebral hemorrhage. *Stroke*. 2011 Nov; 42(11): 3067–74. doi: 10.1161/STROKEAHA.111.617589. Epub 2011 Aug 25. PMID: 21868742; PMCID: PMC3202043.

3   Yeatts SD, Palesch YY, Moy CS, Selim M. High dose deferoxamine in intracerebral hemorrhage (HI-DEF) trial: rationale, design, and methods. *Neurocrit Care*. 2013 Oct; 19(2): 257–66. doi: 10.1007/s12028-013-9861-y. PMID: 23943316; PMCID: PMC3932442.

4   Selim M, Foster LD, Moy CS, Xi G, Hill MD, Morgenstern LB, Greenberg SM, James ML, Singh V, Clark WM, Norton C, Palesch YY, Yeatts SD; i-DEF Investigators. Deferoxamine mesylate in patients with intracerebral haemorrhage (i-DEF): a multicentre, randomised, placebo-controlled, double-blind phase 2 trial. *Lancet Neurol*. 2019 May; 18(5): 428–38. doi: 10.1016/S1474-4422(19)30069-9. Epub 2019 Mar 18. PMID: 30898550; PMCID: PMC6494117.

5   Ginsberg MD, Hill MD, Palesch YY, Ryckborst KJ, Tamariz D. The ALIAS Pilot Trial: a dose-escalation and safety study of albumin therapy for acute ischemic stroke—I: Physiological responses and safety results. *Stroke*. 2006; 37(8): 2100–6. Epub 2006/07/01. doi: 10.1161/01.STR.0000231388.72646.05 PMID: 16809571

6   Ginsberg MD, Palesch YY, Martin RH, Hill MD, Moy CS, Waldman BD, et al. The albumin in acute stroke (ALIAS) multicenter clinical trial: safety analysis of part 1 and rationale and design of part 2. *Stroke*. 2011; 42(1): 119–27. doi: 10.1161/STROKEAHA.110.596072 PMID: 21164127; PubMed Central PMCID: PMC3076742

7   Johnston SC, Easton JD, Farrant M, Barsan W, Conwit RA, Elm JJ, Kim AS, Lindblad AS, Palesch YY; Clinical Research Collaboration, Neurological Emergencies Treatment Trials Network, and the POINT Investigators. Clopidogrel and aspirin in acute ischemic stroke and high-risk TIA. *N Engl J Med*. 2018 Jul 19; 379(3): 215–25. doi: 10.1056/NEJMoa1800410. Epub 2018 May 16. PMID: 29766750; PMCID: PMC6193486.

8   Palma JA, Martinez J, Millar Vernetti P, Ma T, Perez MA, Zhong J, Qian Y, Dutta S, Maina KN, Siddique I, Bitan G, Ades-Aron B, Shepherd TM, Kang UJ, Kaufmann H. mTOR inhibition with sirolimus in multiple system atrophy: a randomized, double-blind, placebo-controlled futility trial and 1-year biomarker longitudinal analysis. *Mov Disord*. 2022 Apr; 37(4): 778–89. doi: 10.1002/mds.28923. Epub 2022 Jan 18. PMID: 35040506; PMCID: PMC9018525.

9   NINDS Exploratory Trials in Parkinson Disease (NET-PD) FS-ZONE Investigators. Pioglitazone in early Parkinson's disease: a phase 2, multicentre, double-blind, randomised trial. *Lancet Neurol*. 2015 Aug; 14(8): 795–803. doi: 10.1016/S1474-4422(15)00144-1. Epub 2015 Jun 23. Erratum in: *Lancet Neurol*. 2015 Oct; 14(10): 979. PMID: 26116315; PMCID: PMC4574625.

10 Simuni T, Fiske B, Merchant K, Coffey CS, Klingner E, Caspell-Garcia C, Lafontant DE, Matthews H, Wyse RK, Brundin P, Simon DK, Schwarzschild M, Weiner D, Adams J, Venuto C, Dawson TM, Baker L, Kostrzebski M, Ward T, Rafaloff G; Parkinson Study Group NILO-PD Investigators and Collaborators. Efficacy of nilotinib in patients with moderately advanced Parkinson disease: a randomized clinical trial. *JAMA Neurol*. 2021 Mar 1; 78(3): 312–20. doi: 10.1001/jamaneurol.2020.4725. Erratum in: JAMA Neurol. 2021 Apr 1;78(4):497. PMID: 33315105; PMCID: PMC7737147.

11 Wittes J, Crowe B, Chuang-Stein C, Guettner A, Hall D, Jiang Q, Odenheimer D, Xia HA, Kramer J. The FDA's final rule on expedited safety reporting: statistical considerations. *Stat Biopharm Res*. 2015 Jul 3; 7(3): 174–90. doi: 10.1080/19466315.2015.1043395. Epub 2015 Oct 9. PMID: 26550466; PMCID: PMC4606817.

12 Crowe B, Brueckner A, Beasley C, Kulkarni P. Current practices, challenges, and statistical issues with product safety labeling. *Stat Biopharm Res*. 2013;5(3):180–93. doi: 10.1080/19466315.2013.791640

13 Farrant M, Easton JD, Adelman EE, Cucchiara BL, Barsan WG, Tillman HJ, Elm JJ, Kim AS, Lindblad AS, Palesch YY, Zhao W, Pauls K, Walsh KB, Martí-Fàbregas J, Bernstein RA, Johnston SC. Assessment of the end point adjudication process on the results of the platelet-oriented inhibition in new TIA and Minor Ischemic Stroke (POINT) Trial: a secondary analysis. *JAMA Netw Open*. 2019 Sep 4; 2(9): e1910769. doi: 10.1001/jamanetworkopen.2019.10769. PMID: 31490536; PMCID: PMC6735409.

14 Johnston SC, Easton JD, Farrant M, Barsan W, Battenhouse H, Conwit R, Dillon C, Elm J, Lindblad A, Morgenstern L, Poisson SN, Palesch Y. Platelet-oriented inhibition in new TIA and minor ischemic stroke (POINT) trial: rationale and design. *Int J Stroke*. 2013 Aug; 8(6): 479–83. doi: 10.1111/ijs.12129. PMID: 23879752; PMCID: PMC4412261.

15 Code of Federal Regulations Title 21 21 CFR 312.32 www.ecfr.gov/current/title-21/chapter-I/subchapter-D/part-312/subpart-B/section-312.32

16 Johnston KC, Bruno A, Pauls Q, et al. Intensive vs standard treatment of hyperglycemia and functional outcome in patients with acute ischemic stroke: the SHINE randomized clinical trial. *JAMA*. 2019; 322(4): 326–35. doi:10.1001/jama.2019.9346

17 Bruno A, Durkalski VL, Hall CE, et al.; SHINE Investigators. The Stroke Hyperglycemia Insulin Network Effort (SHINE) trial protocol: a randomized, blinded, efficacy trial of standard vs intensive hyperglycemia management in acute stroke. *Int J Stroke*. 2014;9(2):246–51. doi:10.1111/ijs.12045

18 Mehrotra DV, Adewale AJ. Flagging clinical adverse experiences: Reducing false discoveries without materially compromising power for detecting true signals. *Stat Med*. 2012; 31:1918–30.

19 Zink RC, Wolfinger RD, Mann G. Summarizing the incidence of adverse events using volcano plots and time intervals. *Clinical Trials* 2013;10:398–406.

20 Writing Group for the NINDS Exploratory Trials in Parkinson Disease (NET-PD) Investigators, Kieburtz K, Tilley BC, Elm JJ, Babcock D, Hauser R, Ross GW, Augustine AH, Augustine EU, Aminoff MJ, Bodis-Wollner IG, Boyd J, Cambi F, Chou K, Christine CW, Cines M, Dahodwala N, Derwent L, Dewey RB Jr, Hawthorne K, Houghton DJ, Kamp C, Leehey M, Lew MF, Liang GS, Luo ST, Mari Z, Morgan JC, Parashos S, Pérez A, Petrovitch H, Rajan S, Reichwein S, Roth JT, Schneider JS, Shannon KM, Simon DK, Simuni T, Singer C, Sudarsky L, Tanner CM, Umeh CC, Williams K, Wills AM. Effect of creatine monohydrate on clinical progression in patients with Parkinson disease: a randomized clinical trial. *JAMA*. 2015 Feb 10;313(6):584–93. doi: 10.1001/jama.2015.120. PMID: 25668262; PMCID: PMC4349346.

14

Bayesian Dynamic Borrowing and Regulatory Considerations

George Chu and Hengrui Sun

13.1 Overview of Bayesian Dynamic Borrowing

Along with the recent rapid surge in real-world data (RWD) sources such as disease/medical product registries, electronic health records (EHRs), claims data, etc., and more accessible historical study datasets, there is an increasing interest and need from investigators and regulatory agencies to leverage all available information to accelerate the development and regulatory decision making for new medical therapies. Due to its flexibility in calibrating uncertainty and handling data heterogeneity and its inherent updating process over time being ideal for synthesizing evidence from multiple data sources, Bayesian inference has regained a huge interest to meet such demand, which is based on a posterior probability distribution for the parameter of interest (e.g., treatment effect) by combining (via Bayes' theorem) a prior probability distribution for the parameter and the observed current data (likelihood function). As compared to the frequentist approach, where the statistical inference is only from the current study, Bayesian inference is basically a weighted average of prior and current, and thus could be heavily influenced by the prior, raising the concern about bias and Type I error rate inflation under confirmatory trial settings when the prior and current study data may not be entirely similar. To address such concern with a more limited borrowing to reduce the chance of overinfluence from the prior, Bayesian dynamic borrowing (BDB) is a statistical approach to account for the inconsistency between the prior datasets and current study by learning how much information to be borrowed. The smaller the drift, the more to be borrowed. The larger the drift, the less to be borrowed, with the Bayesian inference being more dependent on the current study (closer to frequentist inference). In other words, BDB methods, e.g., Bayesian hierarchical modeling and dynamic power prior, allow the incorporation of external data sources (historical clinical trials, RWD) as prior information (i.e., borrow) to support statistical inference from a current clinical trial with the degree of borrowing to be determined based on the similarity between the current and external studies.

Although there are challenges associated with its implementation, such as the selection of appropriate external datasets, data heterogeneity, and prior-current data conflict, clinical trialists and biostatisticians have started to feel more interested and comfortable in the application of BDB methodologies in recent years. This is especially true in the disease areas and medical device areas where there is a high unmet clinical need and a practical difficulty to execute an adequately powered large-scale study, e.g., rare diseases and treating chronic heart failure with preserved ejection fraction (HFpEF) patients using medical devices, due to the regulatory openness for its potential to minimize patient burden, improve study efficiency for the confirmatory trials. The United States Food and Drug Administration (FDA) has recognized the value of Bayesian statistics in medical device trials and issued guidance for their use [1]. Experience with reviewing Bayesian medical device trials has also been documented [2–6].

The concept of such data dynamic borrowing has been around for several decades, with seminal works by Pocock [7] who first proposed a Bayesian method to combine historical control data with data from the control group in a new randomized clinical trial. The proposed method assumed a random variable with zero mean and a specified variance to account for a potential bias in the historical, i.e., the larger the variance, the larger degree of mistrust in the historical control and thus the smaller degree of borrowing. Since Ibrahim and Chen [8] proposed their landmark idea of power prior, various approaches have been proposed for dynamic borrowing in the literature over the last two decades, such as the modified power prior [9, 10], the commensurate prior [11], and the adaptive power prior using empirical Bayesian [12]. Schmidli et al. [13] proposed robust metapredictive priors as an extension of the metaanalytic predictive (MAP) prior [14], where the MAP prior is mixed with a vague distribution, to account for the possibility of shift between historical and current data. For the relationship between some of these dynamic borrowing methods, please refer to Ibrahim and Chen [8], Viele et al. [15], van Rosmalen et al. [16], and Neuenschwander and Schmidli [17].

The above approaches can be used in the context of one or more historical studies. Depending on the number of available historical studies, some alternative methods are proposed. In the situation with one prior dataset, Thompson et al. [18] proposed an adaptive method for dynamic borrowing using a conditional power prior. Instead of using the full set of current data in the final posterior (as done by Haddad et al. [19]), an interim analysis is used to reassess and downgrade the degree of borrowing from the initial prespecified maximum. The final power parameter is to be based on the similarity between a percentage of the current study outcome data available at an interim look and the prior data via the Bayesian posterior probability of outcome similarity within a prespecified clinically appropriate equivalence margin. In addition, the borrowing from the prior only occurs when the difference in sample means between the prior and current data (interim) set is within the similarity margin. Because of this stipulation, similarity is measured not only with respect to the posterior distribution but also with respect to the observed point estimates. When there exist multiple studies (external data sources), Bayesian hierarchical modeling can also be used to combine results to derive MAP as a combined prior "borrowing strength" from multiple external studies. Typically based on the subject level and study level, such multilevel Bayesian model can account for various degrees of between-trial heterogeneity, thus adaptively discounting the external information in proportion to the degree of data conflict. Briefly, patient outcomes within each study are generated from a population with distribution specified by some study-specific parameters, and the study-specific parameters are generated from a common superpopulation that is governed by some hyperparameters whose distribution is further defined by a hyperprior. Through such a multilevel hierarchical structure, the posterior distribution of the parameter of interest can then be derived either using an analytical approach or numerical methods such as Markov chain Monte Carlo (MCMC). It is important to assess the underlying exchangeability assumption at both patient level within each study and study level across the different studies from clinical and engineering perspectives. Note that studies could be conditionally exchangeable when accounting for some difference in observed covariables.

Recent publications have continued to explore the use of Bayesian dynamic borrowing in clinical trial design. One area of focus has been on incorporating propensity scores (PSs) into the borrowing process (for a good literature review on this, please refer to [20] and the External Evidence Methods (EEM) Framework by Medical Device Innovation Consortium (MDIC) [21]). Wang et al. [22] prespecified a maximum for the study-level power parameter (α_{max}) to accommodate a certain level of Type I error rate control with the power parameter of patients in each PS stratum (α_0) being adjusted based on similarity between prior data and current data in terms of baseline covariates. Note that the adjustment of α_0 happens among strata while α_{max} is still used at the study level. This approach may have the following limitations: it usually requires a large sample size of the prior data; patient-level baseline covariates of the prior data may not be adequate or accessible; and similarity of measured baselines may not well ensure a similarity of outcomes. Therefore, since α_{max} is used at the study level, a mild adjustment of α_0 among strata may not fully address the concern of overinfluence from the prior data. As a further improvement to allow for the reduction in the prior effective sample size, Liu et al. [23] proposed the approach to integrate the PS method and Bayesian metaanalytic-predictive (MAP) prior in which PS is applied to select a subset of patients from external data that are similar to those in the current study with regard to key baseline covariates and to stratify the selected patients together with those in the current study into more homogeneous strata.

In summary, Bayesian dynamic borrowing is a powerful tool for incorporating external data into clinical trials and has gained significant traction in the biopharmaceutical industry as well. The development of Bayesian models and guidance from regulatory agencies have facilitated the use of this approach, but careful consideration of the appropriateness and degree of borrowing is critical to ensure the validity of the results. One key issue with any external data borrowing is how to determine the appropriate degree of borrowing while ensuring that any potential bias and Type I error rate inflation will be controlled at an acceptable level. This requires careful consideration of study design, endpoints, patient populations, and other factors that may affect the comparability of the data sources. BDB provides a flexible framework for adjusting the borrowing amount based on these factors determining the similarity between external studies and the current study and linking this similarity measurement to the appropriate amount of borrowing. Sensitivity analyses can also be used to assess the robustness of the results.

Benefits:

1. Improved trial conduct: BDB can improve trial conduct by reducing the need for large sample sizes, shortening trial duration, and reducing costs. This is particularly useful when dealing with small sample sizes or rare diseases, where traditional large-scale RCT cannot be feasible.
2. More efficient use of all available data: BDB potentially allows for the integration of multiple data sources and thus provides improvement in the efficiency of treatment effect estimation when compared to the smaller sample size without any borrowing.
3. More flexible trial design: BDB allows for more flexible trial design, enabling the use of multiple sources of information to guide trial design and decision-making.

Limitations:

1. Complexity: Bayesian dynamic borrowing can be complex and challenging to implement. For example, the required extensive simulations at the study design stage to assess frequentist operation characteristics (power, Type I error rate and

bias) may make it more burdensome for regulatory agencies to evaluate trials at the design stage that use dynamic borrowing.

2. Potential for bias: Dynamic borrowing relies on assumptions about the similarity of historical and current data sources, and these assumptions may not always hold. This could lead to biased estimates of treatment effect if the historical data is not representative of the current population.

3. Availability of data: Dynamic borrowing relies on the availability of high-quality historical data and other relevant sources of information, which may not always be available or reliable. In some cases, historical data may be incomplete or biased, which could impact the validity of the borrowing approach.

4. Interpretability: Bayesian dynamic borrowing may result in complex models that tend to be difficult to interpret and communicate to stakeholders, including regulators, patients, and healthcare providers. This can create challenges in explaining the results of clinical trials and gaining buy-in from key stakeholders.

13.2 Case Studies of Applying Bayesian Dynamic Borrowing in the Regulatory Setting

13.2.1 Medical Device Area That Led to Regulatory Approval

The FDA/CDRH has recognized the potential of Bayesian methods for borrowing information and has encouraged the use of such methods including BDB in medical device trial design and analysis.

Several recent FDA approvals of medical devices have included the use of Bayesian dynamic borrowing as briefly summarized in the EEM Framework by MDIC.

13.2.1.1 Case 1 Using Bayesian Hierarchical Model to Augment Investigational Arm

Cyberonics (LivaNova) VNS Therapy System (P970003/S207) [24] was originally approved for the indication of an adjunctive therapy in reducing the frequency of seizures in adults and adolescents older than 12 years of age with partial-onset seizures that are refractory to antiepileptic medications. In order to obtain an expanded indication to include younger patients of 4–11 years old, a Japanese postapproval study (PAS) was used as the main evidence from which only 30 patients aged 4–11 were available. To augment this small amount of evidence for a reasonable assurance of safety and effectiveness, four premarket clinical studies and the company's Post-Market Surveillance Database served as external information to be leveraged upon. For the primary effectiveness endpoint, a Bayesian hierarchical model was fit to the study-specific 12-month responder rates accounting for age group (4–11 vs. 12+ years). The model allowed the Japanese PAS rate in the 4–11 age group to borrow from all data from all the other studies.

13.2.1.2 Case 2 Using Bayesian Hierarchical Model (to Augment Both Investigational and Control Arms)

Orsiro Sirolimus Eluting Coronary Stent is indicated for improving coronary luminal diameter in patients, including those with diabetes mellitus, symptomatic heart disease, stable angina, unstable angina, non-ST elevation myocardial infarction, or documented silent ischemia due to atherosclerotic lesions in the native coronary arteries (P170030) [25]. Prior to seeking FDA approval, the device system was market-released outside the United States (OUS) since 2011, with more than 1.5 million units sold worldwide through the end of 2018. To establish a reasonable assurance of safety and effectiveness, the sponsor conducted a prospective, international, multicenter, randomized controlled noninferiority trial (RCT: BIOFLOW-V) with another drug-eluting stent as the active control (Xience DES). The primary endpoint is the rate of 12-month target lesion failure (TLF) and was analyzed by employing a Bayesian hierarchical approach in a prospective manner using two historical RCT studies (BIOFLOW-II and BIOFLOW-IV) with the same treatment interventions as BIOFLOW-V. The Bayesian dynamic borrowing to formally incorporate the external historical data used binomial analysis for the presence of a TLF event and a Bayesian model that allowed for bias between the TLF event rates of the BIOFLOW-II and BIOFLOW-IV trials and the TLF event rates of the BIOFLOW-V trial in both the Orsiro and Xience groups.

13.2.2 Drug Development Area That Led to Regulatory Approval or Supported Regulatory Decision-making

We performed an extensive search on currently available drug labels to see if the Bayesian method was applied as the primary analysis that led to the regulatory approvals or played a supportive role in the process of regulatory decision-making and found its use has been rare. Below are several case examples.

13.2.2.1 Case 3 for Preventive Medicine/Vaccine

REBYOTA® was approved by the FDA in 2022, with Bayesian analysis being applied as the primary analysis method. This biologics is a fecal microbiota suspension derived from qualified donor human stool and is indicated for the prevention of recurrence of *Clostridioides difficile* infection (CDI) in adults, following antibiotic treatment for recurrent CDI [26]. Due to enrollment challenges, a single double-blind, randomized, placebo-controlled Phase 3 trial was conducted. The primary efficacy analysis formally integrated information from a double-blind, randomized, placebo-controlled Phase 2 study using a Bayesian hierarchical model. The posterior probability that REBYOTA® was superior to placebo for preventing CDI diarrhea for 8 weeks was 99.1% [26]. The FDA agreed that the two studies were generally exchangeable, and the approach based on Bayesian hierarchical model was acceptable [27]. In addition, other considerations such as seriousness of the disease, unmet medical need, challenges of enrolling placebo-controlled trials for this population, and the supportive results from other nonrandomized trials of REBYOTA® contributed to the decision that REBYOTA® demonstrated substantial evidence of effectiveness [27].

Additionally, the issuance of Emergency Use Authorization (EUA) for the first COVID-19 vaccine, COMIRNATY®, was based on a simple Bayesian approach for the primary efficacy analysis, which showed a vaccine efficacy of 95% with the 95% credible interval being 90.3% to 97.6% [28]. This information was mentioned in the FDA review package for regular approval [29], as well as COMIRNATY® labeling [30].

13.2.2.2 Case 4 for Therapeutic Drug

A post hoc Bayesian dynamic borrowing analysis played a supportive role in the process of regulatory drug approval in the pediatric population. BENLYSTA® (belimumab) was approved for adult patients with active, seropositive lupus erythematosus (SLE) in 2011 [31]. A pediatric ostmarketing study was required under PREA (Pediatric Research Equity Act), which was a randomized, double-blind, placebo-controlled trial that enrolled 93 pediatric subjects 5–17 years of age with active systemic SLE. Due to the rarity of the disease in children, a fully powered study was not feasible. The efficacy was planned to be determined based on pharmacokinetic (PK) and efficacy results from the study based on descriptive analyses. The observed odds ratio (compared to the control group) for the primary endpoint of week 52 response rate of the SLE response index in this pediatric study was 1.5, with a 95% confidence interval of 0.6–3.5 [32].

Since the course of the disease and response to the treatment are believed to be similar between the adults and pediatric patients, a post-hoc Bayesian analysis was requested by FDA to analyze the pediatric data that borrowed information from the completed adult studies. A weighted combination of a skeptical prior and adult treatment effect estimate distribution was used as the prior of pediatric study, with weights on the adult data ranging from 0 to 1 in increments of 0.05. It was reported that a weight of 0.55 and above could achieve at least 97.5% posterior probability for the pediatric study. The FDA review team then evaluated this weight range and deemed it reasonable to support the conclusion of the positive treatment effect of BENLYSTA on pediatric patients [32]. The BENLYSTA® example resembles a reverse process compared to the Bayesian dynamic borrowing approach, where similarities between prior and subsequent data are evaluated and weights are normally determined *a priori*. However, this case shows that, when appropriate, results from Bayesian dynamic borrowing approaches could also facilitate regulatory decision-making as supportive evidence.

13.3 Regulatory Considerations on Bayesian Approaches for Decision-making

13.3.1 Areas or Potential Areas of Application

For medical devices, the first Bayesian approval dates back to April 1999, where a Bayesian multinomial logistic hierarchical model was used to borrow information from two other studies for the evaluation of efficacy of the TransScan T-2000 Multi-frequency Impedance Breast Scanner [33]. In the year 2010, FDA issued a guidance to discuss important statistical issues in Bayesian clinical trials for medical devices [1]. Over the years, many medical devices with Bayesian designs have been approved by the FDA.

For confirmatory drug trials, in addition to the case examples previously introduced, the Bayesian dynamic borrowing approach could potentially be formally planned for pediatric extrapolation, which is an approach to providing evidence in support of effective and safe use of drugs in the pediatric population when the course of the disease and the expected response to the drug is sufficiently similar in the pediatric and adult population [34]. This ensures the protection of the vulnerable pediatric population in that children only participate in clinical trials when necessary and clinical benefit is expected. With pediatric extrapolation, it is hoped that the drug development for children can be expedited and fewer children be exposed to investigational drugs when possible. Therefore, when the adult data are relevant and available, borrowing information from adult trials using a Bayesian approach could be reasonable [34].

Another potential area of application could be for rare disease, which is defined as affecting fewer than 200,000 people in the United States. However, many rare diseases affect far fewer people. Thus, some of the major challenges with rare disease clinical trials are limited sample size and lack of a randomized concurrent control arm. When it is impractical or unethical to enroll adequate number of patients in the randomized control arm, a well-designed and conducted natural history study may provide an external control group for investigational trials [35]. For this situation, Bayesian methods that examine the consistency between the randomized control and external control may be of particular interest. In addition, when treatment effect of the investigational drug from past clinical trial(s) is relevant to the current trial, borrowing information from prior study(ies) using Bayesian approaches could effectively reduce the required sample size at the design stage.

13.3.2 Considerations of Data Borrowing

Rationale for using external data: There are many challenges associated with borrowing information from external studies, for example, the comparability of patient population, the similarity of treatment guidelines over time, the consistency of outcome assessment, etc. Therefore, the fundamental question here is whether it is reasonable to borrow external information. For pediatric extrapolation, it is required that the course of disease and expected response to the treatment are sufficiently similar between the adult and pediatric patient populations [34]. For rare disease, when the disease is serious and there is an unmet medical need, interest in using an external historical control is frequently raised. However, in many situations, the likelihood of credibly demonstrating the effectiveness of a drug with external control is low, and thus a more suitable design should be chosen regardless of the prevalence of disease [36]. Only when conducting a concurrently controlled trial is impractical or unethical and the conditions for the acceptability of external control are met [7] can an external control be considered [35].

Borrowing strength determination: Once we decide that using external data is reasonable and feasible, the next step is to determine how much to borrow. One of the advantages of Bayesian dynamic borrowing is to examine the compatibility between the reference and target data so that more data borrowing will occur if the compatibility is high and less or no borrowing will occur if the compatibility is low. More details can be found in Section 1.

Additionally, depending on the aspects of the data to be examined for compatibility, the borrowing strength is normally determined through the following two directions. One direction is to evaluate the consistency of the outcomes between the reference and target studies, and priors will be constructed so that the degree of prior data discounting represents the degree of inconsistency. The other direction is to assess the similarity of subject baseline characteristics between the reference and target studies using propensity scoring approaches, and then the propensity score–based priors will be incorporated into the Bayesian dynamic borrowing framework to determine the degree of borrowing [20, 22, 23, 37].

The decision of which direction should be chosen needs to be based on the individual trial property. For example, in the case of pediatric extrapolation, because a lot of baseline characteristics of children are expected to be different from adults, outcome-based priors may be of more interest; however, sometimes there exist known differences in the disease severity that can be predicted by baseline covariates, and so the propensity score–based priors may have advantages in establishing population comparability through the collected baseline characteristics. Nonetheless, the two directions are not necessarily totally separate from each other. For example, at the study design stage, the maximum borrowing can be driven by propensity scores as an initial step, and then to address remaining confounding from unobserved confounders not captured in the initial step, outcome-based further-downward tuning via Bayesian dynamic borrowing can be followed.

Simulations: For Bayesian designs and analyses, analytical derived properties may not be feasible and as such, simulations are necessary to determine trial operating characteristics. The key operating characteristics for clinical trials at the design stage include Type I error rate, power, bias, and mean squared error. These design properties are important as they can help us to understand how results will be impacted by applying various data-borrowing approaches. Also, simulations should be based on various scenarios that cover adequate breadth of varying baseline characteristics, model assumptions, parametric versus nonparametric models, proportions of missing data, and possibly more depending on the specific case [38, 39].

Communicating the magnitude of borrowing: It is important to understand that the amount of information being borrowed from the reference population is relative to the amount of data generated in the target population. The effective sample size (ESS), which measures the information gained from the prior in terms of the number of subjects the prior is worth, is a good way to communicate with both the statistical group and among all other stakeholders. However, there are challenges with the use of ESS. For example, for the case of using nonconjugate priors, there is no unique definition of ESS. Also, ESS could be a negative value if the reference and target data conflict exists under the dynamic borrowing framework. This could be hard to understand for nonstatisticians. Another example is that for robust mixture priors, the weight on the reference data should really be interpreted as the probability that the reference data are relevant to the target data instead of ESS. When ESS is not applicable or does not have a clear definition, other matrices can be useful, such as effective supplemental sample size (ESSS, which is a measure of the amount of precision gained from a model that leverages the previous study data over a model that only uses the current trial data) [11], or effective current sample size (ECSS, which quantifies the number of samples to be added or subtracted to the likelihood in order to obtain a posterior inference equivalent to that of a baseline prior model) [40].

Estimand: The ICH E9 (R1) addendum on estimands and sensitivity analysis in clinical trials provides a framework for clinical study planning to ensure alignment between study objectives, design, conduct, and analysis [41]. FDA also emphasized its interest in the application of the principles outlined in this addendum for confirmatory clinical trials and for data integrated across trials with the purpose of generating confirmatory conclusions [42]. The five attributes that construct estimand and define the treatment effect of interest are treatment, population, variable, intercurrent events, and population-level summary.

For clinical trials with Bayesian designs, explicitly specifying details using the estimand framework can increase the clarity of communication and precision in describing a treatment effect of interest. Here are some key elements to be documented in the protocol: whether external data will be used and how those data align with the characteristics of the study population, how treatment is defined and the duration of treatment, what the concomitant medications are and the strategies of handling intercurrent events, whether the endpoints and timing of the endpoint aligned, and details of the statistical plan such as prior distribution, sample size determination, simulations, winning criteria, sensitivity analyses, etc.

Best practice: All the considerations discussed above are essential parts of the best practice when planning for Bayesian trial designs or conducting Bayesian analyses. Several additional things are equally important under the regulatory framework and should be considered:

Transparency – Starting the conversations early among all stakeholders regarding the necessity and practicality of using external data is the first step. Any assumptions, considerations, concerns, and judgment related to study designs and statistical analyses should be fully revealed for stakeholders to consider and critique. Consulting with regulatory agencies early to have an agreed-upon plan will likely save time for the drug development program in the long run.

Prespecification – The study protocol should be finalized before initiating the trial that plans to use external data so that potential bias can be reduced [36]. Specific design elements to be prespecified include but are not limited to the source and relevance of external data being borrowed, baseline eligibility criteria, clinically meaningful endpoints, and details of the data borrowing plan.

Sensitivity analyses – Sensitivity analyses can be useful to test the robustness of trial results and to examine the vulnerability of results to assumptions applied, such as applying priors with different Bayesian dynamic borrowing approaches or conducting a tipping point analysis.

Reevaluating assumptions – After study data are generated, examining the assumptions made for data borrowing and evaluating whether a knowledge gap exists are necessary steps. For example, during the execution of pediatric extrapolation, when the generated pediatric data are different from what were previously expected, the extrapolation concept should be reevaluated [34].

GC authored sections 1 and 2.1; HS authored sections 2.2 and 3.

Disclaimer: Dr. Sun is an employee of the FDA. This book chapter reflects the views of the author and should not be considered to represent FDA's views or policies.

References

1. FDA, Guidance for Industry and FDA Staff: Guidance for the Use of Bayesian Statistics in Medical Device Clinical Trials. 2010. www.fda.gov/media/71512/download.
2. Campbell, G., FDA regulatory acceptance of Bayesian statistics, in E. Lesaffre, G. Baio, & B. Brunolanger (Eds.), *Bayesian Methods in Pharmaceutical Research.* 2020, Chapman and Hall/CRC. pp. 41–51.
3. Pennello, G. and L. Thompson, Experience with reviewing Bayesian medical device trials. *Journal of Biopharmaceutical Statistics*, 2007. 18(1): pp. 81–115.
4. Bonangelino, P., et al., Bayesian approaches in medical device clinical trials: a discussion with examples in the regulatory setting. *Journal of Biopharmaceutical Statistics*, 2011. 21(5): pp. 938–953.
5. Campbell, G., Bayesian statistics in medical devices: innovation sparked by the FDA. *Journal of Biopharmaceutical Statistics*, 2011. 21(5): pp. 871–887.
6. (ACDRS), A.C.o.D.D.a.R.S. Substantial Evidence in 21st Century Regulatory Science: Borrowing Strength from Accumulating Data. 2016 [cited 2023 April 24]; Available from: https://pharmacy.ucsf.edu/events/2016/04/evidence.
7. Pocock, S.J., The combination of randomized and historical controls in clinical trials. *Journal of Chronic Diseases*, 1976. 29(3): pp. 175–88.

8. Ibrahim, J.G. and M.-H. Chen, Power prior distributions for regression models. *Statistical Science*, 2000. 15(1): pp. 46–60.

9. Duan, Y., K. Ye, and E.P. Smith, Evaluating water quality using power priors to incorporate historical information. *Environmetrics*, 2006. 17(1): pp. 95–106.

10. Neuenschwander, B., M. Branson, and D.J. Spiegelhalter, A note on the power prior. *Statistics in Medicine*, 2009. 28(28): pp. 3562–6.

11. Hobbs, B.P., et al., Hierarchical commensurate and power prior models for adaptive incorporation of historical information in clinical trials. *Biometrics*, 2011. 67(3): pp. 1047–1056.

12. Gravestock, I., L. Held, and C.N. consortium, Adaptive power priors with empirical Bayes for clinical trials. *Pharmaceutical Statistics*, 2017. 16(5): pp. 349–360.

13. Schmidli, H., et al., Robust meta-analytic-predictive priors in clinical trials with historical control information. *Biometrics*, 2014. 70(4): pp. 1023–1032.

14. Neuenschwander, B., et al., Summarizing historical information on controls in clinical trials. *Clinical Trials*, 2010. 7(1): pp. 5–18.

15. Viele, K., et al., Use of historical control data for assessing treatment effects in clinical trials. *Pharmaceutical Statistics*, 2014. 13(1): pp. 41–54.

16. van Rosmalen, J., et al., Including historical data in the analysis of clinical trials: Is it worth the effort? *Statistical Methods in Medical Research*, 2018. **27**(10): pp. 3167–3182.

17. Neuenschwander, B. and H. Schmidli, Use of historical data, in E. Lesaffre, G. Baio, & B. Brunolanger (Eds.), *Bayesian Methods in Pharmaceutical Research*. 2020, Chapman and Hall/CRC. pp. 111–137.

18. Thompson, L., et al., Dynamic borrowing from a single prior data source using the conditional power prior. *Journal of Biopharmaceutical Statistics*, 2021. 31(4): pp. 403–424.

19. Haddad, T., et al., Incorporation of stochastic engineering models as prior information in Bayesian medical device trials. *Journal of Biopharmaceutical Statistics*, 2017. 27(6): pp. 1089–1103.

20. Lin, J. and J. Lin, Incorporating propensity scores for evidence synthesis under Bayesian framework: review and recommendations for clinical studies. *Journal of Biopharmaceutical Statistics*, 2022. 32(1): pp. 53–74.

21. (MDIC), M.D.I.C., External Evidence Methods (EEM) Framework. April 2022. https://mdic.org/wp-content/uploads/2022/05/MDIC_EEM_Framework_2022-1.pdf

22. Wang, C., et al., Propensity score-integrated power prior approach for incorporating real-world evidence in single-arm clinical studies. *Journal of Biopharmaceutical Statistics*, 2019. 29(5): pp. 731–748.

23. Liu, M., et al., Propensity-score-based meta-analytic predictive prior for incorporating real-world and historical data. *Statistics in Medicine*, 2021. 40(22): pp. 4794–4808.

24. *VNS Therapy System: Summary of Safety and Effectiveness Data (SSED)*. 2017.

25. *NIQ: Summary of Safety and Effectiveness Data (SSED)*. 2019.

26. *REBYOTA Labeling*. 2022. www.fda.gov/media/163587/download.

27. *REBYOTA Summary Basis for Regulatory Action*. 2022. www.fda.gov/media/163879/download.

28. *Pfizer-BioNTech COVID-19 Vaccine Emergency Use Authorization (EUA) Review Memorandum*. 2020. www.fda.gov/media/144416/download.

29. *COMIRNATY Summary Basis for Regulatory Action* 2021. www.fda.gov/media/151733/download.

30. *COMIRNATY® Labeling*. 2021. www.fda.gov/media/154834/download.

31. *BENLYSTA Labeling*. 2019. www.accessdata.fda.gov/drugsatfda_docs/label/2019/125370s064,761043s007lbl.pdf.

32. *BENLYSTA® Multidisciplinary Review and Evaluation*. 2019. www.fda.gov/media/127912/download.

33. *TransScan T-2000 Multi-frequency Impedance Breast Scanner*. 1999. www.accessdata.fda.gov/cdrh_docs/pdf/P970033b.pdf.

34. ICH, *ICH Guideline E11A on Pediatric Extrapolation*. 2022. www.fda.gov/media/161190/download.

35. FDA, *Draft Guidance for Industry: Rare Diseases: Common Issues in Drug Development*. 2019. www.fda.gov/media/119757/download.

36. FDA, *Draft Guidance for Industry: Considerations for the Design and Conduct of Externally Controlled Trials for Drug and Biological Products*. 2023. www.fda.gov/regulatory-informat ion/search-fda-guidance-documents/considerations-design-and-conduct-externally-con trolled-trials-drug-and-biological-products.

37. Lin, J., M. Gamalo-Siebers, and R. Tiwari, Propensity-score-based priors for Bayesian augmented control design. *Pharmaceutical Statistics*, 2019. 18(2): pp. 223–238.

38. FDA, *Guidance for Industry: Adaptive Designs for Clinical Trials of Drugs and Biologics*. 2019. www.fda.gov/media/78495/download.

39. FDA, *Guidance for Industry: Interacting with the FDA on Complex Innovative Trial Designs for Drugs and Biological Products*. 2020. www.fda.gov/media/130897/download.

40. Wiesenfarth, M. and S. Calderazzo, Quantification of prior impact in terms of effective current sample size. *Biometrics*, 2020. 76(1): pp. 326–336.

41. ICH, *ICH E9 (R1) addendum on estimands and sensitivity analysis in clinical trials to the guideline on statistical principles for clinical trials*. 2019. www.ema.europa.eu/en/documents/scientific-guideline/ich-e9-r1-addendum-estimands-sensitivity-analysis-clinical-trials-guideline-stat istical-principles_en.pdf.

42. FDA, *FDA Guidance for Industry: E9(R1) Statistical Principles for Clinical Trials: Addendum: Estimands and Sensitivity Analysis in Clinical Trials*. 2021. www.fda.gov/media/148473/download.

15

Bayesian Optimal Interval Design

Martin Klein and Jian Wang

Disclaimer: This paper reflects the views of the authors and should not be construed to represent the views and/or policies of the U.S. Food and Drug Administration.

Introduction

The Bayesian Optimal Interval (BOIN) Design is a statistical methodology for designing a dose finding clinical trial where the goal is to identify the maximum tolerated dose of the investigational medicinal product (IMP). The BOIN design was proposed by Liu and Yuan (2015). Liu and Yuan (2015) proposed the local and global BOIN designs, and recommended the local BOIN design for practical use, based on its simplicity for practical implementation, theoretical properties, and the fact that it performed well in simulation studies. The local BOIN design was reviewed by the FDA under the FDA's Drug Development Tools: Fit-for-Purpose Initiative. Details about this review and its findings can be found at the website www.fda.gov/drugs/development-approval-process-drugs/drug-development-tools-fit-purpose-initiative. As a result of the FDA's review, Liu and Yuan (2022) presented some revisions to the original version of the local BOIN design as it appeared in Liu and Yuan (2015). In this paper we present the local BOIN design (henceforth referred to simply as the BOIN design) of Liu and Yuan (2015). We describe the statistical foundations of the BOIN design and provide numerical examples to illustrate its practical application. Our presentation incorporates the revisions of Liu and Yuan (2022).

15.1 Description of the Methodology

15.1.1 General Form of the Design

Assume that a total of J dose levels of the investigational medicinal product (IMP) have been prespecified for use in the trial. Let the dose levels be labeled as $1, 2, \ldots, J$, where the dose labeling is ordered such that dose level $j = 1$ represents the lowest dose of the IMP that will be used in the study, dose level $j = 2$ represents the second lowest dose of the

 DOI: 10.1201/9781003288640-15

IMP that will be used in the study, and so on, with $j = J$ representing the highest dose of the IMP that will be used in the study. It is assumed that the probability that a patient experiences dose limiting toxicity is a monotonically increasing function of the dose level in the mathematical sense that $p_1 \leq p_2 \leq \ldots \leq p_J$ where $p_1, p_2, \ldots, p_J$ denote the (unknown) probabilities that a patient experiences dose limiting toxicity at the dose levels $1, 2, \ldots, J$, respectively. It is also assumed that efficacy monotonically increases with toxicity. Let ϕ represent the prespecified targeted dose toxicity probability. The goal of the trial is to find the maximum tolerated dose (MTD) – the dose under which the probability that a patient experiences dose limiting toxicity (toxicity probability) is closest to the target value ϕ.

The general form of the BOIN design can be described via the decision rules used by the design once the trial is in progress. The trial is conducted such that patients are treated in cohorts with the sample size of each cohort prespecified. Patients in the first cohort of the trial are treated at the dose level 1 (the lowest dose level used in the trial). Once the trial is in progress, suppose that the current cohort of patients in the trial are treated at dose level $j \in \{1, 2, \ldots, J\}$. Because the BOIN design incorporates the dose elimination rule discussed in Section 15.1.3, let $j_{\max} \in \{1, 2, \ldots, J\}$ denote the largest dose level which, at the current stage, has not been eliminated from the trial at any previous stage, and therefore $\{1, 2, \ldots, j_{\max}\}$ denotes the set of all dose levels used in the trial which, at the current stage, were not eliminated from the trial at any previous stage. If, at the current stage of the trial, there are no dose levels that were eliminated at a previous stage, then it would be the case that $j_{\max} = J$; however, because the BOIN design incorporates the dose elimination rule discussed in Section 15.1.3, there exists the possibility of having $j_{\max} < J$. Because patients can no longer be assigned to a dose level after it is eliminated, it must be the case that $j \leq j_{\max}$.

Let n_j represent the total (cumulative) number of patients that have been treated at dose level j, and m_j represent the total (cumulative) number of patients who experienced dose limiting toxicity (DLT) at dose level j. Let $\hat{p}_j = m_j / n_j$ which is the observed proportion of patients experiencing DLT at dose level j. To specify the design, a decision rule is specified to decide on the dose level to use in the next stage of the trial (if the trial is terminated due to the maximum sample size being reached, or because of excessive toxicity, then this action would naturally supersede actions about dose escalation, deescalation, or retainment). The actions under consideration concerning the dose level for the next stage are to escalate the dose to level $j+1$, deescalate to dose level $j-1$, or retain the current dose level j. In the case $j = j_{\max}$ it is not possible to escalate the dose to level $j+1$, and in the case $j = 1$ it is not possible to deescalate to dose level $j-1$. Therefore, the decision rule needs adjustment to handle the $j = j_{\max}$ and $j = 1$ cases. Note that if $j_{\max} = 1$ and the trial is not terminated, the only dosing option is to retain dose level 1.

For $j \in \{2, 3, \ldots, j_{\max} - 1\}$, $j_{\max} \geq 3$, let $\lambda_{1j}(n_j, \boldsymbol{\omega})$ and $\lambda_{2j}(n_j, \boldsymbol{\omega})$ denote escalation and deescalation boundary values for $\hat{p}_j$, respectively, satisfying $\lambda_{1j}(n_j, \boldsymbol{\omega}) \leq \lambda_{2j}(n_j, \boldsymbol{\omega})$. These values can depend on j, n_j, and $\boldsymbol{\omega}$ where $\boldsymbol{\omega}$ represents a vector of known parameters that are prespecified before conducting the trial (including, for instance, the targeted dose toxicity probability ϕ, see Section 15.1.2 for details). If $j = 1$ so that the current dose level

TABLE 15.1

Decision rule used by the BOIN design.

Suppose the trial is in progress. Let $j \in \{1, 2, \ldots, J\}$ denote the dose level used to treat patients in the current stage of the trial. At the current stage of the trial let $j_{\max} \in \{1, 2, \ldots, J\}$ denote the maximum dose level among all dose levels under consideration that were not eliminated at any previous stage. Therefore, at the current stage of the trial $\{1, 2, \ldots, j_{\max}\}$ is the set of dose levels that were not eliminated at any previous stage. Because patients can no longer be assigned to a dose level after it is eliminated, it must be the case that $j \leq j_{\max}$.

Assume $j_{\max} \geq 2$ (If $j_{\max} = 1$ and the trial is not terminated, the only dosing option is to retain dose level 1 for the next cohort of patients.)

For $j \in \{2, 3, \ldots, j_{\max} - 1\}$ and $j_{\max} \geq 3$, let $\lambda_{1j}(n_j, \boldsymbol{\omega})$ and $\lambda_{2j}(n_j, \boldsymbol{\omega})$ denote escalation and deescalation boundary values, respectively, satisfying $\lambda_{1j}(n_j, \boldsymbol{\omega}) \leq \lambda_{2j}(n_j, \boldsymbol{\omega})$.

Define the escalation boundary $\lambda_1^{(1)}(n_1, \boldsymbol{\omega})$ for use when the $j = 1$ and $j_{\max} \geq 2$.

Define deescalation boundary $\lambda_2^{(j_{\max})}(n_j, \boldsymbol{\omega})$ for use when $j = j_{\max}$ and $j_{\max} \geq 2$.

When the current dose level is $j \in \{2, 3, \ldots, j_{\max} - 1\}$ and $j_{\max} \geq 3$:

- If $\hat{p}_j \leq \lambda_{1j}(n_j, \boldsymbol{\omega})$, then escalate the dose to level $j + 1$.
- If $\hat{p}_j > \lambda_{2j}(n_j, \boldsymbol{\omega})$, then deescalate the dose to level $j - 1$.
- If $\lambda_{1j}(n_j, \boldsymbol{\omega}) < \hat{p}_j \leq \lambda_{2j}(n_j, \boldsymbol{\omega})$, then retain the dose level j.

When the current dose level is $j = 1$ and $j_{\max} \geq 2$:

- If $\hat{p}_j \leq \lambda_1^{(1)}(n_1, \boldsymbol{\omega})$, then escalate the dose to level 2.
- If $\hat{p}_1 > \lambda_1^{(1)}(n_1, \boldsymbol{\omega})$, then retain the dose level 1.

When the current dose level is $j = j_{\max}$ and $j_{\max} \geq 2$:

- If $\hat{p}_j > \lambda_2^{(j_{\max})}(n_j, \boldsymbol{\omega})$, then deescalate the dose to level $j - 1$.
- If $\hat{p}_j \leq \lambda_2^{(j_{\max})}(n_j, \boldsymbol{\omega})$, then retain the dose at level j.

The trial ends when the maximum prespecified sample size is reached, or if it is determined that excessive toxicity has occurred based on the dose elimination rule (Section 15.1.3).

Note: The decision rule shown here incorporates the revisions presented by Liu and Yuan (2022).

is the lowest dose of the IMP used in the study, then it is not possible to deescalate the dose level at the next stage and therefore the decision rule can be specified using a single boundary value $\lambda_1^{(1)}(n_1, \boldsymbol{\omega})$. Similarly, if $j = j_{\max}$ so that the current dose level is the highest dose of the IMP used in the study among all dose levels that were not eliminated at a previous stage, then it is not possible to escalate the dose level at the next stage, and therefore the decision rule can be specified using a single boundary value $\lambda_2^{(j_{\max})}(n_j, \boldsymbol{\omega})$. The action to take at the next stage of the trial is determined using the decision rule shown in Table 15.1. The trial ends when the maximum prespecified sample size is reached, or if at any stage it is determined that excessive toxicity has occurred. Next, we will discuss the escalation and deescalation boundaries used by the BOIN design.

15.1.2 Obtaining the Escalation and Deescalation Boundaries

It is clear from Table 15.1 that the BOIN design depends on a set of escalation and deescalation boundaries. The quantities that these boundaries depend on include a set of known parameters that are prespecified before conducting the trial and these parameters have been denoted by the vector $\boldsymbol{\omega}$. Specifically, in the general case, the decision boundaries used by the BOIN design depend on values ϕ, ϕ_1, ϕ_2 satisfying $0 < \phi_1 < \phi < \phi_2 < 1$, as well as prior probabilities π_{0i}, π_{1i}, π_{2i} satisfying $\pi_{0i} + \pi_{1i} + \pi_{2i} = 1$ and $0 < \pi_{0i} < 1$, $0 < \pi_{1i} < 1$, $0 < \pi_{2i} < 1$ for each dose level $i \in \{1,2,...,J\}$. The quantities ϕ, ϕ_1, ϕ_2, and $\pi_{0i}, \pi_{1i}, \pi_{2i}$ for $i \in \{1,2,...,J\}$ are prespecified and fixed before conducting the trial. Among ϕ, ϕ_1, ϕ_2, and $\pi_{0j}, \pi_{1j}, \pi_{2j}$, as we will discuss below, if one chooses to use default values of ϕ_1 and ϕ_2 recommended by Liu and Yuan (2015) (see equation (1) below) and to use the noninformative prior distribution (see equation (5) below), then only ϕ would remain to be specified. We now describe the interpretation of ϕ, ϕ_1, ϕ_2 and $\pi_{0i}, \pi_{1i}, \pi_{2i}$ for $i \in \{1,2,...,J\}$.

Recall that p_i denotes the probability that a patient experiences dose limiting toxicity at the dose level $i \in \{1,2,...,J\}$ and is unknown. The value ϕ represents the targeted dose toxicity probability; the goal of the trial is to find the maximum tolerated dose (MTD) – the dose under which the probability that a patient experiences dose limiting toxicity (toxicity probability) is closest to the target value ϕ. Then, as described by Liu and Yuan (2015), ϕ_1 is interpreted as the largest dose toxicity probability that is considered as subtherapeutic such that the dose should be escalated, while ϕ_2 is interpreted as the smallest dose toxicity probability that is considered overly toxic such that the dose should be deescalated. Liu and Yuan (2015) also describe $\delta_1 = \phi - \phi_1$ and $\delta_2 = \phi_2 - \phi$ as representing the smallest differences of practical interest to be distinguished from the target value ϕ. For general use, Liu and Yuan (2015) recommend default values representing a 40% deviation from the target value ϕ:

$$\phi_1 = \phi - 0.4\phi = 0.6\phi \text{ and } \phi_2 = \phi + 0.4\phi = 1.4\phi. \tag{1}$$

Recall also that the choice of ϕ, ϕ_1, ϕ_2 must satisfy the condition $0 < \phi_1 < \phi < \phi_2 < 1$. One then defines the following point hypotheses for each $i \in \{1,2,...,J\}$.

$$
\begin{aligned}
&H_{0i}: p_i = \phi \text{ (Implies does level } i \text{ is on target.)} \\
&H_{1i}: p_i = \phi_1 \text{ (Implies does level } i \text{ is subtherapeutic.)} \\
&H_{2i}: p_i = \phi_2 \text{ (Implies does level } i \text{ is too toxic.)}
\end{aligned}
\tag{2}
$$

The quantities $\pi_{0i}, \pi_{1i}, \pi_{2i}$ are interpreted in a Bayesian statistical setting as the prior probabilities associated with the point hypotheses in (2), that is,

$$\pi_{0i} = P(H_{0i}) = P(p_i = \phi), \tag{3}$$

$$\pi_{1i} = P(H_{1i}) = P(p_i = \phi_1),$$

$$\pi_{2i} = P(H_{2i}) = P(p_i = \phi_2).$$

As in Section 15.1.1, once the trial is in progress, suppose that patients in the current cohort are treated at dose level $j \in \{1, 2, \ldots, J\}$, and let $j_{\max} \in \{1, 2, \ldots, J\}$ be such that $\{1, 2, \ldots, j_{\max}\}$ represent the set of all dose levels used in the trial which, at the current stage, were not eliminated from the trial at any previous stage. Assume $j_{\max} \geq 2$ (if $j_{\max} = 1$ and the trial is not terminated, the only dosing option is to retain dose level 1 for the next cohort of patients). Under the decision rule shown in Table 15.1, a Bayesian formulation is used to derive an equation for the probability of making an incorrect decision. The derivation of this decision error probability is discussed in Section 15.2. For convenience of notation the escalation and deescalation boundaries and the minimizing values discussed below will be written with the arguments n_j and ω suppressed. The values of the escalation and deescalation boundaries that appear in Table 15.1 are obtained as the values that minimize this decision error probability, for fixed values of j, $j_{\max}$, n_j, and ω. To describe these values, for each $i \in \{1, 2, \ldots, J\}$ define

$$\lambda_{1i}^* = \frac{\log\left(\frac{1-\phi_1}{1-\phi}\right) + n_i^{-1}\log\left(\frac{\pi_{1i}}{\pi_{0i}}\right)}{\log\left(\frac{\phi(1-\phi_1)}{\phi_1(1-\phi)}\right)} \quad \text{and} \quad \lambda_{2i}^* = \frac{\log\left(\frac{1-\phi}{1-\phi_2}\right) + n_i^{-1}\log\left(\frac{\pi_{0i}}{\pi_{2i}}\right)}{\log\left(\frac{\phi_2(1-\phi)}{\phi(1-\phi_2)}\right)}. \tag{4}$$

Case 1: $j \in \{2, 3, \ldots, j_{\max} - 1\}$ and $j_{\max} \geq 3$.

In this case the current dose assignment is neither the lowest dose of IMP used in the study, nor is it the highest dose among doses not eliminated at a previous stage. The decision error probability depends on both an escalation boundary λ_{1j} and deescalation boundary λ_{2j}, and it must be the case that $\lambda_{1j} \leq \lambda_{2j}$ (see Table 15.1). Hence minimization of the decision error probability with respect to λ_{1j} and λ_{2j} must be performed subject to the constraint $\lambda_{1j} \leq \lambda_{2j}$. If $\lambda_{1j}^* \leq \lambda_{2j}^*$ (with λ_{1j}^* and λ_{2j}^* as defined in (4)), then it can be shown that the incorrect decision error probability is minimized with respect to λ_{1j} and λ_{2j}, subject to the constraint $\lambda_{1j} \leq \lambda_{2j}$, at the value $\lambda_{1j} = \lambda_{1j}^*$ and $\lambda_{2j} = \lambda_{2j}^*$. There exist scenarios where (4) will result in values of λ_{1j}^* and λ_{2j}^* such that $\lambda_{1j}^* > \lambda_{2j}^*$, in which case λ_{1j}^* and λ_{2j}^* cannot be used as escalation and deescalation boundaries. In such a scenario, one would need to obtain values of λ_{1j} and λ_{2j} that minimize the decision error probability under the constraint $\lambda_{1j} \leq \lambda_{2j}$. Details on how to handle a situation where $\lambda_{1j}^* > \lambda_{2j}^*$ and the decision error must be minimized under the constraint $\lambda_{1j} \leq \lambda_{2j}$ are presented in Example 2, Example 3, and Example 4 in Section 15.3.

Case 2: $j = 1$ and $j_{\max} \geq 2$.

When $j = 1$ the current dose assignment is the lowest dose of the IMP used in the study, and hence it is not possible to deescalate the dose. Therefore, the decision error probability depends on an escalation boundary $\lambda_1^{(1)}$, but it does not depend on a deescalation boundary as there is no deescalation boundary in this case (see Table 15.1). It can be shown that the decision error probability is minimized with respect to $\lambda_1^{(1)}$ at the value $\lambda_1^{(1)} = \lambda_{11}^*$ with λ_{11}^* defined in (4).

Case 3: $j = j_{\max}$ and $j_{\max} \geq 2$.

When $j = j_{\max}$ the current dose assignment is the highest dose of the IMP used in the study among all dose levels that were not eliminated at a previous stage. Hence it is not possible to escalate the dose. Therefore, the decision error probability depends on a deescalation boundary $\lambda_2^{(j_{\max})}$, but it does not depend on an escalation boundary as there is no escalation boundary in this case (see Table 15.1). It can be shown that the decision error probability is minimized with respect to $\lambda_2^{(j_{\max})}$ at the value $\lambda_2^{(j_{\max})} = \lambda_{2j}^*$ with λ_{2j}^* defined in (4).

Remark. It will be observed in Section 15.2 that, due to the discrete nature of the distribution of m_j, the minimizing values discussed above are not unique minimizing values.

In the BOIN design, often the noninformative prior is used for each of $p_1, p_2, \ldots, p_J$. In this context, the noninformative prior is defined by the condition

$$\pi_{0i} = \pi_{1i} = \pi_{2i} = 1/3 \text{ for } i \in \{1, 2, \ldots, J\}. \tag{5}$$

An advantage of using the noninformative prior is that if (5) holds, then λ_{1i}^* and λ_{2i}^* simplify to $\lambda_{1i}^* = \lambda_1^*$ and $\lambda_{2i}^* = \lambda_2^*$ for all $i \in \{1, 2, \ldots, J\}$ where

$$\lambda_1^* = \frac{\log\left(\dfrac{1-\phi_1}{1-\phi}\right)}{\log\left(\dfrac{\phi(1-\phi_1)}{\phi_1(1-\phi)}\right)} \quad \text{and} \quad \lambda_2^* = \frac{\log\left(\dfrac{1-\phi}{1-\phi_2}\right)}{\log\left(\dfrac{\phi_2(1-\phi)}{\phi(1-\phi_2)}\right)}. \tag{6}$$

The values λ_1^* and λ_2^* do not change as the dose level j changes, nor do they change as n_j changes. Furthermore, it can be shown that the condition $0 < \phi_1 < \phi < \phi_2 < 1$ implies that

$$0 < \phi_1 < \frac{\log\left(\dfrac{1-\phi_1}{1-\phi}\right)}{\log\left(\dfrac{\phi(1-\phi_1)}{\phi_1(1-\phi)}\right)} < \phi < \frac{\log\left(\dfrac{1-\phi}{1-\phi_2}\right)}{\log\left(\dfrac{\phi_2(1-\phi)}{\phi(1-\phi_2)}\right)} < \phi_2 < 1. \tag{7}$$

Thus, the condition $0 < \phi_1 < \phi < \phi_2 < 1$ implies that $0 < \phi_1 < \lambda_1^* < \phi < \lambda_2^* < \phi_2 < 1$ with λ_1^* and λ_2^* as defined in (6). Therefore, while in the general setting it is possible to have $\lambda_{1j}^* > \lambda_{2j}^*$ in which case the decision boundary values in (4) cannot be used; this issue does not occur if the noninformative prior (5) is used. Furthermore, the boundary values in (6) do not depend on the current dose level j, nor do they depend on n_j.

Let us consider Cases 1, 2, and 3 above under the situation when the noninformative prior is used. Suppose the noninformative prior (5) is used; then in Case 1 the decision error probability is minimized with respect to λ_{1j} and λ_{2j} under the constraint $\lambda_{1j} \leq \lambda_{2j}$ when $\lambda_{1j} = \lambda_1^*$ and $\lambda_{2j} = \lambda_2^*$; in Case 2 the decision error probability is minimized with respect to $\lambda_1^{(1)}$ at the value $\lambda_1^{(1)} = \lambda_1^*$; and in Case 3 the decision error probability is minimized with respect to $\lambda_2^{(j_{\max})}$ at the value $\lambda_2^{(j_{\max})} = \lambda_2^*$. Therefore, the noninformative prior (5) leads to a simplification of the design because when the noninformative prior (5) is used, the boundary values in (6) can be used at each stage of the trial.

15.1.3 Dose Elimination Rule for Determination of Excessive Toxicity

The BOIN design also incorporates the following dose elimination rule. As the trial proceeds, suppose that patients are currently being treated at dose level j. The dose elimination rule states that dose levels j and higher are eliminated from the trial if

$$P(p_j > \phi \mid m_j) > 0.95 \text{ and } n_j \geq 3, \tag{8}$$

and if dose level $j = 1$ is eliminated because of (8), then the trial is terminated.

To evaluate the probability that appears in (8), the following Bayesian model is assumed:

$$
\begin{aligned}
m_j \mid p_j &\sim \text{Binomial}(n_j, p_j) \\
p_j &\sim \text{Beta}(1, 1) \left[\text{equivalently, } p_j \sim \text{Uniform}(0,1)\right].
\end{aligned}
\tag{9}
$$

Note that n_j, the total number of patients treated at current dose level j, is treated as fixed (nonrandom) throughout. Under the model (9) it follows that

$$p_j \mid m_j \sim \text{Beta}(m_j + 1, \; n_j - m_j + 1). \tag{10}$$

Hence the probability $P(p_j > \phi \mid m_j)$ that appears in (8) can be calculated as

$$P(p_j > \phi \mid m_j) = 1 - F_{\text{Beta}}\left(\phi; m_j + 1, n_j - m_j + 1\right) \tag{11}$$

where $F_{\text{Beta}}(x; a, b)$ denotes cumulative distribution function of the $\text{Beta}(a, b)$ distribution for $a > 0, b > 0$ (thus, $F_{\text{Beta}}(x; a, b) = P(X \leq x)$ where $X \sim \text{Beta}(a, b)$).

Observe from (3) that the prior distribution specified for p_j to obtain the decision rule escalation and deescalation boundaries states that p_j takes values ϕ, ϕ_1, ϕ_2 with probabilities $\pi_{0j}, \pi_{1j}, \pi_{2j}$. The prior distribution specified for p_j to evaluate the dose elimination rule is the $\text{Beta}(1,1)$ distribution as displayed in (9) (the $\text{Beta}(1,1)$ distribution is equivalent to the $\text{Uniform}(0,1)$ distribution). Therefore, comparing (3) and (9) it is seen that the prior distribution specified for p_j to obtain the decision rule escalation and deescalation boundaries differs from the prior distribution specified for p_j to evaluate the dose elimination rule.

15.1.4 Selecting the Maximum Tolerated Dose

Once the trial is complete Liu and Yuan (2015) suggest using the data obtained from the trial to obtain isotonic estimates of the toxicity probabilities $p_1, p_2, \ldots, p_J$ using the pooled adjacent violators algorithm (Barlow et al., 1972) and selecting as the MTD the dose having estimated toxicity probability closest to the target value ϕ. If there are ties among the doses having estimated toxicity probability closest to ϕ, then Liu and Yuan (2015) suggest selecting either the highest or lowest dose among the ties depending on whether the tied estimated toxicity probabilities are less than ϕ or greater than ϕ, respectively. An approach to selecting the MTD in case there are tied estimated toxicity probabilities equal to ϕ can also be prespecified before conducting the trial. The BOIN package (Yan et al., 2020) of the R software (R Core Team, 2022) provides a function called select.mtd which performs tasks related to this step, including computation of the isotonic estimates of toxicity probabilities and MTD selection based on the estimated toxicity probabilities. The documentation for the BOIN R package mentions that other approaches such as an approach based on logistic regression could be used to select the MTD once the trial is complete and that selecting the MTD and the decision rule for dose escalation/deescalation are viewed as independent components of the BOIN design.

15.2 Theoretical Basis for the Decision Boundaries

As in the previous section, once the trial is in progress, suppose that the current cohort of patients in the trial are treated at dose level $j \in \{1, 2, \ldots, J\}$, and let $j_{\max} \in \{1, 2, \ldots, J\}$ be such that $\{1, 2, \ldots, j_{\max}\}$ represents the set of all dose levels used in the trial which, at the current stage, were not eliminated from the trial at any previous stage. Assume that $j_{\max} \geq 2$ because if $j_{\max} = 1$ and the trial is not terminated, the only dosing option is to retain dose level 1 for the next cohort of patients. Consider the three hypotheses in (2) where the parameter space for p_j is $\{\phi, \phi_1, \phi_2\}$. The action space consists of the set of three actions {Retain, Escalate, De-escalate} which are defined as follows.

- R = Retain: Retain the same dose level, meaning dose level j will be assigned to patients during the next stage of the trial.
- E = Escalate: Escalate the dose by one level, meaning dose level $j+1$ will be assigned to patients during the next stage of the trial. (When $j = j_{\max}$ this action cannot be implemented, and the decision rule [see Table 15.1] excludes this action in that case.)
- D = De-escalate: Deescalate the dose by one level, meaning dose level $j-1$ will be assigned to patients during the next stage of the trial. (When $j = 1$ this action cannot be implemented, and the decision rule [see Table 15.1] excludes this action in that case.)

The actions Retain, Escalate, De-escalate about the dose level to use for the next stage of the trial are associated with the unknown parameter p_j via the hypotheses in (2) as follows.

- When the hypothesis $H_{0j}{:}p_j = \phi$ is true, the correct action is R, an incorrect action would be either E or D.
- When the hypothesis $H_{1j}{:}p_j = \phi_1$ is true, the correct action is E, an incorrect action would be either R or D.
- When the hypothesis $H_{2j}{:}p_j = \phi_2$ is true, the correct action is D, an incorrect action would be either E or R.

The decision boundaries are determined by minimizing the probability of making an incorrect decision about the dosing level assignment for the next stage of the trial. This probability is derived using a Bayesian framework as shown below. In this framework, j, j_{max}, and n_j are treated as fixed (nonrandom) and it is assumed that the conditional distribution of m_j given p_j is Binomial(n_j, p_j). The prior distribution of p_j is the discrete distribution where p_j takes values ϕ, ϕ_1, ϕ_2 with probabilities $\pi_{0j}, \pi_{1j}, \pi_{2j}$ (see (2) and (3)). The cumulative distribution function of the Binomial(n, p) distribution for $n \in \{1, 2, 3, ...\}$, $p \in [0,1]$ is denoted by $F_{\text{Bin}}(x; n, p)$ (thus, $F_{\text{Bin}}(x; n, p) = P(X \le x)$ where $X \sim$ Binomial(n, p)). Also define the following functions for each $i \in \{1, 2, ..., J\}$ (it will be seen that these expressions appear in the decision error probability).

$$\alpha_{1i}(\lambda_1) = \pi_{0i} F_{\text{Bin}}(n_i \lambda_1; n_i, \phi) - \pi_{1i} F_{\text{Bin}}(n_i \lambda_1; n_i, \phi_1) \tag{12}$$

$$\alpha_{2i}(\lambda_2) = \pi_{2i} F_{\text{Bin}}(n_i \lambda_2; n_i, \phi_2) - \pi_{0i} F_{\text{Bin}}(n_i \lambda_2; n_i, \phi)$$

Case 1: $j \in \{2, 3, ..., j_{max} - 1\}$ and $j_{max} \ge 3$.
In this case the decision rule for choosing among the actions $\{E, D, R\}$ is described in Table 15.1 and can be written as the following function.

$$\delta_j(\hat{p}_j) = \begin{cases} E & \text{if} & \hat{p}_j \le \lambda_{1j} \\ D & \text{if} & \hat{p}_j > \lambda_{2j} \\ R & \text{if} & \lambda_{1j} < \hat{p}_j \le \lambda_{2j} \end{cases}$$

Then the probability of making an incorrect decision can be obtained as follows.

$$P\{\delta_j(\hat{p}_j) \ne R \text{ and } H_{0j}\} + P\{\delta_j(\hat{p}_j) \ne E \text{ and } H_{1j}\} + P\{\delta_j(\hat{p}_j) \ne D \text{ and } H_{2j}\} \tag{13}$$

$$= P\{\delta_j(\hat{p}_j) \ne R \mid H_{0j}\} P\{H_{0j}\} + P\{\delta_j(\hat{p}_j) \ne E \mid H_{1j}\} P\{H_{1j}\} + P\{\delta_j(\hat{p}_j) \ne D \mid H_{2j}\} P\{H_{2j}\}$$

$$= P\{\hat{p}_j \le \lambda_{1j} \text{ or } \hat{p}_j > \lambda_{2j} \mid H_{0j}\} P\{H_{0j}\} + P\{\hat{p}_j > \lambda_{1j} \mid H_{1j}\} P\{H_{1j}\} + P\{\hat{p}_j \le \lambda_{2j} \mid H_{2j}\} P\{H_{2j}\}$$

$$= \left\{ F_{\text{Bin}}(n_j \lambda_{1j}; n_j, \phi) + 1 - F_{\text{Bin}}(n_j \lambda_{2j}; n_j, \phi) \right\} \pi_{0j} + \left\{ 1 - F_{\text{Bin}}(n_j \lambda_{1j}; n_j, \phi_1) \right\} \pi_{1j} \\ + \left\{ F_{\text{Bin}}(n_j \lambda_{2j}; n_j, \phi_2) \right\} \pi_{2j}$$

$$= \left\{ \pi_{0j} F_{\text{Bin}}(n_j \lambda_{1j}; n_j, \phi) - \pi_{1j} F_{\text{Bin}}(n_j \lambda_{1j}; n_j, \phi_1) \right\} + \left\{ \pi_{2j} F_{\text{Bin}}(n_j \lambda_{2j}; n_j, \phi_2) - \pi_{0j} F_{\text{Bin}}(n_j \lambda_{2j}; n_j, \phi) \right\} \\ + \pi_{0j} + \pi_{1j}$$

$$= \alpha_{1j}(\lambda_{1j}) + \alpha_{2j}(\lambda_{2j}) + \pi_{0j} + \pi_{1j}$$

Case 2: $j = 1$ and $j_{\max} \geq 2$.

In this case the decision rule for choosing among the actions $\{E, R\}$ is described in Table 15.1 and can be written as the following function.

$$\delta_1(\hat{p}_1) = \begin{cases} E & \text{if} \quad \hat{p}_1 \leq \lambda_1^{(1)} \\ R & \text{if} \quad \hat{p}_1 > \lambda_1^{(1)} \end{cases}$$

Then the probability of making an incorrect decision can be obtained as follows.

$$P\left\{\delta_1(\hat{p}_1) \neq R \text{ and } H_{01}\right\} + P\left\{\delta_1(\hat{p}_1) \neq E \text{ and } H_{11}\right\} + P\left\{\delta_1(\hat{p}_1) \neq D \text{ and } H_{21}\right\}$$

$$= P\left\{\delta_1(\hat{p}_1) \neq R \mid H_{01}\right\} P\{H_{01}\} + P\left\{\delta_1(\hat{p}_1) \neq E \mid H_{11}\right\} P\{H_{11}\}$$
$$+ P\left\{\delta_1(\hat{p}_1) \neq D \mid H_{21}\right\} P\{H_{21}\}$$

$$= P\left\{\hat{p}_1 \leq \lambda_1^{(1)} \mid H_{01}\right\} P\{H_{01}\} + P\left\{\hat{p}_1 > \lambda_1^{(1)} \mid H_{11}\right\} P\{H_{11}\} + P\{H_{21}\} \tag{14}$$

$$= F_{\text{Bin}}\left(n_1 \lambda_1^{(1)}; n_1, \phi\right) \pi_{01} + \left\{1 - F_{\text{Bin}}\left(n_1 \lambda_1^{(1)}; n_1, \phi_1\right)\right\} \pi_{11} + \pi_{21}$$

$$= \left\{\pi_{01} F_{\text{Bin}}\left(n_1 \lambda_1^{(1)}; n_1, \phi\right) - \pi_{11} F_{\text{Bin}}\left(n_1 \lambda_1^{(1)}; n_1, \phi_1\right)\right\} + \pi_{11} + \pi_{21}$$

$$= \alpha_{11}\left(\lambda_1^{(1)}\right) + \pi_{11} + \pi_{21}$$

Case 3: $j = j_{\max}$ and $j_{\max} \geq 2$.

In this case the decision rule for choosing among the actions $\{D, R\}$ is described in Table 15.1 and can be written as the following function.

$$\delta_j^{(j_{\max})}(\hat{p}_j) = \begin{cases} D & \text{if} \quad \hat{p}_j > \lambda_2^{(j_{\max})} \\ R & \text{if} \quad \hat{p}_j \leq \lambda_2^{(j_{\max})} \end{cases}$$

Then the probability of making an incorrect decision can be obtained as follows.

$$P\left\{\delta_j^{(j_{\max})}(\hat{p}_j) \neq R \text{ and } H_{0j}\right\} + P\left\{\delta_j^{(j_{\max})}(\hat{p}_j) \neq E \text{ and } H_{1j}\right\} + P\left\{\delta_j^{(j_{\max})}(\hat{p}_j) \neq D \text{ and } H_{2j}\right\}$$

$$= P\left\{\delta_j^{(j_{\max})}(\hat{p}_j) \neq R \mid H_{0j}\right\} P\{H_{0j}\} + P\left\{\delta_j^{(j_{\max})}(\hat{p}_j) \neq E \mid H_{1j}\right\} P\{H_{1j}\}$$
$$+ P\left\{\delta_j^{(j_{\max})}(\hat{p}_j) \neq D \mid H_{2j}\right\} P\{H_{2j}\}$$

$$= P\left\{\hat{p}_j > \lambda_2^{(j_{\max})} \mid H_{0j}\right\} P\{H_{0j}\} + P\{H_{1j}\} + P\left\{\hat{p}_j \leq \lambda_2^{(j_{\max})} \mid H_{2j}\right\} P\{H_{2j}\} \tag{15}$$

$$= \left\{ 1 - F_{\text{Bin}}\left(n_j \lambda_2^{(j_{\max})}; n_j, \phi \right) \right\} \pi_{0j} + \pi_{1j} + \left\{ F_{\text{Bin}}\left(n_j \lambda_2^{(j_{\max})}; n_j, \phi_2 \right) \right\} \pi_{2j}$$

$$= \left\{ \pi_{2j} F_{\text{Bin}}\left(n_j \lambda_2^{(j_{\max})}; n_j, \phi_2 \right) - \pi_{0j} F_{\text{Bin}}\left(n_j \lambda_2^{(j_{\max})}; n_j, \phi \right) \right\} + \pi_{0j} + \pi_{1j}$$

$$= \alpha_{2j}\left(\lambda_2^{(j_{\max})} \right) + \pi_{0j} + \pi_{1j}$$

Liu and Yuan (2022, Supplementary Materials) show that the function $\alpha_{1i}(\lambda_1)$ is minimized with respect to λ_1 (with the other quantities $n_i, \pi_{0i}, \pi_{1i}, \phi, \phi_1$ that appear in this function held fixed) when λ_1 is contained in the following interval:

$$\left\{ \begin{array}{ll} \left[1 - \dfrac{I\left(y_i^* = n_i \right)}{n_i}, \ \infty \right) & \text{if} \quad y_i^* \geq n_i \\[3mm] \left[\dfrac{\lceil y_i^* \rceil - 1}{n_i}, \ \dfrac{\lfloor y_i^* \rfloor + 1}{n_i} \right) & \text{if} \quad 0 < y_i^* < n_i \\[3mm] \left(-\infty, \ \dfrac{I\left(y_i^* = 0 \right)}{n_i} \right) & \text{if} \quad y_i^* \leq 0 \end{array} \right\} \tag{16}$$

where

$$y_i^* = \frac{n_i \log\left(\dfrac{1-\phi_1}{1-\phi} \right) + \log\left(\dfrac{\pi_{1i}}{\pi_{0i}} \right)}{\log\left(\dfrac{\phi(1-\phi_1)}{\phi_1(1-\phi)} \right)}.$$

Furthermore, one specific value that is contained in the interval (16) is

$$\lambda_{1i}^* = \frac{y_i^*}{n_i} = \frac{\log\left(\dfrac{1-\phi_1}{1-\phi} \right) + n_i^{-1} \log\left(\dfrac{\pi_{1i}}{\pi_{0i}} \right)}{\log\left(\dfrac{\phi(1-\phi_1)}{\phi_1(1-\phi)} \right)}$$

which is the value defined previously in (4).

Similarly, using the fact that the functions $\alpha_{1i}(\lambda_1)$ and $\alpha_{2i}(\lambda_2)$ have similar form (differing only in the values of the fixed quantities), Liu and Yuan (2022, Supplementary Materials) show that the function $\alpha_{2i}(\lambda_2)$ is minimized with respect to λ_2 (with the other quantities $n_i, \pi_{2i}, \pi_{0i}, \phi_2, \phi$ that appear in this function held fixed) when λ_2 is contained in the following interval:

$$\left\{ \begin{array}{ll} \left[1 - \dfrac{I\left(y_i^{**} = n_i\right)}{n_i}, \quad \infty \right) & \text{if} \quad y_i^{**} \geq n_i \\[2ex] \left[\dfrac{\lceil y_i^{**} \rceil - 1}{n_i}, \dfrac{\lfloor y_i^{**} \rfloor + 1}{n_i} \right) & \text{if} \quad 0 < y_i^{**} < n_i \\[2ex] \left(-\infty, \dfrac{I\left(y_i^{**} = 0\right)}{n_i} \right) & \text{if} \quad y_i^{**} \leq 0 \end{array} \right\} \tag{17}$$

where

$$y_i^{**} = \frac{n_i \log\left(\dfrac{1-\phi}{1-\phi_2}\right) + \log\left(\dfrac{\pi_{0i}}{\pi_{2i}}\right)}{\log\left(\dfrac{\phi_2(1-\phi)}{\phi(1-\phi_2)}\right)}.$$

Furthermore, one specific value that is contained in the interval (17) is

$$\lambda_{2i}^* = \frac{y_i^{**}}{n_i} = \frac{\log\left(\dfrac{1-\phi}{1-\phi_2}\right) + n_i^{-1} \log\left(\dfrac{\pi_{0i}}{\pi_{2i}}\right)}{\log\left(\dfrac{\phi_2(1-\phi)}{\phi(1-\phi_2)}\right)}.$$

which is the value defined previously in (4). These results lead to the following conclusions.

Case 1: $j \in \{2, 3, \dots, j_{\max} - 1\}$ and $j_{\max} \geq 3$.

In this case the probability of making an incorrect decision is given by (13) as $\alpha_{1j}\left(\lambda_{1j}\right) + \alpha_{2j}\left(\lambda_{2j}\right) + \pi_{0j} + \pi_{1j}$. Because of the requirement that $\lambda_{1j} \leq \lambda_{2j}$, the minimization of (13) with respect to λ_{1j} and λ_{2j} must be performed under the constraint $\lambda_{1j} \leq \lambda_{2j}$. The global minimization of $\alpha_{1j}\left(\lambda_{1j}\right) + \alpha_{2j}\left(\lambda_{2j}\right) + \pi_{0j} + \pi_{1j}$ can be performed by separately minimizing $\alpha_{1j}\left(\lambda_{1j}\right)$ with respect to λ_{1j} and $\alpha_{2j}\left(\lambda_{2j}\right)$ with respect to λ_{2j}. Therefore, in view of the results above, the global minimization of $\alpha_{1j}\left(\lambda_{1j}\right) + \alpha_{2j}\left(\lambda_{2j}\right) + \pi_{0j} + \pi_{1j}$ occurs when λ_{1j} is in the interval (16) and λ_{2j} is in the interval (17). One choice of minimizing values is $\lambda_{1j} = \lambda_{1j}^*$ and $\lambda_{2j} = \lambda_{2j}^*$ as defined in (4). If it turns out that $\lambda_{1j}^* \leq \lambda_{2j}^*$, then (being a global minimum) this choice also minimizes $\alpha_{1j}\left(\lambda_{1j}\right) + \alpha_{2j}\left(\lambda_{2j}\right) + \pi_{0j} + \pi_{1j}$ under the condition $\lambda_{1j} \leq \lambda_{2j}$. However, if $\lambda_{1j}^* > \lambda_{2j}^*$ then one must obtain minimizing values of λ_{1j}

and λ_{2j} under the constraint $\lambda_{1j} \leq \lambda_{2j}$. Numerical examples illustrating minimization of $\alpha_{1j}(\lambda_{1j}) + \alpha_{2j}(\lambda_{2j}) + \pi_{0j} + \pi_{1j}$ under the constraint $\lambda_{1j} \leq \lambda_{2j}$ when $\lambda_{1j}^* > \lambda_{2j}^*$ are presented in Example 2, Example 3, and Example 4 in Section 15.3. While in general, it is possible that $\lambda_{1j}^* > \lambda_{2j}^*$, if $\pi_{0j} = \pi_{1j} = \pi_{2j} = 1/3$ then it will not be possible to have $\lambda_{1j}^* > \lambda_{2j}^*$ (because the condition $0 < \phi_1 < \phi < \phi_2 < 1$ [which must hold by definition of ϕ_1, ϕ, and ϕ_2] implies that the inequality (7) holds). Thus, when the noninformative prior (5) is used, the boundaries (6), namely $\lambda_{1j} = \lambda_1^*$ and $\lambda_{2j} = \lambda_2^*$, can be used, and if $\lambda_{1j} = \lambda_1^*$ and $\lambda_{2j} = \lambda_2^*$, then it will be the case that $\lambda_{1j} \leq \lambda_{2j}$.

Case 2: $j = 1$ and $j_{\max} \geq 2$.
In this case the probability of making an incorrect decision is given by (14) as $\alpha_{11}(\lambda_1^{(1)}) + \pi_{11} + \pi_{21}$ and this probability is minimized with respect to $\lambda_1^{(1)}$ when $\lambda_1^{(1)}$ is in the interval (16). One choice of minimizing value is $\lambda_{1j} = \lambda_{1j}^*$ as defined in (4). Recall that when the noninformative prior (5) is used, λ_{1j}^* simplifies to λ_1^* as defined in (6).

Case 3: $j = j_{\max}$ and $j_{\max} \geq 2$.
In this case the probability of making an incorrect decision is given by (15) as $\alpha_{2j}(\lambda_2^{(j_{\max})}) + \pi_{0j} + \pi_{1j}$ and this probability is minimized with respect to $\lambda_2^{(j_{\max})}$ when $\lambda_2^{(j_{\max})}$ is in the interval (17). One choice of minimizing value is $\lambda_2^{(j_{\max})} = \lambda_{2j}^*$ as defined in (4). Recall that when the noninformative prior (5) is used, λ_{2j}^* simplifies to λ_2^* as defined in (6).

15.3 Example Scenarios

Example 1
Consider a scenario where the current dose level is $j \in \{1, 2, , \ldots, J\}$ the noninformative prior (5) is used and $n_j = 3$, $\phi = 0.25$, $\phi_1 = 0.15$, $\phi_2 = 0.35$. Let $j_{\max} \in \{1, 2, \ldots, J\}$ be such that $\{1, 2, \ldots, j_{\max}\}$ represents the set of all dose levels used in the trial which, at the current stage, were not eliminated from the trial at any previous stage. Assume $j_{\max} \geq 2$.

Applying (4) we obtain $\lambda_{1j}^* \approx 0.1968$ and $\lambda_{2j}^* \approx 0.2984$ which will minimize $\alpha_{1j}(\lambda_1)$ and $\alpha_{2j}(\lambda_2)$, respectively. In this case, because the noninformative prior is used, we can also apply (6) to obtain $\lambda_1^* = \lambda_{1j}^* \approx 0.1968$ and $\lambda_2^* = \lambda_{2j}^* \approx 0.2984$. As discussed in Section 15.2, the function $\alpha_{1j}(\lambda_1)$ is minimized with respect to λ_1 when λ_1 is contained in the interval (16), and the function $\alpha_{2j}(\lambda_2)$ is minimized with respect to λ_2 when λ_2 is contained in the interval (17). To apply (16), observe that $y_j^* \approx 0.5904$, and therefore by (16), $\alpha_{1j}(\lambda_1)$ is minimized when λ_1 is in the interval $\left[\dfrac{\left\lceil y_j^* \right\rceil - 1}{n_j}, \dfrac{\left\lfloor y_j^* \right\rfloor + 1}{n_j}\right) = \left[\dfrac{\lceil 0.5904 \rceil - 1}{3}, \dfrac{\lfloor 0.5904 \rfloor + 1}{3}\right) = \left[\dfrac{1-1}{3}, \dfrac{0+1}{3}\right) = \left[0, \dfrac{1}{3}\right).$ To

apply (17), observe that $y_j^{**} \approx 0.8952$, and therefore by (17), $\alpha_{2j}(\lambda_2)$ is minimized when λ_2 is

in the interval $\left[\dfrac{\left\lceil y_j^{**} \right\rceil - 1}{n_j}, \dfrac{\left\lfloor y_j^{**} \right\rfloor + 1}{n_j}\right) = \left[\dfrac{\lceil 0.8952 \rceil - 1}{3}, \dfrac{\lfloor 0.8952 \rfloor + 1}{3}\right) = \left[\dfrac{1-1}{3}, \dfrac{0+1}{3}\right) = \left[0, \dfrac{1}{3}\right).$ If

$j \in \{2, 3, \ldots, j_{max} - 1\}$ and $j_{max} \geq 3$, then for $\lambda_1 \leq \lambda_2$, the function $\alpha_{1j}(\lambda_1) + \alpha_{2j}(\lambda_2) + \pi_{0j} + \pi_{1j}$ represents the decision error probability as a function of λ_1 and λ_2. This function is minimized with respect to λ_1 and λ_2, under the constraint that $\lambda_1 \leq \lambda_2$, when $0 \leq \lambda_1 \leq \lambda_2 < \dfrac{1}{3}$. To illustrate the minimizing values discussed above, Table 15.2 presents numerical evaluation of the functions $\alpha_{1j}(\lambda_1)$ and $\alpha_{2j}(\lambda_2)$, and Table 15.3 presents numerical evaluation of the function $\alpha_{1j}(\lambda_1) + \alpha_{2j}(\lambda_2) + \pi_{0j} + \pi_{1j}$.

Table 15.2 demonstrates that $\alpha_{1j}(\lambda_1)$ is minimized when $\lambda_1 \in \left[0, \dfrac{1}{3}\right)$ and $\alpha_{2j}(\lambda_2)$

is minimized when $\lambda_2 \in \left[0, \dfrac{1}{3}\right)$ (and the minimum values of $\alpha_{1j}(\lambda_1)$ and $\alpha_{2j}(\lambda_2)$ are

shown in Table 15.2 as -0.0641 and -0.0491, respectively). The shaded cells in Table 15.3 correspond to subsets of the domain of the function of $\alpha_{1j}(\lambda_1) + \alpha_{2j}(\lambda_2) + \pi_{0j} + \pi_{1j}$ where there exist values λ_1 and λ_2 satisfying $\lambda_1 \leq \lambda_2$ (for some of the subsets corresponding to the shaded cells all values of λ_1 and λ_2 in the subset satisfy $\lambda_1 \leq \lambda_2$, and for others some but not all values of λ_1 and λ_2 in the subset satisfy $\lambda_1 \leq \lambda_2$). Therefore, the minimizing

TABLE 15.2

Numerical evaluation of the functions $\alpha_{1j}(\lambda_1)$ and $\alpha_{2j}(\lambda_1)$ for the scenario of Example 1. These functions take the constant value given in the table over each interval shown. Function values were rounded to four decimal places when necessary.

λ_1	$\alpha_{1j}(\lambda_1)$	λ_2	$\alpha_{2j}(\lambda_2)$
$\lambda_1 \in (-\infty, 0)$	0	$\lambda_2 \in (-\infty, 0)$	0
$\lambda_1 \in \left[0, \dfrac{1}{3}\right)$	-0.0641	$\lambda_2 \in \left[0, \dfrac{1}{3}\right)$	-0.0491
$\lambda_1 \in \left[\dfrac{1}{3}, \dfrac{2}{3}\right)$	-0.0318	$\lambda_2 \in \left[\dfrac{1}{3}, \dfrac{2}{3}\right)$	-0.0418
$\lambda_1 \in \left[\dfrac{2}{3}, 1\right)$	-0.0041	$\lambda_2 \in \left[\dfrac{2}{3}, 1\right)$	-0.0091
$\lambda_1 \in [1, \infty)$	0	$\lambda_2 \in [1, \infty)$	0

TABLE 15.3

Numerical evaluation of the function $\alpha_{1j}(\lambda_1) + \alpha_{2j}(\lambda_2) + \pi_{0j} + \pi_{1j}$ for the scenario of Example 1. This function takes the constant value given in the table over each subset of $\mathbb{R}^2$ indicated by the combination of row and column. The shaded cells correspond to subsets of $\mathbb{R}^2$ on which the function $\alpha_{1j}(\lambda_1) + \alpha_{2j}(\lambda_2) + \pi_{0j} + \pi_{1j}$ is constant and there exist values λ_1 and λ_2 satisfying $\lambda_1 \leq \lambda_2$. Function values were rounded to four decimal places when necessary.

	$\lambda_2 \in (-\infty, 0)$	$\lambda_2 \in \left[0, \frac{1}{3}\right)$	$\lambda_2 \in \left[\frac{1}{3}, \frac{2}{3}\right)$	$\lambda_2 \in \left[\frac{2}{3}, 1\right)$	$\lambda_2 \in [1, \infty)$
$\lambda_1 \in (-\infty, 0)$	0.6667	0.6176	0.6248	0.6576	0.6667
$\lambda_1 \in \left[0, \frac{1}{3}\right)$	0.6026	0.5535	0.5608	0.5935	0.6026
$\lambda_1 \in \left[\frac{1}{3}, \frac{2}{3}\right)$	0.6348	0.5858	0.5930	0.6258	0.6348
$\lambda_1 \in \left[\frac{2}{3}, 1\right)$	0.6626	0.6135	0.6207	0.6535	0.6626
$\lambda_1 \in [1, \infty)$	0.6667	0.6176	0.6248	0.6576	0.6667

value of $\alpha_{1j}(\lambda_1) + \alpha_{2j}(\lambda_2) + \pi_{0j} + \pi_{1j}$ subject to the constraint $\lambda_1 \leq \lambda_2$ can be found numerically by locating the smallest value among the shaded cells in Table 15.3. Thus, we find that $\alpha_{1j}(\lambda_1) + \alpha_{2j}(\lambda_2) + \pi_{0j} + \pi_{1j}$ is minimized, subject to the constraint $\lambda_1 \leq \lambda_2$, when $0 \leq \lambda_1 \leq \lambda_2 < \frac{1}{3}$ (and the minimum value of $\alpha_{1j}(\lambda_1) + \alpha_{2j}(\lambda_2) + \pi_{0j} + \pi_{1j}$ under the constraint $\lambda_1 \leq \lambda_2$ is shown in Table 15.3 as 0.5535, which is the global minimum value of the function in this scenario). Note that the numerical results coincide with the results discussed above obtained using (16) and (17).

Thus, the decision error probability in (13) (which requires $\lambda_{1j} \leq \lambda_{2j}$) is minimized when $0 \leq \lambda_{1j} \leq \lambda_{2j} < \frac{1}{3}$ (hence the choice $\lambda_{1j} = \lambda_1^* \approx 0.1968$ and $\lambda_{2j} = \lambda_2^* \approx 0.2984$ is in this set of minimizing values); the decision error probability in (14) is minimized when $\lambda_1^{(1)} \in \left[0, \frac{1}{3}\right)$ (hence the choice $\lambda_1^{(1)} = \lambda_1^* \approx 0.1968$ is in this set of minimizing values); and the decision error probability in (15) is minimized when $\lambda_2^{(j_{\max})} \in \left[0, \frac{1}{3}\right)$ (hence the choice $\lambda_2^{(j_{\max})} = \lambda_2^* \approx 0.2984$ is in this set of minimizing values). In this scenario, since $\hat{p}_j$ takes values in the set $\left\{0, \frac{1}{3}, \frac{2}{3}, 1\right\}$, these minimizing values lead to the following decision rule.

Case 1: $j \in \{2,3,\ldots,j_{\max}-1\}$ and $j_{\max} \geq 3$.

- If $\hat{p}_j = 0$, then escalate the dose to level $j+1$.

- If $\hat{p}_j \in \left\{\dfrac{1}{3},\dfrac{2}{3},1\right\}$, then deescalate the dose to level $j-1$.

Case $j = 1$:

- If $\hat{p}_1 = 0$, then escalate the dose to level 2.

- If $\hat{p}_j \in \left\{\dfrac{1}{3},\dfrac{2}{3},1\right\}$, then retain dose level 1.

Case $j = j_{\max}$:

- If $\hat{p}_j \in \left\{\dfrac{1}{3},\dfrac{2}{3},1\right\}$, then deescalate the dose to level $j-1$.

- If $\hat{p}_j = 0$, then retain dose level j.

Dose Elimination Rule: As discussed in Section 15.1.3 the BOIN design adds an additional component based on the dose elimination rule defined in (8). To apply the dose elimination rule as defined in (8), we use (11) to calculate the probability $P(p_j > \phi \mid m_j)$. In this scenario, this probability approximately equals 0.3164, 0.7383, 0.9492, and 0.9961, when m_j equals 0, 1, 2, and 3, respectively. Thus, when $m_j = 3$, $P(p_j > \phi \mid m_j) > 0.95$, so in this scenario (recall $n_j = 3$ in this example) if $\hat{p}_j = \dfrac{3}{3} = 1$, then dose levels j and higher (that is, dose levels $j, j+1, \ldots, J$) would be eliminated from the trial. If $j = 1$ and $\hat{p}_1 = 1$, then the trial would be terminated (this action of terminating the trial would supersede the action to "retain" given by the decision rule above). As discussed by Liu and Yuan (2015) the dose elimination rule does not actually need to be evaluated in real time during conduct of the trial; instead, the dose elimination boundaries can be calculated and enumerated prior to conducting the trial as a function of n_j.

Remark. Each of the following examples has $\phi = 0.25$ and $n_j = 3$, and therefore the calculations of the probability $P(p_j > \phi \mid m_j)$ that appear in the dose elimination rule (8) are the same as in Example 1. Thus, in the following examples, applying the dose elimination rule defined in (8) leads to the following. If $\hat{p}_j = 1$, then the dose levels j and higher (that is, dose levels $j, j+1, \ldots, J$) would be eliminated from the trial. The following examples assume that j does not equal 1, so the action of terminating the trial does not appear.

TABLE 15.4

Numerical evaluation of the functions $\alpha_{1j}(\lambda_1)$ and $\alpha_{2j}(\lambda_2)$ for the scenario of Example 2. These functions take the constant value given in the table over each interval shown. Function values were rounded to four decimal places when necessary.

λ_1	$\alpha_{1j}(\lambda_1)$	λ_2	$\alpha_{2j}(\lambda_2)$
$\lambda_1 \in (-\infty, 0)$	0	$\lambda_2 \in (-\infty, 0)$	0
$\lambda_1 \in \left[0, \frac{1}{3}\right)$	-0.0577	$\lambda_2 \in \left[0, \frac{1}{3}\right)$	-0.0167
$\lambda_1 \in \left[\frac{1}{3}, \frac{2}{3}\right)$	-0.0286	$\lambda_2 \in \left[\frac{1}{3}, \frac{2}{3}\right)$	0.0342
$\lambda_1 \in \left[\frac{2}{3}, 1\right)$	-0.0037	$\lambda_2 \in \left[\frac{2}{3}, 1\right)$	0.0875
$\lambda_1 \in [1, \infty)$	0	$\lambda_2 \in [1, \infty)$	0.1

Example 2

Consider a scenario where the current dose level is $j \in \{2, 3, \ldots, j_{\max} - 1\}$ and $j_{\max} \geq 3$, and

$n_j = 3,$	$\pi_{0j} = 0.3,$	$\pi_{1j} = 0.3,$	$\pi_{2j} = 0.4,$	$\phi = 0.25,$	$\phi_1 = 0.15,$	$\phi_2 = 0.35.$

Applying (4) we obtain $\lambda_{1j}^* \approx 0.1968$ and $\lambda_{2j}^* \approx 0.0984$ which do not satisfy the condition $\lambda_{1j}^* \leq \lambda_{2j}^*$. Numerical evaluation of the functions $\alpha_{1j}(\lambda_1)$ and $\alpha_{2j}(\lambda_2)$ (defined in (12)) is shown in Table 15.4. Numerical evaluation of $\alpha_{1j}(\lambda_1) + \alpha_{2j}(\lambda_2) + \pi_{0j} + \pi_{1j}$, which, when $\lambda_1 \leq \lambda_2$, represents the probability of making an incorrect decision as a function of λ_1 and λ_2 (see (13)) is shown in Table 15.5.

The minimizing values of $\alpha_{1j}(\lambda_1)$ and $\alpha_{2j}(\lambda_2)$ can be found numerically using Table 15.4. Specifically, Table 15.4 demonstrates that $\alpha_{1j}(\lambda_1)$ is minimized when $\lambda_1 \in \left[0, \frac{1}{3}\right)$ and $\alpha_{2j}(\lambda_2)$ is minimized when $\lambda_2 \in \left[0, \frac{1}{3}\right)$ (and the minimum values of $\alpha_{1j}(\lambda_1)$ and $\alpha_{2j}(\lambda_2)$ are shown in Table 15.4 as -0.0577 and -0.0167, respectively). These intervals for λ_1 and λ_2 on which the functions $\alpha_{1j}(\lambda_1)$ and $\alpha_{2j}(\lambda_2)$ are minimized could also be obtained using (16) and (17), respectively. To apply (16), observe that $y_j^* \approx 0.5904$, and therefore by (16), $\alpha_{1j}(\lambda_1)$ is minimized when λ_1 is in the interval

$$\left[\frac{\lceil y_j^* \rceil - 1}{n_j}, \frac{\lfloor y_j^* \rfloor + 1}{n_j}\right) = \left[\frac{\lceil 0.5904 \rceil - 1}{3}, \frac{\lfloor 0.5904 \rfloor + 1}{3}\right) = \left[\frac{1-1}{3}, \frac{0+1}{3}\right) = \left[0, \frac{1}{3}\right) \quad \text{which}$$

coincides with the minimizing interval found numerically using Table 15.4. To apply (17),

TABLE 15.5

Numerical evaluation of the function $\alpha_{1j}(\lambda_1) + \alpha_{2j}(\lambda_2) + \pi_{0j} + \pi_{1j}$ for the scenario of Example 2. This function takes the constant value given in the table over each subset of $\mathbb{R}^2$ indicated by the combination of row and column. The shaded cells correspond to subsets of $\mathbb{R}^2$ on which the function $\alpha_{1j}(\lambda_1) + \alpha_{2j}(\lambda_2) + \pi_{0j} + \pi_{1j}$ is constant and there exist values λ_1 and λ_2 satisfying $\lambda_1 \leq \lambda_2$. Function values were rounded to four decimal places when necessary.

	$\lambda_2 \in (-\infty, 0)$	$\lambda_2 \in \left[0, \frac{1}{3}\right)$	$\lambda_2 \in \left[\frac{1}{3}, \frac{2}{3}\right)$	$\lambda_2 \in \left[\frac{2}{3}, 1\right)$	$\lambda_2 \in (1, \infty)$
$\lambda_1 \in (-\infty, 0)$	0.6	0.5833	0.6342	0.6875	0.7
$\lambda_1 \in \left[0, \frac{1}{3}\right)$	0.5423	0.5256	0.5765	0.6299	0.6423
$\lambda_1 \in \left[\frac{1}{3}, \frac{2}{3}\right)$	0.5714	0.5546	0.6055	0.6589	0.6714
$\lambda_1 \in \left[\frac{2}{3}, 1\right)$	0.5963	0.5796	0.6305	0.6839	0.6963
$\lambda_1 \in [1, \infty)$	0.6	0.5833	0.6342	0.6875	0.7

observe that $y_j^{**} \approx 0.2953$, and therefore by (17), $\alpha_{2j}(\lambda_2)$ is minimized when λ_2 is in the

interval $\left[\dfrac{\lceil y_j^{**}\rceil - 1}{n_j}, \dfrac{\lfloor y_j^{**}\rfloor + 1}{n_j}\right) = \left[\dfrac{\lceil 0.2953\rceil - 1}{3}, \dfrac{\lfloor 0.2953\rfloor + 1}{3}\right) = \left[\dfrac{1-1}{3}, \dfrac{0+1}{3}\right) = \left[0, \dfrac{1}{3}\right)$

which coincides with the minimizing interval found numerically using Table 15.4.

The minimizing value of $\alpha_{1j}(\lambda_1) + \alpha_{2j}(\lambda_2) + \pi_{0j} + \pi_{1j}$ (which, when $\lambda_1 \leq \lambda_2$ represents the probability of making an incorrect decision as a function of the escalation boundary λ_1 and deescalation boundary λ_2) subject to the constraint $\lambda_1 \leq \lambda_2$ can be found numerically using Table 15.5. The shaded cells in Table 15.5 correspond to subsets of the domain of the function of $\alpha_{1j}(\lambda_1) + \alpha_{2j}(\lambda_2) + \pi_{0j} + \pi_{1j}$ where there exist values λ_1 and λ_2 satisfying $\lambda_1 \leq \lambda_2$ (for some of the subsets corresponding to the shaded cells all values of λ_1 and λ_2 in the subset satisfy $\lambda_1 \leq \lambda_2$, and for others some but not all values of λ_1 and λ_2 in the subset satisfy $\lambda_1 \leq \lambda_2$). Therefore, the minimizing value of $\alpha_{1j}(\lambda_1) + \alpha_{2j}(\lambda_2) + \pi_{0j} + \pi_{1j}$ subject to the constraint $\lambda_1 \leq \lambda_2$ can be found numerically by locating the smallest value among the shaded cells in Table 15.5. Thus, we find that $\alpha_{1j}(\lambda_1) + \alpha_{2j}(\lambda_2) + \pi_{0j} + \pi_{1j}$ is minimized, subject to the constraint $\lambda_1 \leq \lambda_2$, when $0 \leq \lambda_1 \leq \lambda_2 < \dfrac{1}{3}$ (and the minimum value of $\alpha_{1j}(\lambda_1) + \alpha_{2j}(\lambda_2) + \pi_{0j} + \pi_{1j}$ under the constraint $\lambda_1 \leq \lambda_2$ is shown in Table 15.5 as 0.5256).

Note that in this example, the values $\lambda_{1j}^* \approx 0.1968$ and $\lambda_{2j}^* \approx 0.0984$ did not satisfy $\lambda_{1j}^* \leq \lambda_{2j}^*$; however, because $\alpha_{1j}(\lambda_1)$ is minimized when $\lambda_1 \in \left[0, \frac{1}{3}\right)$ and $\alpha_{2j}(\lambda_2)$ is minimized when $\lambda_2 \in \left[0, \frac{1}{3}\right)$, any values of λ_1 and λ_2 satisfying $0 \leq \lambda_1 \leq \lambda_2 < \frac{1}{3}$ will globally minimize $\alpha_{1j}(\lambda_1) + \alpha_{2j}(\lambda_2) + \pi_{0j} + \pi_{1j}$ while also satisfying the constraint $\lambda_1 \leq \lambda_2$. Thus, although in this example we do not have $\lambda_{1j}^* \leq \lambda_{2j}^*$, here there still exist values of λ_1 and λ_2 that globally minimize $\alpha_{1j}(\lambda_1) + \alpha_{2j}(\lambda_2) + \pi_{0j} + \pi_{1j}$ and satisfy $\lambda_1 \leq \lambda_2$. Finally note that in this example $\hat{p}_j$ takes values in the set $\left\{0, \frac{1}{3}, \frac{2}{3}, 1\right\}$ and decision boundaries λ_1 and λ_2 satisfying $0 \leq \lambda_1 \leq \lambda_2 < \frac{1}{3}$ will result in the following decision rule for this scenario.

- If $\hat{p}_j = 0$, then escalate the dose to level $j+1$.

- If $\hat{p}_j \in \left\{\frac{1}{3}, \frac{2}{3}, 1\right\}$, then deescalate the dose to level $j-1$.

As there is no value $\hat{p}_j \in \left\{0, \frac{1}{3}, \frac{2}{3}, 1\right\}$ satisfying $0 \leq \lambda_1 < \hat{p}_j \leq \lambda_2 < \frac{1}{3}$, the action of retaining the current dose level j has probability zero in this scenario.

Example 3
Consider a scenario where the current dose level is $j \in \{2, 3, \ldots, j_{max} - 1\}$ and $j_{max} \geq 3$, and

$n_j = 3$,	$\pi_{0j} = 0.25$,	$\pi_{1j} = 0.50$,	$\pi_{2j} = 0.25$,	$\phi = 0.25$,	$\phi_1 = 0.15$,	$\phi_2 = 0.35$.

Applying (4) we obtain $\lambda_{1j}^* \approx 0.5601$ and $\lambda_{2j}^* \approx 0.2984$ which do not satisfy the condition $\lambda_{1j}^* \leq \lambda_{2j}^*$. Numerical evaluation of the functions $\alpha_{1j}(\lambda_1)$ and $\alpha_{2j}(\lambda_2)$ (defined in (12)) is shown in Table 15.6. Numerical evaluation of $\alpha_{1j}(\lambda_1) + \alpha_{2j}(\lambda_2) + \pi_{0j} + \pi_{1j}$, which, when $\lambda_1 \leq \lambda_2$, represents the probability of making an incorrect decision as a function of λ_1 and λ_2 (see (13)) is shown in Table 15.7.

Table 15.6 demonstrates that $\alpha_{1j}(\lambda_1)$ is minimized when $\lambda_1 \in \left[\frac{1}{3}, \frac{2}{3}\right)$ and $\alpha_{2j}(\lambda_2)$ is minimized when $\lambda_2 \in \left[0, \frac{1}{3}\right)$ (and the minimum values of $\alpha_{1j}(\lambda_1)$ and $\alpha_{2j}(\lambda_2)$ are shown in Table 15.6 as -0.2587 and -0.0368, respectively). These intervals for λ_1 and λ_2 on which the functions $\alpha_{1j}(\lambda_1)$ and $\alpha_{2j}(\lambda_2)$ are minimized could also

TABLE 15.6

Numerical evaluation of the functions $\alpha_{1j}(\lambda_1)$ and $\alpha_{2j}(\lambda_1)$ for the scenario of Example 3. These functions take the constant value given in the table over each interval shown. Function values were rounded to four decimal places when necessary.

λ_1	$\alpha_{1j}(\lambda_1)$	λ_2	$\alpha_{2j}(\lambda_2)$
$\lambda_1 \in (-\infty, 0)$	0	$\lambda_2 \in (-\infty, 0)$	0
$\lambda_1 \in \left[0, \frac{1}{3}\right)$	-0.2016	$\lambda_2 \in \left[0, \frac{1}{3}\right)$	-0.0368
$\lambda_1 \in \left[\frac{1}{3}, \frac{2}{3}\right)$	-0.2587	$\lambda_2 \in \left[\frac{1}{3}, \frac{2}{3}\right)$	-0.0314
$\lambda_1 \in \left[\frac{2}{3}, 1\right)$	-0.2522	$\lambda_2 \in \left[\frac{2}{3}, 1\right)$	-0.0068
$\lambda_1 \in [1, \infty)$	-0.25	$\lambda_2 \in [1, \infty)$	0

be obtained using (16) and (17), respectively. To apply (16), observe that $y_j^* \approx 1.6803$, and therefore by (16), $\alpha_{1j}(\lambda_1)$ is minimized when λ_1 is in the interval

$$\left[\frac{\lceil y_j^*\rceil - 1}{n_j}, \frac{\lfloor y_j^*\rfloor + 1}{n_j}\right) = \left[\frac{\lceil 1.6803 \rceil - 1}{3}, \frac{\lfloor 1.6803 \rfloor + 1}{3}\right) = \left[\frac{2-1}{3}, \frac{1+1}{3}\right) = \left[\frac{1}{3}, \frac{2}{3}\right)$$ which

coincides with the minimizing interval found numerically using Table 15.6. To apply (17), observe that $y_j^{**} \approx 0.8952$, and therefore by (17), $\alpha_{2j}(\lambda_2)$ is minimized when λ_2 is in the

interval $\left[\frac{\lceil y_j^{**}\rceil - 1}{n_j}, \frac{\lfloor y_j^{**}\rfloor + 1}{n_j}\right) = \left[\frac{\lceil 0.8952 \rceil - 1}{3}, \frac{\lfloor 0.8952 \rfloor + 1}{3}\right) = \left[\frac{1-1}{3}, \frac{0+1}{3}\right) = \left[0, \frac{1}{3}\right)$

which coincides with the minimizing interval found numerically using Table 15.6.

The minimizing value of $\alpha_{1j}(\lambda_1) + \alpha_{2j}(\lambda_2) + \pi_{0j} + \pi_{1j}$ subject to the constraint $\lambda_1 \leq \lambda_2$ can be found numerically by locating the smallest value among the shaded cells in Table 15.7. Thus, we find that $\alpha_{1j}(\lambda_1) + \alpha_{2j}(\lambda_2) + \pi_{0j} + \pi_{1j}$ is minimized, subject to the constraint $\lambda_1 \leq \lambda_2$, when $\frac{1}{3} \leq \lambda_1 \leq \lambda_2 < \frac{2}{3}$ (and the minimum value of $\alpha_{1j}(\lambda_1) + \alpha_{2j}(\lambda_2) + \pi_{0j} + \pi_{1j}$

under the constraint $\lambda_1 \leq \lambda_2$ is shown in Table 15.7 as 0.4599).

Note that in this example, the minimum value of $\alpha_{1j}(\lambda_1) + \alpha_{2j}(\lambda_2) + \pi_{0j} + \pi_{1j}$ under the constraint $\lambda_1 \leq \lambda_2$ differs from the global minimum of $\alpha_{1j}(\lambda_1) + \alpha_{2j}(\lambda_2) + \pi_{0j} + \pi_{1j}$

which occurs when $\lambda_1 \in \left[\frac{1}{3}, \frac{2}{3}\right)$ and $\lambda_2 \in \left[0, \frac{1}{3}\right)$. Finally note that in this example $\hat{p}_j$

takes values in the set $\left\{0, \frac{1}{3}, \frac{2}{3}, 1\right\}$ and any decision boundaries λ_1 and λ_2 satisfying

$\frac{1}{3} \leq \lambda_1 \leq \lambda_2 < \frac{2}{3}$ will result in the following decision rule for this scenario.

TABLE 15.7

Numerical evaluation of the function $\alpha_{1j}(\lambda_1) + \alpha_{2j}(\lambda_2) + \pi_{0j} + \pi_{1j}$ for the scenario of Example 3. This function takes the constant value given in the table over each subset of $\mathbb{R}^2$ indicated by the combination of row and column. The shaded cells correspond to subsets of $\mathbb{R}^2$ on which the function $\alpha_{1j}(\lambda_1) + \alpha_{2j}(\lambda_2) + \pi_{0j} + \pi_{1j}$ is constant and there exist values λ_1 and λ_2 satisfying $\lambda_1 \le \lambda_2$. Function values were rounded to four decimal places when necessary.

	$\lambda_2 \in (-\infty, 0)$	$\lambda_2 \in \left[0, \frac{1}{3}\right)$	$\lambda_2 \in \left[\frac{1}{3}, \frac{2}{3}\right)$	$\lambda_2 \in \left[\frac{2}{3}, 1\right)$	$\lambda_2 \in [1, \infty)$
$\lambda_1 \in (-\infty, 0)$	0.75	0.7132	0.7186	0.7432	0.75
$\lambda_1 \in \left[0, \frac{1}{3}\right)$	0.5484	0.5116	0.5170	0.5416	0.5484
$\lambda_1 \in \left[\frac{1}{3}, \frac{2}{3}\right)$	0.4913	0.4545	0.4599	0.4845	0.4913
$\lambda_1 \in \left[\frac{2}{3}, 1\right)$	0.4978	0.4610	0.4664	0.4910	0.4978
$\lambda_1 \in [1, \infty)$	0.5	0.4632	0.4686	0.4932	0.5

- If $\hat{p}_j \in 0$, then escalate the dose to level $j+1$.

- If $\hat{p}_j \in \left\{\frac{1}{3}, \frac{2}{3}, 1\right\}$, then deescalate the dose to level $j-1$.

As there is no value $\hat{p}_j \in \left\{0, \frac{1}{3}, \frac{2}{3}, 1\right\}$ satisfying $\frac{1}{3} \le \lambda_1 < \hat{p}_j \le \lambda_2 < \frac{2}{3}$, the action of retaining the current dose level j has probability zero in this scenario.

Example 4

Consider a scenario where the current dose level is $j \in \{2, 3, \ldots, j_{\max}\}$ and $j_{\max} \ge 3$, and

$n_j = 3,$	$\pi_{0j} = 0.25,$	$\pi_{1j} = 0.25,$	$\pi_{2j} = 0.50,$	$\phi = 0.25,$	$\phi_1 = 0.15,$	$\phi_2 = 0.35.$

Applying (4) we obtain $\lambda_{1j}^* \approx 0.1968$ and $\lambda_{2j}^* \approx -0.1834$ which do not satisfy the condition $\lambda_{1j}^* \le \lambda_{2j}^*$. Numerical evaluation of the functions $\alpha_{1j}(\lambda_1)$ and $\alpha_{2j}(\lambda_2)$ (defined in (12)) is shown in Table 15.8. Numerical evaluation of $\alpha_{1j}(\lambda_1) + \alpha_{2j}(\lambda_2) + \pi_{0j} + \pi_{1j}$, which, when $\lambda_1 \le \lambda_2$, represents the probability of making an incorrect decision as a function of λ_1 and λ_2 (see (13)) is shown in Table 15.9.

Table 15.8 demonstrates that $\alpha_{1j}(\lambda_1)$ is minimized when $\lambda_1 \in \left[0, \frac{1}{3}\right)$ and $\alpha_{2j}(\lambda_2)$ is minimized when $\lambda_2 \in (-\infty, 0)$ (and the minimum values of $\alpha_{1j}(\lambda_1)$ and

TABLE 15.8

Numerical evaluation of the functions $\alpha_{1j}(\lambda_1)$ and $\alpha_{2j}(\lambda_2)$ for the scenario of Example 4. These functions take the constant value given in the table over each interval shown. Function values were rounded to four decimal places when necessary.

λ_1	$\alpha_{1j}(\lambda_1)$	λ_2	$\alpha_{2j}(\lambda_2)$
$\lambda_1 \in (-\infty, 0)$	0	$\lambda_2 \in (-\infty, 0)$	0
$\lambda_1 \in \left[0, \frac{1}{3}\right)$	−0.0481	$\lambda_2 \in \left[0, \frac{1}{3}\right)$	0.0318
$\lambda_1 \in \left[\frac{1}{3}, \frac{2}{3}\right)$	−0.0239	$\lambda_2 \in \left[\frac{1}{3}, \frac{2}{3}\right)$	0.1482
$\lambda_1 \in \left[\frac{2}{3}, 1\right)$	−0.0031	$\lambda_2 \in \left[\frac{2}{3}, 1\right)$	0.2325
$\lambda_1 \in [1, \infty)$	0	$\lambda_2 \in [1, \infty)$	0.25

TABLE 15.9

Numerical evaluation of the function $\alpha_{1j}(\lambda_1) + \alpha_{2j}(\lambda_2) + \pi_{0j} + \pi_{1j}$ for the scenario of Example 4. This function takes the constant value given in the table over each subset of $\mathbb{R}^2$ indicated by the combination of row and column. The shaded cells correspond to subsets of $\mathbb{R}^2$ on which the function $\alpha_{1j}(\lambda_1) + \alpha_{2j}(\lambda_2) + \pi_{0j} + \pi_{1j}$ is constant and there exist values λ_1 and λ_2 satisfying $\lambda_1 \leq \lambda_2$. Function values were rounded to four decimal places when necessary.

	$\lambda_2 \in (-\infty, 0)$	$\lambda_2 \in \left[0, \frac{1}{3}\right)$	$\lambda_2 \in \left[\frac{1}{3}, \frac{2}{3}\right)$	$\lambda_2 \in \left[\frac{2}{3}, 1\right)$	$\lambda_2 \in [1, \infty)$
$\lambda_1 \in (-\infty, 0)$	0.5	0.5318	0.6482	0.7325	0.75
$\lambda_1 \in \left[0, \frac{1}{3}\right)$	0.4519	0.4838	0.6001	0.6844	0.7019
$\lambda_1 \in \left[\frac{1}{3}, \frac{2}{3}\right)$	0.4761	0.5080	0.6243	0.7086	0.7261
$\lambda_1 \in \left[\frac{2}{3}, 1\right)$	0.4969	0.5288	0.6451	0.7294	0.7469
$\lambda_1 \in [1, \infty)$	0.5	0.5318	0.6482	0.7325	0.75

$\alpha_{2j}(\lambda_2)$ are shown in Table 15.8 as −0.0481 and 0, respectively). These intervals for λ_1 and λ_2 on which the functions $\alpha_{1j}(\lambda_1)$ and $\alpha_{2j}(\lambda_2)$ are minimized could also be obtained using (16) and (17), respectively. To apply (16), observe that $y_j^* \approx 0.5904$, and therefore by (16), $\alpha_{1j}(\lambda_1)$ is minimized when λ_1 is in the interval

$$\left[\frac{\lceil y_j^* \rceil - 1}{n_j}, \frac{\lfloor y_j^* \rfloor + 1}{n_j}\right) = \left[\frac{\lceil 0.5904 \rceil - 1}{3}, \frac{\lfloor 0.5904 \rfloor + 1}{3}\right) = \left[\frac{1-1}{3}, \frac{0+1}{3}\right) = \left[0, \frac{1}{3}\right)$$ which

coincides with the minimizing interval found numerically using Table 15.8. To apply (17), observe that $y_j^{**} \approx -0.5502$, and therefore by (17), $\alpha_{2j}(\lambda_2)$ is minimized when λ_2 is in the

interval $\left(-\infty, \dfrac{I(y_j^{**}=0)}{n_j}\right) = (-\infty, 0)$ which coincides with the minimizing interval found

numerically Table 15.8.

The minimizing value of $\alpha_{1j}(\lambda_1) + \alpha_{2j}(\lambda_2) + \pi_{0j} + \pi_{1j}$ subject to the constraint $\lambda_1 \leq \lambda_2$ can be found numerically by locating the smallest value among the shaded cells in Table 15.9. Thus, we find that $\alpha_{1j}(\lambda_1) + \alpha_{2j}(\lambda_2) + \pi_{0j} + \pi_{1j}$ is minimized, subject to the constraint $\lambda_1 \leq \lambda_2$, when $0 \leq \lambda_1 \leq \lambda_2 < \dfrac{1}{3}$ (and the minimum value of $\alpha_{1j}(\lambda_1) + \alpha_{2j}(\lambda_2) + \pi_{0j} + \pi_{1j}$ under the constraint $\lambda_1 \leq \lambda_2$ is shown in Table 15.9 as 0.4838).

Note that in this example, the minimum value of $\alpha_{1j}(\lambda_1) + \alpha_{2j}(\lambda_2) + \pi_{0j} + \pi_{1j}$ under the constraint $\lambda_1 \leq \lambda_2$ differs from the global minimum of $\alpha_{1j}(\lambda_1) + \alpha_{2j}(\lambda_2) + \pi_{0j} + \pi_{1j}$ which occurs when $\lambda_1 \in \left[0, \dfrac{1}{3}\right)$ and $\lambda_2 \in (-\infty, 0)$. Finally note that in this example $\hat{p}_j$ takes values in the set $\left\{0, \dfrac{1}{3}, \dfrac{2}{3}, 1\right\}$ and any decision boundaries λ_1 and λ_2 satisfying $0 \leq \lambda_1 \leq \lambda_2 < \dfrac{1}{3}$ will result in the following decision rule for this scenario.

- If $\hat{p}_j = 0$, then escalate the dose to level $j+1$.

- If $\hat{p}_j \in \left\{\dfrac{1}{3}, \dfrac{2}{3}, 1\right\}$, then deescalate the dose to level $j-1$.

As there is no value $\hat{p}_j \in \left\{0, \dfrac{1}{3}, \dfrac{2}{3}, 1\right\}$ satisfying $0 \leq \lambda_1 < \hat{p}_j \leq \lambda_2 < \dfrac{1}{3}$, the action of retaining the current dose level j has probability zero in this scenario.

15.4 Illustration of the Decision Rule under the Noninformative Prior

Consider a hypothetical scenario where the noninformative prior (5) is used and $\phi = 0.25$, $\phi_1 = (0.6)(0.25) = 0.15$, $\phi_2 = (1.4)(0.25) = 0.35$ (which were also the values used in Example 1 in Section 15.3). Further, suppose that $J = 5$ and the maximum sample size is 15 in 5 cohorts each of size 3.

Because the noninformative prior is used in this scenario, we can use (6) to obtain escalation and deescalation boundaries $\lambda_1^* \approx 0.1968$ and $\lambda_2^* \approx 0.2984$ that can be used at each stage of the trial. Hence with decision boundaries $\lambda_1^* \approx 0.1968$ and $\lambda_2^* \approx 0.2984$ used throughout, the decision rule in Table 15.1 gives the following in this scenario.

When the current dose level is $j \in \{2, 3, \ldots, j_{\max} - 1\}$ and $j_{\max} \geq 3$:

- If $\hat{p}_j \leq 0.1968$, then escalate the dose to level $j+1$.
- If $\hat{p}_j > 0.2984$, then deescalate the dose to level $j-1$.
- If $0.1968 < \hat{p}_j \leq 0.2984$, then retain the dose level j.

When the current dose level is $j = 1$ and $j_{\max} \geq 2$:

- If $\hat{p}_j \leq 0.1968$, then escalate the dose to level 2.
- If $\hat{p}_j > 0.1968$, then retain the dose level 1.

When the current dose level is $j = j_{\max}$ and $j_{\max} \geq 2$:

- If $\hat{p}_j > 0.2984$, then deescalate the dose to level $j-1$.
- If $\hat{p}_j \leq 0.2984$, then retain the dose level j.

To apply the dose elimination rule as defined in (8), we use (11) to calculate the probability $P(p_j > \phi \mid m_j)$ in this scenario. The values of the probability $P(p_j > \phi \mid m_j)$ for $\phi = 0.25$, $m_j = 0, 1, \ldots, n_j$, and $n_j = 3, 6, 9, 12, 15$ are shown in Table 15.10 and cells in the

TABLE 15.10

Values of the probability $P(p_j > \phi \mid m_j)$ (for $\phi = 0.25$, $m_j = 0, 1, \ldots, n_j$, and $n_j = 3, 6, 9, 12, 15$) that appear in the dose elimination rule (8) calculated using (11) and rounded to four decimal places. Cells containing values greater than 0.95 are shaded.

m_j	n_j				
	3	6	9	12	15
0	0.3164	0.1335	0.0563	0.0238	0.0100
1	0.7383	0.4449	0.2440	0.1267	0.0635
2	0.9492	0.7564	0.5256	0.3326	0.1971
3	0.9961	0.9294	0.7759	0.5843	0.405
4	-	0.9871	0.9219	0.794	0.6302
5	-	0.9987	0.9803	0.9198	0.8103
6	-	0.9999	0.9965	0.9757	0.9204
7	-	-	0.9996	0.9944	0.9729
8	-	-	1.000	0.999	0.9925
9	-	-	1.000	0.9999	0.9984
10	-	-	-	1.000	0.9997
11	-	-	-	1.000	1.000
12	-	-	-	1.000	1.000
13	-	-	-	-	1.000
14	-	-	-	-	1.000
15	-	-	-	-	1.000

TABLE 15.11

Summary of dose decision rule and dose elimination rule in the example scenario where $\phi = 0.25$, $\phi_1 = 0.15$, $\phi_2 = 0.35$ using the noninformative prior (5) and the maximum sample size is 15 in 5 cohorts each of size 3 (assuming $j_{max} \geq 2$).[1] In this table the action of retaining the dose level j is viewed as the default action to use if the dose is neither escalated nor deescalated.

			n_j		
	3	6	9	12	15
[2]Escalate dose to level $j+1$ if m_j is less than or equal to:	0	1	1	2	2
[3]Deescalate dose to level $j-1$ if m_j is greater than or equal to:	1	2	3	4	5
Eliminate the current dose and any higher doses if m_j is greater than or equal to:	3	4	5	6	7

[1] If $j_{max} = 1$ and the trial is not terminated, the only dosing option is to retain dose level 1 for the next cohort of patients.

[2] In the situation where the dose cannot be escalated because $j = j_{max}$, this action changes to retain dose level j.

[3] In the situation where the dose cannot be deescalated because $j = 1$, this action changes to retain dose level j.

table containing values greater than 0.95 are shaded; thus the dose elimination boundaries are obtained from this table. That is,

- if $n_j = 3$ eliminate the current dose and any higher doses if $m_j = 3$;
- if $n_j = 6$ eliminate the current dose and any higher doses if $m_j \geq 4$;
- if $n_j = 9$ eliminate the current dose and any higher doses if $m_j \geq 5$;
- if $n_j = 12$ eliminate the current dose and any higher doses if $m_j \geq 6$;
- if $n_j = 15$ eliminate the current dose and any higher doses if $m_j \geq 7$.

The decision rule for determining the dose level to use for the next stage of the trial and the dose elimination rule can be summarized in the form shown in Table 15.11. The values of $\lambda_1^* \approx 0.1968$ and $\lambda_2^* \approx 0.2984$ and other information shown in Table 15.11 can be readily obtained using the function get.boundary in the BOIN package (Yan et al., 2020) of the R software (R Core Team, 2022). The get.boundary function in the BOIN R package also gives a table like Table 15.11 for each value $n_j = 1, 2, 3, \ldots$ up to the maximum sample size (which is 15 in this scenario). Information on the BOIN R package can be found in Yan et al. (2020). Ananthakrishnan et al. (2022) discuss the BOIN R package and other software packages implementing the BOIN design. Table 15.11 illustrates how, under the noninformative prior (5), the decision rules of the BOIN design take on a simple form.

15.5 Discussion and Conclusion

Liu and Yuan (2015) present simulation studies evaluating the performance of the BOIN design and comparing its performance with some other available designs for dose finding clinical trials. Other simulation-based evaluations of BOIN that compare it with some other available designs for dose finding clinical trials include Ruppert et al. (2018) and Zhou et al.

(2018). The simulation studies have generally found that the BOIN design performed well in the scenarios considered. Discussion of some of these simulation results also appears in the FDA's statistical review of the BOIN design (FDA, Drug Development Tools: Fit-for-Purpose Initiative). In this paper we have presented the BOIN design and its statistical foundations. This paper focused on the original BOIN design proposed by Liu and Yuan (2015) while incorporating the revisions of Liu and Yuan (2022). Several extensions to the original BOIN design have been proposed as described by Ananthakrishnan et al. (2022).

References

Amy S. Ruppert and Abigail B. Shoben. (2018). Overall Success Rate of a Safe and Efficacious Drug: Results Using Six Phase 1 Designs, Each Followed by Standard Phase 2 and 3 Designs. *Contemporary Clinical Trials Communications*, 12: 40–50.

Fangrong Yan, Liangcai Zhang, Yanhong Zhou, Haitao Pan, Suyu Liu, and Ying Yuan (2020). BOIN: An R Package for Designing Single-Agent and Drug-Combination Dose-Finding Trials Using Bayesian Optimal Interval Designs. *Journal of Statistical Software*, 94(13): 1–32.

FDA. (2022). Drug Development Tools: Fit-for-Purpose Initiative. www.fda.gov/drugs/development-approval-process-drugs/drug-development-tools-fit-purpose-initiative

Heng Zhou, Ying Yuan, and Lei Nie. (2018). Accuracy, Safety, and Reliability of Novel Phase I Trial Designs. *Clinical Cancer Research*, 24(18): 4357–4364.

R Core Team (2022). R: A Language and Environment for Statistical Computing. R Foundation for Statistical Computing, Vienna, Austria. www.R-project.org/.

R. E. Barlow, D.J. Bartholomew, J.M. Bremmer, H.D. Brunk (1972). *Statistical Inference Under Order Restrictions*. Wiley.

Revathi Ananthakrishnan, Ruitao Lin, Chunsheng He, Yanping Chen, Daniel Li, and Michael LaValley (2022). An Overview of the BOIN Design and its Current Extensions for Novel Early-Phase Oncology Trials. *Contemporary Clinical Trials Communications*, 28: 100943.

Suyu Liu and Ying Yuan. (2015). Bayesian Optimal Interval Designs for Phase I Clinical Trials. *Journal of the Royal Statistical Society*, Series C, 64(3): 507–523.

Suyu Liu and Ying Yuan (2022). Erratum: Bayesian Optimal Interval Designs for Phase I Clinical Trials. *Journal of the Royal Statistical Society*, Series C, 71: 491–492.

16

Project Management in Innovative Clinical Trial Design

Doray Sitko

This chapter focuses on the essential considerations of project management as it relates to efforts of designing innovative clinical trials. This chapter draws upon the principles of project management that are contained in the seventh edition of the Project Management Institute's *Project Management Body of Knowledge* (PMBOK®), which is the guiding document that Project Management Professionals® (PMPs) learn from and refer to in obtaining their certification and practicing as Project Managers. There are twelve principles that are included in this edition of the PMBOK® Guide, and each makes an appearance in this chapter. Six of these, indicated by bold in the list below, are focused on more extensively, given their importance in the context of innovative clinical trial design efforts. The remainder are discussed briefly at the end of the chapter.

1. Principle One: Stewardship – Be a diligent, respectful, and caring steward.
2. **Principle Two: Team – Build a culture of accountability and respect.**
3. **Principle Three: Stakeholders – Engage stakeholders to understand their interests and needs.**
4. Principle Four: Value – Focus on value.
5. **Principle Five: Holistic Thinking – Recognize and respond to systems' interactions.**
6. **Principle Six: Leadership – Motivate, influence, coach, and learn.**
7. Principle Seven: Tailoring – Tailor the delivery approach based on context.
8. Principle Eight: Quality – Build quality into processes and results.
9. **Principle Nine: Complexity – Address complexity using knowledge, experience, and learning.**
10. Principle Ten: Opportunities & Threats – Address opportunities and threats.
11. Principle Eleven: Adaptability & Resilience – Be adaptable and resilient.
12. Principle Twelve: Change Management – Enable change to achieve the envisioned future state.

16.1 Principle Versus Process

This chapter focuses on a principle-driven, rather than process-driven, methodology. Process-driven methodology requires a particular set of steps in a particular order without exception, whereas principle-driven methodology instead focuses on the overarching goal

DOI: 10.1201/9781003288640-16

or outcome achieved. This important distinction is especially valuable in situations where processes are too prescriptive and restrictive and/or become outdated quickly as the industry and work rapidly evolves. To illustrate this notion, consider a bleeding wound. Focusing on principle-driven methodology, one seeks to stop the bleeding by whatever means are available and appropriate. At home, this might mean a kitchen towel with direct pressure over a cut. On a battlefield, this may mean a tourniquet and, in the hospital, perhaps a suture or surgical intervention. The important outcome, of course, is to preserve the circulation of blood within the body.

As one can imagine, principle-driven methodology makes for a compelling case in the design of innovative clinical trials given that what is innovative today may soon become standard practice and new innovations will emerge. This approach also allows for the Project Manager and other key personnel to select from a range of practical steps that can reflect differences among projects such as industry/entity type, timelines, regulatory bodies providing oversight, and scopes and budgets of all sizes. Perhaps just as important, the principle-driven methodology can reflect the realities of the most dynamic of all aspects of any project – the people working on it. Whereas guidelines and standard operating procedures (SOPs) are useful and even required at times, the management of projects, and thus people, benefit greatly from a more flexible approach. For example, if the goal is meeting a deadline on time, a keen Project Manager will ascertain which team members may need frequent and early "soft deadlines" versus those that perform best when given more absolute "hard deadlines."

Because principles of project management are imparted in the certification of PMP®, those with the credential are sure to be familiar with and able to implement these practices, thus making a compelling case for engaging a PMP® in projects. However, it is recognized that many other management personnel are also capable of understanding and implementing these principles. In this chapter, where the phrase Project Manager is used, it is understood that this may also be a person with another title acting in the role of Project Manager, such as when a Statistician or Clinical Trialist is tapped to lead the design project.

16.2 Vignettes

To help illustrate the principles in action, this chapter includes several vignettes and references to various types of project arrangements. Note that the term project is often used interchangeably in the chapter with the term trial design or effort, since this chapter focuses on the design of a trial or collection of trials.

Vignette One: A small biopharmaceutical company with one key asset suitable for multiple indications is seeking to develop an adaptive clinical trial for its product in a leading indication. The company engages external resources to augment internal staffing and this project spans approximately 2 years from design initiation to the start of patient enrollment. Stakeholders include key opinion leaders, an advisory board, and the company's own personnel including statisticians, executive leadership, and clinicians. The trial is submitted to the Food and Drug Administration (FDA) and will be operationally implemented by a clinical research organization (CRO). The small company engages its personnel in every effort undertaken, and thus each employee is at least familiar with, if not directly involved in, each trial designed by or for the organization. This design effort includes a dedicated Project Manager for the external resource and a dedicated executive leader for the biopharmaceutical company.

In this vignette, we will explore the first and second principles of project management. Principle One is "Stewardship: Be a diligent, respectful, and caring steward." Of special note related to this principle is preserving ethics in an undeniably competitive industry. Much literature and entire courses are devoted to this topic, and it is mentioned here to highlight the importance and acknowledge the difficulties inevitably faced. As Dr. Agnes V. Klein, a Drug Information Association (DIA) volunteer and Senior Medical Advisor for Health Canada, noted in her editorial for Pharma Focus Asia[1]:

> The design of a study is critical in the ethical consideration of the trial. It has generally been recognised that, if the design of a trial is not sound so that the probability of a meaningful outcome (whether positive or negative) cannot be achieved and as a result the hypothesis being tested cannot be proven or disproven, it is generally considered unethical. It is because the human beings enrolled in a trial will have been subjected to potential or real risks for no benefit to either themselves or even to society.

With respect to this vignette, it was clear that the innovative design increased the ethicality of the trial as compared to a traditional or fixed design, given that it would require fewer patients overall and ensure more of them could be allocated to the new therapy. While the ethical design of the trial is the domain of the scientists designing it, for Project Managers involved in these projects it is still necessary to constantly reflect on this principle of stewardship and ensure that actions of the team and collaborators are ethical and caring. This is especially important considering the reality that many trials will ultimately fail to produce a new approval. The definition of success in the project instead focuses on the information gleaned from the attempt.

This principle also applies to the integrity and compliance aspects of managing the design of an innovative clinical trial. Integrity in the context of this vignette included the Project Manager querying their project records before beginning the work to ensure there were no conflicts of interest. In the later stages when confidential trial data was available, the Project Manager worked with the team to account for implementing and adhering to pertinent firewalls so that interim trial data remained confidential.

Consider now Principle Two: "Team: Build a culture of accountability and respect." The design of an innovative clinical trial is likely to include a multidisciplinary team including statisticians, clinicians, data scientists, clinical trialists, a Project Manager, and other personnel. Between the biotech company and the external resource, the vignette included a Project Manager, Human Resource representative, Director of Clinical Trial Execution, Director of Consulting, Senior Statistical Scientist, and Statistical Scientist, as well as other support staff. An important aspect of the team culture is ensuring there is clear authority, accountability, and a sense of responsibility held by each team member. This enables work to progress, enables decision making to occur, and fosters the necessary collaboration of team members that contributes to quality and timeliness. In this vignette, the Project Manager created opportunities for the team members to earn respect of their peers at the biopharmaceutical organization by supporting the creation of a shared code library with adjacent presentations discussing what it contained. The code library was also an accountability activity as it required the author of the code to not only share the code but to examine it as an outsider and create corresponding notes and documentation for its use.

An important project management consideration regarding team members is risk management. There is always a high degree of risk when placing a dependency on a given team member, and this decision must be weighed against considerations such as resources available, in terms of both people and budget, the duration of the project where longer durations increase the likelihood of temporary or permanent loss of a team member, and the complexity and criticality of the effort. Complex and critical projects merit more redundancy in staffing and measures for risk management. This forethought can help weather turnover. The small biotech company in this vignette had a statistician depart the project midway through. However, continuity in the external resource team ensured no disruption to the project and in fact helped to transition the new statistician onto the project by way of knowledge transfer.

Vignette Two: A United States government entity is seeking to develop a platform trial to test multiple treatments for a single indication. This project spans multiple years, costs millions of dollars to develop, and includes many collaborators including the government entity, an intermediary consortium, a CRO, multiple pharmaceutical sponsors, a consulting company, and various regulatory/oversight organizations including the FDA and the Human Research Protection Office (HRPO). The government entity has a dedicated team of assigned personnel, and they are aware of and involved with all aspects of the effort and in direct communication with all the collaborators. There is a dedicated Project Manager for many of the collaborators and the government entity is led by a Sponsor Office Technical Representative (SOTR).

This vignette illustrates Principle Three, "Stakeholders: Engage stakeholders to understand their interests and needs." Perhaps one of the most crucial aspects of Project Management is defining the scope. In innovative clinical trial design, the scope can vary based on the phase of the trial, the type of innovation(s) contemplated, and how much work is already done either by the Sponsor or other researchers. For example, in this vignette, a new clinical endpoint was proposed, and evaluating that endpoint added to the scope and timeline. If the trial is going to be submitted to a regulatory body such as the FDA, the scope will need to reflect the related regulatory activities that are required, such as a briefing book and likely multiple meetings with the Agency.

A Project Manager must ensure that as much detail as possible is understood about the interests and needs of the stakeholders upfront to plan appropriate resources, communicate the information to the team, and confirm that interested stakeholders are kept informed throughout the design process. There is a tendency by many parties involved in clinical trial design to hold separate meetings with clinical personnel, statistical personnel, operations, funders, etc. This causes a silo effect for the groups instead of creating an important cross-functional dialogue. The most successful clinical trial design projects, and in fact most projects in general, are those in which multidisciplinary parties communicate at and even before key decision points. Discussions must be arranged such that pertinent team members are in fact granted access to important conversations. Here the Project Manager played a crucial role in arranging meetings and advocating for the scientific design team to ensure that they were able to fully participate in sharing information with and collecting feedback from all stakeholders. This helps avoid the common challenge of information being misunderstood or miscommunicated along the way. This also expedites the process by eliminating the need for multiple meetings or communications to convey information to all parties. Further, it helps to reinforce other principles such as respect, accountability, and leadership including education.

In some cases, a written communication plan is appropriate and can be a helpful tool for documenting communication expectations. The government entity required such a plan, and it was updated as necessary during the project to reflect changes to personnel or to add or remove communication activities and channels as conditions changed. Even where a formal written plan is not created, it can help to have an internally defined set of standard practices. The specifics of these practices will vary from organization to organization and perhaps even project to project, but identifying and consistently using communication tools (e.g., Slack, Microsoft Teams, email) and holding regular communication forums (e.g., a twice-monthly team meeting, a weekly one on one, a daily standup) are good practices to foster communication within a team and with other stakeholders. These can also provide a means of early detection of any potential challenges or even identify when work is progressing faster than anticipated and whether additional tasks can be initiated sooner than planned.

This vignette also illustrates Principle Five, "Holistic Thinking: Recognize and respond to systems' interactions." Here the Project Manager in innovative clinical trial design projects will need to understand the ways in which the organization and trial fit into the larger picture. For instance, in this vignette, the trial is just one of many that the government entity was funding to address various health conditions faced by a target population served by the same. Moreover, in addition to creating a design that satisfies the government organization, it must also comply with HRPO requirements, meet FDA approval, be attractive to potential pharmaceutical partners, be able to be implemented by the CRO, and be able to recruit and retain patients in the trial. Innovative designs often have aspects that are more desirable to patients, such as 2:1 randomization, a cross-over design, or the potential to transition to a new regimen if a treatment is not effective. At the same time, the design must pass muster for regulatory approval and must capture data that is adequate for a valid analysis. Recognizing these interactions and needs helps create realistic designs that are viable, which preserve integrity, and help sustain a demand for innovative designs.

Vignette Three: A large multinational pharmaceutical company with hundreds of different products for many different indications is simultaneously developing several innovative and traditional clinical trials in various stages of development. This entity combines in-house resources with various sources of external support and each project has a unique timeline, scope, budget, and team and may have different regulatory oversight including FDA, European Medicines Agency (EMA), and other government bodies as well as Internal Review Boards (IRBs), advisory boards, key opinion leaders, and other stakeholders. Because of the large nature of this organization and its extensive portfolio, there is often a lack of awareness or involvement of the pharmaceutical company's personnel across projects. However, a single point of contact provides executive oversight to all the innovative trial design projects that are undertaken with the support of a given external resource, and a dedicated Project Manager at the external resource oversees all efforts undertaken by personnel there. The relationship between the pharmaceutical company and the external support from a given resource spans multiple years and encompasses more than 15 different trial design projects.

Here we will turn to Principle Six, "Leadership: Motivate, influence, coach, and learn." In innovative clinical trial design, there is a persistent need to ensure that those who best understand the latest innovative approaches are not only carrying out the work of designing the trials but also are intentionally and indirectly providing education of other team members, stakeholders, partners, regulators, patients, clinicians, and even the public. The point of contact from the large pharmaceutical company in this vignette, for example, not only influenced those personnel at that company but later went on to introduce an entirely new organization to innovative designs when hired by a different company. This organic process can account for much of the spread in the interest and understanding of adaptive designs, especially as personnel change employers, receive promotional advances, and regularly expand their collaborators in the course of their duties.

The process of designing a trial that is accepted by a sponsor, enrolled in by patients, approved by a regulator, and delivers data that can be successfully analyzed and from which conclusions can be drawn will inherently inform and enlighten those who participate in the design, implementation, analysis, and result sharing. Likely this will also influence those who were involved with it to consider innovative designs for future needs. However, it is not sufficient to educate only passively. Perhaps the most obvious means of furthering knowledge of what innovative clinical trials are, how they can be used, where they are most or least useful, and how well they deliver the desired outcomes is through established professional networks. Some good examples of networks and groups that have and continue to promote these learnings include DIA, the National Institute of Neurological Disorders and Stroke Clinical Trials Methodology Course (CTMC), the Society of Clinical Trials (SCT), American Statistical Association (ASA) Biopharmaceutical Section, and working groups from government agencies including FDA, Health and Human Services, and others. The National Heart, Lung, and Blood Institute funded an effort to provide access to educational materials related to innovative clinical trial design called the Innovative Clinical Trial Resource. This initiative included an in-person short course, recorded webinars and videos, and live question-and-answer opportunities.[2] The intent of these materials was to educate not only those interested in designing innovative trials but also those who review grant applications, provide regulatory oversight, and serve on Data Safety Monitoring Boards (DSMBs).

There is a need to use empathy and flexibility to bridge the gap from what is already known and understood by an audience to new material that well explains innovative design elements. Those recognized as skilled in translating complex material into an understandable format should be identified and called upon as often as possible. For example, the Principal Investigator supporting this effort for the given resource was able to conduct a web-based informational learning session early in the project, with attendance by representatives from the large pharmaceutical company. Efforts such as this are crucial, and Project Managers should actively seek out opportunities for team members to participate in educational outreach so that innovative designs are welcomed and even requested in appropriate situations.

The last of our key principles, Principle Nine, is "Complexity: Address complexity using knowledge, experience, and learning." The overarching theme of this chapter, and in fact this book, is that innovative clinical trials are or tend to be perceived as complex, and that all persons responsible for their design and implementation must use knowledge, experience, and learning to address that complexity. Like all projects, too, the size of the projects is larger, usually but not always, correlating to the size of the eventual clinical trial. In addition, the more innovative aspects of the design, the more complex it will be to conceive, evaluate, and execute. Higher-value or pressure projects like a novel therapy for a fatal disease that is in the confirmatory phase of development or those that reflect incredible societal need such as a treatment for Ebola during an acute large-scale outbreak may also face additional complexities with increased pressures on timelines, or more media/public interest. And, of course, anything that is considered "new" in an industry, which is much of what innovative designs are, at least for some introductory period, is inherently considered more complex. Publications such as case studies, journal articles, and other media can help cast light on positive experiences that provide further assurance. Project Managers should support publication efforts, conference/speaking engagements, and other such activities that address complexity. Not to be overlooked is the education of patients as well. Patient advocacy groups can be a great source of information sharing for this purpose.

A crucial need that must be ascertained by the Project Manager is related to the timeline for efforts. Sponsors often have desires related to timelines that may reflect funding opportunities, demands from executive leadership, and goals for trial enrollment/start dates, among other priorities. In innovative clinical trial design, much of the design timeline is dependent on the iterative nature of the work. While fixed and traditional designs also have various decision points and require communication to proceed, the complex nature of innovative designs and the typical modeling and simulation work involved often require more intense iteration. It is not unusual for an innovative design to undergo multiple permutations as options are simulated, presented, debated, and considered. In fact, even when decisions are made rapidly, the process can take weeks to months, and this can vary with the amount of labor available to contribute. Some innovative trial designs will require custom computer coding and extensive simulations. Coding requires time and even with an ample supply of labor, improvements in computing power, or the reuse of some existing code, there is a certain amount of time that cannot be expedited as hundreds, thousands, or even tens of thousands of simulations are run.

The COVID-19 pandemic presented an unprecedented scenario in which essentially the world was immediately united in quickly finding effective treatments. Even in this case where resources were available in typically unheard-of abundance, the designs for a platform trial testing multiple therapies could only be expedited to be open for enrollment in, at best, a matter of weeks. Even then, changes continued to occur as the trial was enrolling, partly because of new information becoming available and partly because some decisions were necessarily delayed allowing the trial to begin enrollment faster. The regulatory review period is variable as well, both within a regulatory agency and between them (e.g., FDA versus EMA). Of course, this timeline is also relative to the phase of the trial being submitted, with exploratory and early phase trials experiencing generally faster review than confirmatory trials. Further, special programs such as the FDA's Complex Innovative Trial Design program or the orphan drug designation may affect timelines, negatively or positively, and occurrences such as a global pandemic may help expedite reviews of relevant trials while other trials may be unusually delayed as a result.

16.3 Other PMBOK(r) Principles

The remaining six PMBOK® principles are described briefly here.

16.3.1 Principle Four: Value – Focus on Value

This principle relates to the value of an innovative clinical trial design, such as the financial business case and societal and public health value. These are not as imperative for Project Managers to act on but are important to recognize and understand as they often serve as the basis for decision makers to select innovative designs over more traditional ones.

16.3.2 Principle Seven: Tailoring – Tailor the Delivery Approach Based on Context

As has been alluded to in other principles, a savvy Project Manager uses professional judgment to tailor the approach based on context. This is also a continual process, and the Project Manager and team members must react to changes and realities in the present. For example, if new regulatory guidance is issued or if real-world conditions shift such as an approval for a new therapy for an indication under study in other trials, this must be accounted for in the design and management of the project.

16.3.3 Principle Eight: Quality – Build Quality into Processes and Results

When working in innovative clinical trial designs, where every action is a teachable opportunity and, in an industry, where oversight is in abundance, quality cannot be compromised. Custom clinical trial designs also mean that some processes and approaches to quality control may require modification or special provisions. For instance, validating code that is complex or in a programming language that is not familiar to those usually responsible for such tasks may require new resources, new processes, and education.

16.3.4 Principle Ten: Opportunities & Threats – Address Opportunities and Threats

Innovative clinical trial designs offer an opportunity to provide for better clinical trials – that is, they may improve the ethicality, or they may reduce costs or provide other benefits. Conversely, they also may threaten existing and accepted approaches. Stakeholders or regulators may demand traditional approaches as a means of risk aversion or simply because of a lack of understanding. And, of course, inherent in the clinical trial landscape is the threat of competition, both between industry organizations and within an indication when trials are enrolling from the same patient population at the same time. Threats should be considered opportunities for paradigm changes and Project Managers can contribute to such activities.

16.3.5 Principle Eleven: Adaptability & Resilience – Be Adaptable and Resilient

A hallmark of innovative trial design is the adaptability and resilient nature of the designs. More frequent analyses with prespecified rules, for example, allow for midtrial adjustments. The management of these trial designs should be equally as adaptive and resilient!

16.3.6 Principle Twelve: Change Management – Enable Change to Achieve the Envisioned Future State

Change management is a critical component of managing any project, and this is especially important in the landscape of clinical trial design. The Project Manager must enable yet manage change, considering limits imposed by budget, timeline, and available resources as well as reflective of the stakeholder and, where applicable, regulatory tolerance. Most crucial, Project Managers need to consider impact on the team when change is considered. Being adaptable and resilient is desirable, but so is avoiding chaos, burnout, frustration, and fatigue that can accompany constant change.

Conclusion

Following the PMBOK® Guide's 12 principles of Project Management in the design of innovative clinical trials can help PMPs®, Project Managers, or anyone serving in a management capacity to ensure the highest chance for a successful project that is completed on time, within scope, and within budget. These principles play a critical role in acting as a guide to effectively managing projects, offering a direction for applying knowledge, skills, tools, and techniques that exist or become available over time. These principles also help identify needs, goals, resources, and other elements required to define the project scope, budget, and timeline. They represent person-focused, learning-centered approaches. Further, they offer direction for how to carry out the scope and for addressing inevitable challenges along the way. A Project Manager who acts with these principles in mind is much more likely to find success in project completion, satisfaction from the client, and contentment among the team.

Notes

1 www.pharmafocusasia.com/clinical-trials/ethics-clinical-trials
2 https://innovativeclinicaltrial.org/about-ictr/

Reference

The Guide to the Project Management Body of Knowledge. 7th ed. Project Management Institute (PMI®); 2021.

Index

283

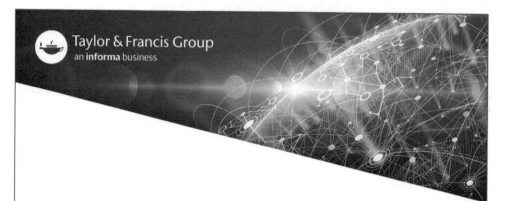
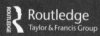
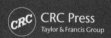